D0493172

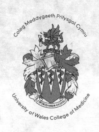

The Sir Herbert Duthie Library
University of Wales College of Medicine
Heath Park, Cardiff
Tel: (029) 2074 2875

This loan may be renewed

A Compendium of Effective, Evidence-Based Best Practices in Prevention of Neurotrauma

Every year, thousands of people suffer neurotrauma due to motor vehicle accidents, sports and playground injuries, and farm and occupational injuries. Although injury reduction targets have been established and indicators have been developed to measure progress in prevention, no method of examining and evaluating effective injury prevention practices has been readily available.

This compendium aims to fill this gap by portraying exemplars that have the potential to reduce the incidence of these injuries, and by providing a detailed methodology that is effective in identifying innovative best practices. The intention of this work is not to be encyclopedic; rather, the authors have reviewed the twenty-eight best and promising practices, taking into consideration the complexity of injury dynamics, and analysed what constitutes a best practice as the shift is made from individual clinical practice to the collective practice associated with policy implementation at the community level. They have also provided unique coverage of age-specific practices, an up-to-date bibliography, and a directory of the major programs and professionals. The first worldwide assessment of its kind, this work is an important contribution to the emerging field of unintentional-injury prevention.

RICHARD VOLPE is Professor of Human Development and Applied Psychology at the University of Toronto.

JOHN H. LEWKO is Director of the Centre for Research in Human Development at Laurentian University.

ANGELA BATRA is a Research Associate in the Department of Human Development and Applied Psychology at the University of Toronto.

A Compendium of Effective, Evidence-Based Best Practices in Prevention of Neurotrauma

Richard Volpe,
John Lewko,
and Angela Batra

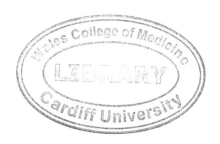

UNIVERSITY OF TORONTO PRESS
Toronto Buffalo London

© University of Toronto Press Incorporated 2002
Toronto Buffalo London
Printed in Canada

ISBN 0-8020-3617-1

Printed on acid-free paper

National Library of Canada Cataloguing in Publication Data

Volpe, Richard
    A compendium of effective, evidence-based best practices in
    prevention of neurotrauma

    ISBN 0-8020-3617-1

    1. Nervous system – Wounds and injuries – Prevention.
    2. Accidents – Prevention.   I. Lewko, John.   II. Batra, Angela, 1974–
    III. Title.

    RA645.T73V67 2002   617.4'804452   C2002-900418-7

University of Toronto Press acknowledges the financial assistance to
its publishing program of the Canada Council for the Arts and the
Ontario Arts Council.

University of Toronto Press acknowledges the financial support for
its publishing activities of the Government of Canada through the
Book Publishing Industry Development Program (BPIDP).

This publication is the result of research supported by a grant from the
Ontario Neurotrauma Foundation. Funding for the publication of this
volume was also provided by the SMARTRISK Foundation.

LIFE SPAN ADAPTATION PROJECTS
UNIVERSITY OF TORONTO

A Compendium of Effective, Evidence-Based Best Practices
in Prevention of Neurotrauma

Editors

Richard Volpe, PhD, Professor and Projects Director, Life Span
Adaptation Projects, and Co-Director of the Institute of Child Study,
Department of Human Development and Applied Psychology (OISE),
Graduate Department of Community Health, Faculty of Medicine,
University of Toronto

John Lewko, PhD, Professor and Director, Centre for Research in Human Development, Laurentian University. Member of the Board of the
NTF and Chair of the Research Committee, SMARTRISK Foundation

Angela Batra, MSW, Project Coordinator of this project and the current
LSAP international survey of integrated services

Research Team, Life Span Adaptation Projects, University of Toronto

Jeannette L. Amio, MA, PhD Candidate
Claire Howard, MA
Janice Ketley, BA
Carly Leung , BSc
Donna Louie, BS
Julie Michelangelo, BSc
Susan McNab, BA, MA Candidate
Susan Murphy, BA, DCS, MA Candidate
Nathaniel Paul, BA, MA Candidate
Vera Roberts, MA, PhD Candidate
Dara Sikljovan, MA, PhD Candidate
C. Shawn Tracy, BA, MA
Man Sang Wong, BA, Bcom

Consortium Members
Burton L. Borthwick, PhD, President/Director of Education/
    Consultation Evaluation & Research (E-CER) at the Bloorview
    MacMillan Centre

Geoffrey Roy Fernie, PhD, MIMech E, CEng, PEng, CCE, Director at
the Centre for Studies in Aging, Sunnybrook and Women's College
Health Sciences Centre; a Professor in the Department of Surgery,
University of Toronto; and Director of Research in Aging, Sunny-
brook and Women's College Health Sciences Centre
Gretchen Kerr, PhD, Associate Professor and Associate Dean, Faculty
of Physical Education and Health at the University of Toronto
Yves Lajoie, PhD, Assistant Professor at the School of Human Kinetics,
Laurentian University
Geraldine A. Macdonald , EdD, Lecturer, Faculty of Nursing, Univer-
sity of Toronto
C. William L. Pickett, PhD, Assistant Professor in the Community
Health and Epidemiology Department, and Emergency Medicine
Queen's University
Peter G. Rumney, MD, F.R.C.P.C. is Physician Director of the Neuro
Rehabilitation Program and Staff Paediatrician, Bloorview Mac-
Millan Centre
David A. Wolfe, PhD, ABPP, Professor, Department of Psychology, and
the Department of Psychiatry, University of Western Ontario

Partners
William Adair, Executive Director, Canadian Paraplegic Association
Ontario
Brian Hayday, Executive Director, Canadian Health Network
David Steen, President and CEO, Society for Manitobans with
Disabilities
John Kumpf, Executive Director, Ontario Brain Injury Association
Jennifer Norquay, Executive Assistant, Ontario Brain Injury Asso-
ciation

Contents

Foreword

Unintentional injuries are the leading cause of death for Canadians aged 1 to 44, and outnumber all other causes of death combined for Canada's children. In 1995, 6,170 Canadians died of unintentional injuries, of which nearly 30% had suffered neurotrauma or spinal cord injuries.[1] In the same year 37,494 Canadians were hospitalized for their injuries, with over one-third of these cases resulting from neurotrauma and spinal cord injuries.[2] While many have called this a silent epidemic, and lamented the fact that little is being done to curb these incidents, the issue has nevertheless received considerable attention.

SMARTRISK and a number of local partner organizations have extended the methodology developed in the 1998 study entitled *Economic Burden of Unintentional Injury in Canada*. Studies of the economic burden of unintentional injuries in British Columbia, Ontario, and Saskatchewan have been completed as of the writing of this foreword, while studies for Alberta, Manitoba, and Atlantic Canada are under way. The results are striking. To cite just one example, in 1998 preventable injuries cost the people of British Columbia $2.1 billion or $513 for every citizen.[3] These Canadian studies are part of a growing international literature of investigations of the costs of injury. Indeed a movement has begun among European economists to attempt to standardize some of the terminology and methodology of this literature to facilitate international comparisons and ultimately to help set transnational agendas.

1 SMARTRISK (1998), *The Economic Burden of Unintentional Injury in Canada*, Table III.5.
2 Ibid., Table III.12.
3 SMARTRISK (2001), *Economic Burden of Unintentional Injury in British Columbia*, p. 9.

When people become aware of the enormity of the social costs associated with injury, both in terms of direct health care costs and the loss of human capital, they are often motivated to take action. As a result, there have been periodic episodes of frenetic activity aimed at the prevention of injuries. Yet in many cases there has been little or no improvement in the incidence rates of such serious injuries as neurotrauma or spinal cord injuries. The problem has always been that while all of the prevention activities undertaken have been well intended, they have not all been founded on a solid evidence base.

That is why this volume is so important. *A Compendium of Effective Evidence-Based Best Practices in Prevention of Neurotrauma* is the first effort to systematically compile success stories in injury prevention programming. The creation of this evidence base will serve two important purposes: it will facilitate the often difficult task of decision-making in regard to resource allocation and, perhaps more important, provide the foundations for the next generation of injury prevention programming.

The book can serve both these functions because of its methodological rigour. A creative evaluative framework, the BRIO model (Background, Resources, Implementation, and Outcome), is presented, as well as selection criteria for the various phases of analysis each investigated program was subject to. The BRIO framework provides not only a consistent metric for comparing existing programs, but also a template for the designers of new injury prevention programming, urging them to think about areas they might not otherwise consider. In short, the model helps raise the bar for the next generation of neurotrauma and other injury prevention initiatives by encouraging practitioners to take an evaluative stance from the planning phase onwards.

More significant than the mere production of such criteria and frameworks is the way in which they were produced. The criteria for selection of best practices are not the results of armchair speculation. They were developed from surveying the field itself, and in consultation with many key stakeholders. Such stakeholder involvement is the hallmark of good action research, a methodology that is increasingly being recognized as important for the production of useful research results in complex interdisciplinary domains.

The field of injury prevention is certainly complex. Indeed, it is the very complexity of the dynamic interplay of causes leading to an injury that demands a multifaceted approach to prevention, yet frustrates many attempts to develop consistent evaluation strategies or clear comparisons between prevention programs. That is one reason why the richness of the data contained in the case studies within this book is so important. The authors acknowledge that it is impossible to evaluate programs for injury prevention by any single, simple metric, and instead provide detailed descriptions of each program, arranged according to the BRIO framework. A program's Background is assessed, including its central vision, initial assessment of needs, any legal mandate, and ongoing planning processes. The Resources and structuring of a program are assessed, including the nature of any assets the program may have and the strategies chosen and, perhaps equally important, not chose. Implementation is described in terms of ongoing priority setting, management, and feedback procedures employed – in short, the operationalization of the vision. Finally Outcomes are discussed not only in terms of impact and effectiveness, but also in terms of a program's transportability – the potential for recycling or extending what works into other contexts. While this is an international compendium, albeit largely restricted to the English-speaking world, it is noteworthy that a section is included about the potential applicability of a given program to the Canadian, and especially Ontarian, context.

The selection criteria for best practices also explicitly embrace the complexity of the subject matter. First of all, a program must demonstrate a commitment to prevention at both the primary (pre-event) and secondary (event) phases according to Haddon's typology, and even within this framework must show innovation in recognizing the interplay of host, agent, and environment in the injury process. Accordingly, the second and third criteria require a multidisciplinary framework or approach, including both environmental and behavioural strategies. Given the importance of matching appropriate program strategies with target audiences, a program must demonstrate a developmental approach to the issue of prevention. No matter how passive an intervention may seem on paper, there is always a "buy-in" requirement: at some level a program must involve the fostering of broad-based community support and capacity building to be considered a best practice. Finally, while there is no universally applicable framework for evaluating individual progams, a program must engage in some sort of implementation and outcome evaluation as well as cost analysis if it is to be considered part of the evidence-based best practices in the field.

Canada has long been considered a leader in health policy, in health promotion programming, and in population health research. In recent years, there have been those in the international community who have been looking to Canada for leadership in the field of injury prevention as well. However, as the many American, Australian, and British initiatives found in this volume show, Canada has as much or more to learn from other countries about this issue than it has to offer. For Canada, this compendium represents both a major opportunity for learning and a major contribution to the world. In conclusion, the publication of this volume is an important step towards a truly evidence-based strategic response to the international epidemic of unintentional injuries.

Dr. Robert Conn, FRCSC
President and CEO
SMARTRISK Foundation
Toronto, Ontario
November 2001

Introduction

Introduction

The enormous social and personal cost of preventable unintentional injury has been well documented in terms of societal well-being and individual life prospects (see SMARTRISK, 1998). The Public Health Branch of the Ontario Ministry of Health recently completed the creation of injury control objectives in 1997, through the Mandatory Health Programs and Services Guidelines. However, while injury reduction targets were set and indicators established to measure progress, the guidelines do not provide an overall strategy identifying best practice and innovative injury prevention (SMARTRISK, 1998). Our *Compendium* attempts to fill this gap by portraying exemplars that have the potential to reduce the incidence of unintentional neurotrauma injuries and by providing a detailed methodology for identifying innovative best practices. The review focuses on prevention initiatives that target the leading causes of brain and spinal cord injury. Given the recent creation of a Secretariat for Injury Prevention and Control, in the Environmental Health Directorate of Health Canada, publication of an up-to-date and comprehensive compendium of effective, evidence-based injury prevention initiatives is timely.

The *Compendium* is the result of a worldwide systematic survey of people and programs. An interinstitutional consortium of co-investigators from the Bloorview MacMillan Centre, Laurentian University, Queen's University, the University of Western Ontario, and the University of Toronto was assembled to implement this project and an interdisciplinary project team was created to carry out the survey. Referrals and selection criteria emerged from a consultation process that involved consumers, providers, and evaluators (see appendices for the contacts directory and profiles of project team members, consortium members, and partners).

Aims of Project

Our goal in producing this *Compendium* was to provide a casebook of best practices and a portal to the general area of unintentional brain injury prevention. The case studies cover the life span and we have included an up-to-date bibliography as well as a directory of major programs and professionals. Our intention, however, was not to be encyclopedic or exhaustive. Rather, we sought to be discriminating and highly selective. Our review of possible programs used a worldwide network, the Cochrane Collaboration, primary research reports, literature summaries, and meta-analyses. We sought works that would provide meaningful examples of best practice; moreover, we sought to be open about the winnowing process, delineating the criteria utilized in selecting 30 case presentations from among 300 candidates. The combination of systematic review and case analysis is designed to increase the usefulness of the *Compendium* for other evaluation researchers, academics, scientists, administrators, policy analysts, planners, engineers, health care specialists, evaluators, traffic and safety specialists, and public health workers. We expect that this work will be relevant beyond North America to prevention efforts in other developed countries.

This project aimed to: (1) survey the range of neurotrauma prevention strategies and programs; (2) identify examples of effective, evidence-based practice; (3) describe, analyse, and evaluate these in terms of their effectiveness for diverse age groups; (4) develop and strengthen networks by mobilizing public support and encouraging the participation of stakeholders; (5) provide a compendium of exemplary, evidence-based neurotrauma prevention efforts; and (6) create an electronic means of distributing the *Compendium*, resource documents, and a directory of contacts in this field.

In reviewing universal (primary) and targeted (secondary and tertiary) prevention efforts in this area since the 1990s, it became clear that, in spite of good intentions, knowledge of effective strategies for reducing the incidence of unintentional neurotrauma is scattered across diverse scientific fields and literatures. While no panacea has been found, there is consensus that effective programs are multifaceted. Recognition of the need for multifaceted approaches in addressing multiple prevention levels has been both a source of strength for the field and an impediment to scientific communication, paralysing effective action (Bonnie, Fulco, and Liverman, 1999). It is also apparent that neurotrauma has a different face for each stage of human development. Understanding unintentional neurotrauma in terms of lifespan development is a key to organizing prevention programs and central to the application of this knowledge.

Facets of Unintentional Injury Prevention

Successful adoption of any strategy to prevent neurotrauma depends to a large extent upon well-formulated theory, understanding of the phenomena, politics, and adequate funding. Scientific inquiry has transformed long-standing perceptions of injury as the consequence of unavoidable occurrences to the result of events that are predictable and amenable to prevention. The concept of unintentional injury implies that prevention efforts must go beyond merely strengthening the host and take into account human intention and agency. In order to capture this complexity, a model was developed to organize and analyse best practices uncovered in the survey. The model draws on the work of Haddon (1980), Bronfenbrenner (1979), Volpe (1992), and Rutter (1987).

The Ontario Neurotrauma Foundation defines injuries as the result of an externally caused transfer of energy or absence of oxygen that affects the functioning of the brain or spinal cord. Among the 5 types of energy that can result in fatal or nonfatal damage to the body (i.e., deaths or hospitalizations), kinetic energy is the most predominant one for neurotrauma-related injuries (Health Canada, 1997; SMARTRISK, 1998). The Haddon matrix (1980) provides a framework for examining such injury events. Rooted in the Haddon matrix are potential risk factors that interact over pre-event and event time to cause neurotrauma injuries: the host, the agent, and the environment. Due to their co-presence at multiple levels within the causal chain, multiple interventions can be considered at various points, once hazardous exposures and circumstances are known.

Haddon (1980) identified 10 logically distinct technical strategies for injury prevention: (1) prevent the creation of the hazard in the first place; (2) reduce the amount of the hazard brought into being; (3) prevent the release of the hazard that already exists; (4) modify the rate or spatial distribution of release of the hazard from its source; (5) separate, in time or space, the hazard and that which is to be protected; (6) separate the hazard and that which is to be protected by interposition of a material barrier; (7) modify basic relevant qualities of the hazard; (8) make what is to be protected more resistant to damage from the hazard; (9) begin to counter the damage already done by the environmental hazard; and (10) stabilize, repair, and rehabilitate the object of the damage. He noted that any of the 10 countermeasures that reduce energy exchanges beyond human tolerance will reduce injury severity, regardless of the factors that increased the probability of the event. The more proximate a risk factor is to the energy exchanges, the greater the likelihood that changing the risk factor would have an effect on injuries.

The Haddon matrix has proven to be a successful tool for analysing injury-producing events and identifying factors important to injury prevention. In developing a specific neurotrauma injury model, however, it is necessary to take into account strategies that have evolved for inducing the best adaptive fit (Volpe, 1992). Altering the environment with the goal of reducing the risk for 1 type of injury may set the stage for increased risks of another kind. The changing nature of environments creates additional possibilities for new kinds of injuries (Garling, 1985).

In order to increase the likelihood of success, a variety of complementary intervention approaches is often necessary. Although some passive interventions (e.g., engineering: roadway design changes) are within the realm of provincial or local injury prevention programs, most of the practices that these programs imply are active to 1 degree or other, such as the legislative enactment of speed limits (Bonnie, Fulco, & Liverman, 1999). Active interventions, like education, by definition require people to adopt and maintain new behaviour in old environments, as well as to change these environments by their actions and to construct the bases for potentially new kinds of life events (which also include injuries). Thus, in practice, interventions are usually a mix of the three Es: legislation/enforcement/*Enactment*, health/*Education*/behaviour change, and *Engineering*/technology/environment, which complement each other and thereby increase their potential effectiveness.

Unintentional Head and Spinal Cord Injuries Across the Lifespan

Neurotrauma in Childhood

Among the seven countries (i.e., the United States, Japan, France, Germany, Italy, the United Kingdom, and Sweden) selected for comparison by Health Canada (1997), Canada had some of the highest rates of injury-related deaths among children and youth for suicide, homicides, and fires. Canada also ranked within the top 4 countries in motor vehicle injuries and falls. Motor vehicle crashes were most likely associated with injuries to the spinal cord, internal, organs, and the brain/skull; falls were related to injuries to the lower extremities, followed by those related to spinal cord, the brain/skull, and the internal organs (SMARTRISK, 1998). Thus, both motor vehicle crashes and falls were notably related to brain and spinal cord injuries, indicating long-lasting injuries and complex recoveries (SMARTRISK, 1998). Brain/skull injuries were more prevalent in children under the age of 10 (21%) while spinal cord injuries increased from 11 years of age and over.

According to the Center for Disease Control, unintentional injuries in traffic crashes are the principal cause of morbidity and mortality among children. Motor Vehicle Occupant (MVO) injuries occur when the occupant comes into contact or collides with the interior vehicle or another passenger, or is thrown from the vehicle. Restraint systems make the child an integral part of the vehicle and have been shown to reduce injury, and the chance of death, by 40% (Health Canada, 1997). Seat belts can be effective if used properly, but they may also cause injury in 4–10 year olds as they are not designed to fit children of this size. Likewise, air bags have been shown to reduce head and neck injury in adult passengers but pose risks of injury and even death to children.

Helmets and paved road shoulders are 2 of many preventative measures that can be implemented to reduce risk of bicycling injuries. Examination of police reports has shown that in many Ontario cases (70%), the child or youth cyclist was responsible for the accident. Most neurotrauma-related injuries incurred by riders of motorized bikes were due to either loss of control or collision (Health Canada, 1997).

Canadian statistics show that 5–9 year olds are especially susceptible to pedestrian injuries, that is, those caused by any moving road vehicle. In 1990–1992, for example, 1,318 children under the age of 14 suffered pedestrian injuries, and 82 of these children died of their injuries. As with motor and other vehicle injuries, boys had a higher rate of death and injury than girls.

Falls have been documented as the leading cause of injury-related hospitalization among children (Health Canada, 1997). Forty per cent of these hospitalizations are due to falls from playground equipment or stairs, during sports activities, from a chair or bed, or from a building.

Younger children tend to fall at home whereas fall-related injuries in older children occur during sport or at school. Although for infants falls occur most commonly from a resting position, older children tend to be active when they fall. In falls, the head and neck are commonly injured areas. Indeed, after unintentional injuries suffered in motor vehicle settings, the second leading cause of traumatic head injury is falling. Once again, the rate of death and injury was greater for boys than girls.

Climbers, swings, and slides seem to be the pieces of equipment on which children most often injure themselves. In the majority of cases (77%), the injury was fracture or dislocation, and was the result of a fall from the equipment on which the child was playing (Health Canada, 1997). The percentage of injuries to the head and neck declined with age and was usually related to a fall from another level. In 1–4 year olds, the percentage of head injuries following a collision with a swing seat or a fall from a swing or slide was greater in public playgrounds than at home. Once again, boys were more often injured than girls.

Most recent data show that the preventable water-related death rate in Ontario decreased in 1997 to the lowest measured rate yet achieved in the province (Byers, 1999). This is the first time the death rate has dropped below the rate of 1.5 in 11 years for all age groups, particularly in northern Ontario, the Golden Horseshoe, and across southwest, central, and eastern Ontario. Once again, boys had higher rates of both death and injury. Death and hospitalization rates were highest among toddlers (1–4-year-old children). In this age group, drowning accounted for more than 20% of injury-related deaths and, after motor vehicle injuries, was the second major cause of death through injury. It should be mentioned that the long-term consequences of a near-drowning can be serious. Six per cent of individuals who experience a near-drowning are the victims of severe brain injury (Health Canada, 1997).

The consequences of serious head injuries on children's cognitive and behavioural functions have been well described; those of minor head injuries may include problems with memory, language, and spatial orientation several months after the event. There is good reason to greatly intensify current efforts to prevent fall-related injuries across the lifespan.

Rates of hospitalization for agricultural machinery–related injuries in Ontario were higher than the Canadian average. Pre-school children are at particular risk for severe farm injury, particularly related to head and neck (45.6% in the 0–4 age group). Inadequate supervision is often a risk factor in these injuries (Health Canada, 1997), and entanglement in moving parts of various types of farm machinery, such as tractors, was by far the leading cause of injury identified for Ontario children and youth (Health Canada, 1997).

Neurotrauma in Youth

For Canadian children and youth under the age of 20, unintentional injuries were the leading cause of death and the second most frequent cause of hospitalization (Health Canada, 1997). Youth, 15–19 years, as defined by Health Canada, is the under-20 age group with the highest rates of death and hospitalization for all injury categories in Canada for the 1990–1992 period. Compared to females, males were more than three times at risk for injury-related death and at higher risk for injury-related hospitalization. Ontario ranked lowest in the rate of injury-related deaths and second to Quebec in injury-related hospitalizations.

Motor vehicles and other road vehicles were the leading cause of injury-related deaths for this age group, and the brain and the skull were the major body regions affected in motor vehicle crashes (SMARTRISK, 1998). According to SMARTRISK Foundation (1998), brain injury accounted for 15.5% of all injuries for this age group while spinal cord injury accounted for a further 3.5%. According to Health Canada (1997), head and neck injuries accounted for 18% of all injuries, trunk injuries 7.2%, and systemic/special injuries accounted for 5.2% of all injuries for youth aged 15–19.

Neurotrauma in Adults

Rates of unintentional injury to the brain/skull resulting in death peak during adolescence and early adulthood (11 to 20 years) and decrease about one-third at 21 to 60 years (SMARTRISK, 1998). In comparison, the number of adult (21 to 60 years) deaths resulting from unintentional spinal cord injury was the lowest of all the age groups (SMARTRISK, 1998). High death rates in young adults are partly attributable to alcohol use (Baker et al., 1992). Generally, men have higher rates of death and hospitalization due to unintentional injuries than women, with the exception of injuries related to falls (SMARTRISK, 1998). Risk-taking behaviour may be a factor in the disproportionate rates of injury between men and women (Zigler & Capen, 1998).

When considering rates of hospitalization due to unintentional injuries, adults aged 21 to 40 and 41 to 60 account for the highest and second highest rates of unintentional injuries to the spinal cord (SMART-RISK, 1998). Falls are the leading agent of injury resulting in hospitalization for adults aged 21 to 60 years, while motor vehicle crashes are the leading agents of injury resulting in death (SMARTRISK, 1998). Legislation enforcing seat-belt use and prohibiting alcohol use have lowered the incidence of vehicle-related spinal trauma (Zigler & Capen, 1998).

Neurotrauma in Older Adults

The problem of unintentional injury as it relates to older adults is largely unrecognized (Horan and Little, 1998). Although clearly overshadowed by degenerative diseases, unintentional injury is a major cause of death for older adults. Motor vehicle crashes are the leading cause of preventable death between the ages of 55 and 79. Falls are the second leading cause of deaths in this age group. After the age of 80, falls take the lead (Walker, 1995). Falls and motor vehicle crashes account for most head and spinal cord injuries in the older population.

For every death among seniors, there are 100 injuries that require hospitalization. Many of those who suffer the longest periods of recovery and rehabilitation are older adults. Moreover, a disproportionate number of older adults who suffer head and spinal cord injuries suffer permanent disability. Although the progressive loss of brain volume due to ageing increases the protective distance from the skull and may provide protection from contusions, it contributes to an increased chance that head injury will produce subdural haematomas. Likewise, intra-arenchymal haemorrhage is more frequent in older people (Jennett, 1996).

There is a slight increase in the incidence of neurotrauma after age 60. Men are more commonly injured than women even into very old age. Because of the preponderance of women surviving into old age, Horan and Little (1998) note that figures unadjusted for sex may underestimate the significance of head injuries among older adults. Older people appear to have poorer outcomes after even minor head injuries. This outcome may be due to factors such as co-morbidity and less-than-optimal care and management, as well as the likelihood of complications, all of which possibly reduce recovery capability of older brains (Voilmer, 1991).

Prevention of brain and spinal cord injury has received increased attention in the last decade. Proven preventive outcomes have resulted from the application of knowledge in self-care education and training programs for those who serve older adults (Walker, 1995).

Evaluation Framework and the BRIO Case Study Model

Our challenge was to jointly develop criteria for best practice and produce exemplar case studies. The case study method is an effective way to examine and compare prevention practices. The organization of the diverse data yielded by this method, however, requires a multi-dimensional evaluation model. The BRIO model is such a model. It provides a simple means of organizing complex information collected through a number of methods (Volpe, 1998).

The BRIO Model is particularly appropriate for this survey for 3 main reasons. First, the framework facilitates a comparative analysis of the disparate programs/models by providing a consistent set of dimensions to explore and evaluate. Past applications of BRIO have proven the framework highly effective in comparing a range of prevention initiatives delivered across the lifespan and within a variety of settings (e.g., schools, communities). This model was used as the basis for the worldwide OECD Best Practices Survey of Integrated Services for At Risk Children and Youth (Volpe, 1998). Second, the description derived from the model is comprehensive in that it explores additional relevant information such as program aims, structure, process, and product, which are critical to replicating the best practices. Moreover, the BRIO framework involves an investigation of outcome and process measures, demographic target groups for injury prevention, program settings, and the evaluation methodology of each prevention initiative.

The BRIO Model was inspired by Stufflebeam's (1974) attempt to provide descriptions of context, input, process, and product evaluations (CIPP) and thus move evaluation research away from a narrow focus on whether programs achieved their stated objectives to a more constructive emphasis on the general information needed for decision making. The fundamental premise on which the model is based is that "the purpose of program evaluation is not to prove but to improve." Stufflebeam went so far as to define evaluation as "the process of delineating, obtaining, and providing useful information for judging decision alternatives" (Stufflebeam, 1974). From this perspective, evaluation is a means to make programs work better for those they intend to serve. This position was one of the early expressions of naturalistic inquiry that eventually became the basis of fourth generation evaluation research (Guba & Lincoln, 1989). The first generation was dominated by measurement, the second by description, the third by judgment, and the fourth by responsive, participative, constructivist, action-oriented inquiry. The rendering of the model provided here is the outcome of numerous applications in the evaluation of integrated services (Volpe, 1988a, 1998b, 1998c, 1999). Although following the intent of Stufflebeam, our use of the BRIO model does not serve 4 separate classes of decision making as he prescribed. Rather, we use the BRIO model as a general framework in which to elaborate the details of a whole case (Volpe, 1994b, 1998a). Based on the case study description, links between each program's evaluation criteria and our best practice criteria were clarified in addition to specifying best practice guidelines/principles from each exemplar.

The 4 categories of evaluation in the BRIO model are Background, Resources, Implementation, and Outcome (BRIO). It is noteworthy that the BRIO model parallels the VanLeer Foundation Evaluation Model, the components of which involve programs being described in terms of their philosophy, activities, effects, and results. In both models the nature of services must be portrayed, significant others or partners delineated, the process of integration captured in terms of salient facilitators/obstacles, and consequent outcomes of the program noted. The emphasis of these evaluation models is on describing means/ends and intended/actual dimensions of program delivery.

Background includes program objectives; the environment and events surrounding the development and implementation of a program, such as previous research and evaluation studies; socio-political occurrences; and community reactions. Described under this heading is all that is of relevance to a particular program, such as the apparent need, the legal mandates that exist in a given community, the preparation and practice traditions of associated professionals, and the existence of special funding opportunities. The primary objective is to describe the history and background of a program. For the case study, it is important to note how the program has been and is currently perceived by clients, associated professionals, and sponsors. The intended ends of the program are determined in association with the needs, issues, and opportunities available to the program designers. These decisions are usually articulated as goals and objectives.

Resources refers to the nature and kind of assets developed for and allocated to the program. Under this heading, the choice of strategies employed in the program is captured. In this dimension, it is useful to note any alternative programs or strategies. Policy guidelines for program activities and protocols should also be made clear.

Implementation refers to the ongoing project or program management, such as feedback and priority setting and the provision of service. This section determines how the program is guided at the operational level, what sort of checks on implementation have been made, and what evidence exists as to the relation between what was intended in a program design and what actually exists. The monitoring of programs provides feedback and enables adjustments between what is intended and what actually happens.

Outcome includes the impact and effectiveness of programs and strategies. At this phase, an evaluative examination is made of the practices of both professionals and clients. This component asks how practitioners, participants, and observers judge the attainments of the program. Included here are the actual outcomes of programs. Both long- and short-term outcomes are of interest. Legitimate vantage points for measurement, interpretation, and judgment can be achieved by obtaining information from both individuals and aggregates of stake-holders. Also important is the need to examine the relation of intended ends and unanticipated positive and negative outcomes. Further, this phase provides summative analysis, interpretation, conclusions, and recommendations derived from the obtained data.

The BRIO model is founded on a premise that includes both implementation and outcome measures, gathering data that may aid decision making and improve the program in question. Acquiring information to facilitate decision making is possible throughout the evaluation process. Not only does the BRIO framework facilitate the evaluation of best practices, it provides the kind of information that may assist programs in improving their current level of functioning. "Background" informs planning, "resources" serves structuring efforts, "implementation" deals with operationalizing programs, and "outcome" focuses on recycling or extending the program to other jurisdictions.

Methodology

The Project Team gathered information by interviewing program representatives (called main key informants) in face-to-face, telephone, and internet situations. Further collection of information was obtained from multiple methods through a variety of sources (see Volpe, 1993). Description of the application of this methodology is divided into 3 parts in accordance with the various phases of the process itself. Phase A outlines the nomination criteria established. Phase B describes the selection criteria and the key informant interview. Phase C outlines best practice selection criteria.

Nomination Phase

The aim of the nomination phase was to form a broad picture of programs that seemed promising and deserving of further investigation. Only programs that satisfied collaboratively agreed-upon criteria were investigated and ultimately evaluated for the *Compendium*. The following nomination criteria were employed during this phase of the project:

1 Credibility of source: a rating of the authority of the source in the field.
2 Community reputation: a rating of the program's standing among members of the field.
3 Frequency of referral: the number of times a specific program is nominated by different referral agents.
4 Country and region: the geographical location of the program.
5 Position and demonstrated experience: length and degree of experience of the program since its inception.
6 Consumer participation: the extent to which consumers have roles in the program.

In order to uncover published neurotrauma programs/models on an international scale, referrals were garnered both through literature reviews and key informants. Specifically, systematic literature reviews were obtained from the Cochrane Collaboration, as well as from journals (e.g., *Journal of Head Trauma Rehabilitation, Injury Prevention, Sports Medicine, Canadian Journal of Public Health, American Journal of Epidemiology, Accident Analysis and Prevention, Journal of Occupational and Environmental Medicine*), key databases (e.g., National Centre for Injury Prevention and Control), websites (e.g., Canadian Standards Organization), and books (e.g., *A Community Guide for Injury Prevention*). The literature search was facilitated by access to the research centres of the 5 consortium institutions, namely: Bloorview-MacMillan Centre, Laurentian University, Queen's University, the University of Western Ontario, and the University of Toronto.

Two types of key informants were used. First, a reference group was established to nominate unpublished national and international programs for possible investigation. Recruitment of the reference group relied on the contacts of our interdisciplinary consortium members. The reference group included consumers, community leaders, non-governmental organizations, government agencies, field practitioners, consultants, and researchers. Second, referrals from nominated programs were also investigated. Past experience in the evaluation of best practices for other projects (e.g., Volpe, 1998), taught us that knowledge of unpublished yet worthwhile programs is often gained by networking with program personnel.

The various prevention strategies identified through these processes (the term strategies includes prevention efforts at all levels, whether legislative, environmental, community, or individual) that met our nomination criteria were contacted. In this phase, key informant contacts were identified and/or established, program documents such as annual reports and evaluations were requested, and further referral information was obtained. As information was received and key informants and strategies were identified, the second phase of selection criteria began.

Second Phase: Selection Criteria and Key Informant Interview

Documented information received from programs that met our nomination criteria was further examined to determine if the programs met our selection criteria. The purpose of this second set of criteria was to help further develop a profile of what constitutes best practice and what strategies exhibit this potential. This set of criteria was created by the combined research knowledge and expertise of the research team and contacts established within the unintentional injury prevention field. The selection criteria included:

• replicability and adaptability to Ontario;
• availability of sufficient documented information providing a solid, descriptive, evidence base;
• innovative strategies; and
• cooperative, multiple referrals.

Those programs that met both our nomination and selection criteria were contacted for further investigation using a semi-structured questionnaire, primarily through telephone interviews. (See Appendix A for a copy of the Interview Guide used during this process.)

Information obtained from each interview was formed into a case study program description. In addition, any literature (e.g., program descriptions, evaluations, year-end reports) and other forms of media (e.g., video) that could further inform the case study were collected and reviewed. A project archive was established at the University of Toronto to store all pertinent documentation and correspondence related to the project. The BRIO model provided a consistent way of describing each case so that a comprehensive yet succinct understanding of the program's structure and operation could be made explicit.

Third Phase: Best Practice Selection Criteria

In the final phase, best practices were identified. A descriptive analysis of each case study facilitated the evaluation of the nominated strategy against a set of collaboratively generated best practice criteria.

Criteria were derived from the team's professional experience, partners of this research initiative, and published literature in the broader field of prevention, and more specifically from successful neurotrauma injury prevention practices and programs. The 7 criteria utilized in this phase are outlined below.

1   *Avowed Support of Neurotrauma Prevention: Is the program*
    committed to prevention at the primary and secondary level
    (i.e., at the pre-event and event phases)?
As outlined previously, the Haddon matrix (1980) has proven to be a successful tool for analysing injury-producing events and facilitating the recognition of practices important to injury prevention. The 3 factors identified by Haddon as playing a role in the transfer of energy, the host, the agent, and the environment, must be considered in 3 phases (pre-event, event, and post-event). As criteria for best practice, programs that address prevention must take into account the interplay of these factors at the pre-event and event phases. Hence, in accordance with this model, which suggests that events leading to the injury are separate from the injury itself, a program's commitment to prevention at the primary and secondary levels is paramount.

2   *Multidisciplinary Framework and Multilevel Approaches: Does the*
    program use a multidisciplinary framework or approach?
Developmental stress on the relation between the person and the environment across the lifespan has resulted in the recognition that a synthesis of perspectives from multiple disciplines is needed to understand

the multilevel integration involved in neurotrauma injury prevention. A collaborative commitment to expanding the scientific foundation of injury prevention from different disciplines is required. Effective measures often necessitate participation by a variety of disciplines, such as economics, engineering, epidemiology, law, medicine, psychology, and social work (Durlak, 1997).

As academics, researchers, and practitioners, we understand and emphasize the importance of multilevel intervention, using a comprehensive framework of health in implementing preventative programs. This conceptual framework, which connects different aspects of mental, physical, social, and academic health, should be adapted when designing and evaluating prevention programs (Durlak, 1997). Multidisciplinary collaboration and coordination are essential to the more comprehensive programs required to meet the changing and diverse needs of the population. Best practices must address how this multilevel approach is managed; for example, identifying what practices and policies are in place to deal with the differences that arise within the multifaceted and multidisciplinary context in which injury prevention is practised.

3 *Environmental and Behavioural Strategies: Does the program employ a combination of environmental and behavioural strategies? Does it create new injury risks?*
Neither environmental nor behavioural strategies can ensure safety. Together, however, they may improve the chances for safer outcomes. The transactional nature of childhood injuries and their prevention prescribes to childcaregivers and social policy makers an emphasis on the combined use of environmental and behavioural means to reduce risks. The home-based nature of many programs may be critical. Families given home training are in a better position to change because intervention is individualized, and, as a result, specific interventions can have a high degree of ecological validity. Incentives for behavioural change in the form of free or discounted safety products, for instance, are particularly beneficial (Durlak, 1997).

4 *Developmental Approaches – Flexibility and Adaptability: Does the program incorporate a developmental perspective?*
Program flexibility and adaptability within a developmental framework spanning the entire life course are important features contributing to best practices. The populations served by these programs are

diverse and their changing needs are often challenging to meet if a program is not readily able to adapt to and address change. The risk for different types of injury varies with age, illustrating the importance of incorporating a developmental perspective to prevention (Durlak, 1997; Valsiner & Lightfoot, 1987). Further, specific intervention may work with one type of group and one type of injury but not for other injuries of younger or older populations. Personal and social change can result in the emergence of new phenomena in the course of development. A developmental perspective on the prevention of unintentional injuries is thus essential.

5 Implementation and Outcome Evaluation: Is the program's methodology grounded in credible and appropriate research? Can the program be defined in terms of its implementation?

Successful efforts by a given society to prevent neurotrauma injuries depend to a large extent upon well-formulated theory and descriptions of the phenomena. A specific plan, a methodology to execute the program(s) and policies, and informed and appropriate approaches to measure outcomes are required to establish sustainability, reliability, and replicability. Program objectives need to be informed by previous research or local epidemiological data. Grounding in credible and appropriate research helps the implementation process by identifying what types of injuries are occurring, where they are occurring, and who are most affected (Durlak, 1997). To understand the process of change involved in the relations between individual and context, both descriptive and explanatory research must be conducted within the ecology of people's lives.

Success in prevention efforts can be evaluated in terms of fewer instances, rather than the complete disappearance, of particular accident types. However, before any conclusions about the impact of a particular injury prevention program are articulated, how the program is conducted, the internal structure of the program, and what strategies are in place to implement best practices must all be understood. Implementation refers to how a proposed program of intervention is put into practice and has been alternatively described as treatment adherence, fidelity or integrity, process research or process evaluation. Information on implementation is critical to the validity of program evaluations (Durlak & Ferrari, 1998) and generates guidelines for identifying what in particular in the delivery of a program is most effective in meeting the goals of prevention and thus can be translated into best practices. Durlak & Ferrari (1998) divided evaluation of implementation into 4 steps: 1) define active program ingredients, 2) use well-grounded methodology to assess implementation, 3) monitor implementation, and 4) relate implementation to outcome. In the case of nonstandardized interventions that cannot be predetermined by number and sequence of activities, a combination of overlapping strategies is used. Examples include coalition building, empowerment, capacity building, media advocacy, and participatory research (Durlak, 1997).

6 Broad-Based Community Support and Capacity Building: Does the program have active community support?

To ensure broad-based public support, community coalitions need to be formed involving local agencies and citizen groups. If many community members participate, social norms develop around promoting injury prevention, resulting in an increase in public awareness. Modifying social norms helps ensure long-term benefits in the attitudes regarding the importance and benefits of prevention. Critical to any effort at capacity building is determining whether the program is responsive to community needs and how these needs are to be assessed. In order to ensure longevity and strengthen social impact, it is also necessary to determine whether community partnerships are formed and active.

7 Cost-Effectiveness Analyses: Does the program employ a cost analysis? Can it adopt one with a long term-perspective?

Another criteria that can be used in evaluating a program are cost analyses, which compare the benefits and costs of an intervention program. All relevant costs and benefits must be considered, and participants need to be followed for a long enough period to assess preventative effects. Few cost evaluations of preventative programs have been reported. However, results suggest that prevention is a worthwhile social investment. For example, legislation requiring bicycle helmets yielded a benefit to cost at a ratio of 3.01 to 1 ($3 in benefits achieved for every dollar spent, 5-year projection). According to Durlak (1997), when evaluating programs based on cost analysis certain issues must be addressed:

- most health and social interventions have not been subjected to cost analyses;
- a standard procedure for cost analyses does not exist; therefore, it is

- a standard procedure for cost analyses does not exist; therefore, it is important to examine procedures and assumptions that guide cost analyses;
- cost analyses are context specific; and
- money should not be the only criteria when evaluating programs.

It is useful to adopt a long-term perspective when conducting cost analyses because costs and benefits occur at different times. This perspective ties in with our approach to prevention. Benefit-cost analyses and cost-effectiveness results are not reduced to a single summary statistic, but involve a listing of different costs and benefits. Some costs and benefits are described in monetary terms; others are quantified without estimating economic value. Cost-effectiveness analyses can accommodate more personal benefits, especially those that do not translate into and cannot be measured solely in monetary terms. The inclusive nature of cost-effective analyses renders them a useful criteria for examining best practices in prevention programs. Unfortunately, there have not yet been any detailed cost-effectiveness analyses of prevention programs (Durlak, 1997).

Implementation of Best Practices Survey

Throughout the investigation, research was conducted in a manner consistent with the principles of collaboration and democratic participation. In particular, our research process assumes an empowerment orientation by emphasizing meaningful consumer involvement throughout the span of the research. As a result of our participatory vision, aspects of our research design were not finalized (e.g., best practice criteria) at the beginning of the project.

Collaboration and democratic participation guided the decision making of the interdisciplinary consortium and reference group. Consensus-building strategies were employed to determine the nomination, selection, and best practice criteria, as well as what programs satisfy these parameters. Although we wished to finalize the criteria at the outset of the project, we recognized that our commitment to a collaborative approach and the unknowns about the nature of the programs rendered a predetermined set of criteria inadequate. The proposal offered tentative sets of criteria that were reworked during the research process to better reflect our interdisciplinary, stakeholder-based team. A collaborative rather than authoritarian approach pervaded the relationship between researchers and participants from the nominated neurotrauma programs, shifting the notion of burden from one of imposition to one of consensus.

We recognized the experiential knowledge that neurotrauma consumers, consumer survivors, and their family members possess. The Ontario Brain Injury Association, CPA Ontario, and other groups were asked to review products and provide consultation in various phases of the project. We acknowledge the awareness and sensitivity they bring to the neurotrauma project that non-consumers cannot contribute. Thus, we endeavoured to meaningfully involve consumers in all aspects of the research.

Trustworthiness of the Data

Multiple methods were used to determine the validity of the program description and the choice of best practices for the *Compendium*. A form of investigator triangulation was the primary means of assuring the trustworthiness of the data. Consensus building across members from multiple disciplines and service sectors minimized the bias inherent in allowing a single approach to neurotrauma prevention to determine the best practice programs. Our interdisciplinary team, which includes neurotrauma consumers and consumer survivors, produced evaluation criteria and best practice program nominations grounded in experiential knowledge and informed by multiple perspectives of avoiding and reducing the incidence of neurotrauma (e.g., engineering, psychology, epidemiology, public health). What emerged throughout the project was an ability to achieve subjectivity in relating and cooperating with key informants, and a process of obtaining objectivity through group processes and the judgments of the larger community (i.e., the reference group). To ensure the validity of the case study descriptions, a preliminary feedback circle was established that allowed key informants to review their respective case studies and adjust the descriptions if necessary. Prior to publication of the final *Compendium*, the interdisciplinary partners, consumers, and co-investigators reviewed the document to offer their input.

Reliability and Validity

The multiple data sources developed in this project included verbal accounts, behavioural observations, and a variety of attitudinal and demographic measures. In this situation, words/deeds discrepancies can be expected, and the study was designed to reveal and cross-check any discrepancies through the sharing of observational activities in round robin research meetings within and between partner projects. The task of the research team was to achieve objectivity through opening our methods to public witness and making our findings accessible to others. Moreover, the entire enterprise was theory driven and related to previous research. Face, criterion, convergence, and construct validity were achievable through these means. The importance of comparison is also central to the question of reliability. Reliability in the case of this project depends on the explicitness with which observations can be described. Only after events, situations, and processes are characterized can their consistency be assessed. Moreover, the demand characteristics of a study such as this required that we know what comprised the expected behaviours and answers. With this understanding, we determined the stability of findings through time and the similarity of findings within the same time period across situations.

Summary of Criteria

In summary, the systematic worldwide review of neurotrauma prevention strategies required the development and application of several sets of selection criteria. In the first phase of obtaining nominations of potential best practices, the following criteria were employed: credibility of source, community reputation, frequency of referral, country and region, position and demonstrated experience, and consumer participation. In the second phase, nominated programs were sorted and sifted by applying another set of criteria: replicability and adaptability to Ontario, availability of sufficiently documented information providing a solid, descriptive evidence base; innovative strategies; and cooperative, multiple referrals. In the third and final phase, case studies were evaluated in terms of these criteria: avowed support of neurotrauma prevention; multidisciplinary framework and multilevel approaches; environmental and behavioural strategies; developmental approaches; implementation and outcome evaluations; broad-based community support and capacity building; and cost-effectiveness analyses.

Moreover, intervention programs were divided into best and promising practices. Intervention programs qualified as best practices when they incorporated at least two of the three Es (education, engineering, and enactment). These three Es have been found to be necessary elements in effective prevention. Although the promising programs did not meet all of the criteria, they exhibited significant potential. In many instances, these strategies were not adequately resourced either to become fully implemented as multilevel approaches or to be properly evaluated. Our purpose in profiling these promising prevention efforts, in addition to the best practices, was to draw attention to some very innovative and adaptable strategies that may develop into important ways of advancing injury prevention.

Prologue to the Case Studies

The prevention programs and strategies profiled in the following sections are organized according to the leading causes of neurotrauma, across the lifespan. (See Appendix B for the Summary Table of events most likely to lead to neurotrauma injury across the lifespan.) These unintentional injury producing areas include: asphyxiation-related injuries; motor vehicle- and other road vehicle-related injuries; sports, playground, and recreation injuries; farm-related and occupational injuries; and falls-related injuries. A section that encompasses comprehensive, community-based strategies aimed at preventing more than one type of unintentional injury is also included. Many of the aforementioned injuries are not age specific; however, they do occur more frequently within an identified age group. See Appendix C for a summary of each of the best practice strategies profiled in this *Compendium*.

Case Studies

Prevention of Asphyxiation-Related Injuries

The human organism cannot function without enough energy. The absence of oxygen to sustain endogenous energy conversion, called asphyxiation, causes damage to essential cells in the brain and heart within minutes. Without oxygen for more than 4 minutes, brain damage or even death may occur. Causal subgroups of asphyxiation include suffocation, choking, and strangulation.

Suffocation is related to oxygen deprivation from mechanical causes (e.g., plastic bags, refrigerator entrapment, or fallen earth). In other words, suffocation is caused by an environmental deficiency in oxygen. Choking, on the other hand, results from the interruption of breathing due to obstruction or compression of the upper airway. In children, choking is typically due to a foreign body such as a piece of food lodged in the upper airway (e.g., candies, nuts, grapes, coins, undersized pacifiers, small toys, latex balloons). Strangulation occurs when there is mechanical pressure on the trachea (e.g., drapery cords, clothing drawstrings).

As "acute unintentional obstruction of the respiratory tract associated with external causes," choking or suffocation was the leading cause of unintentional death and the second leading cause of unintentional injury–related hospitalizations for infants.

The most common fatal form of asphyxia from acute exposure to external sources, counted as injury, is water in the lungs, usually labelled as drowning or near-drowning. This section profiles the implementation of pool fencing as an effective strategy that incorporates education, environmental changes, and the enforcement of legislation to prevent unintentional brain injury related to drowning.

Best Practices

- Pool Fencing: Effectiveness of Legislation and Education

Pool Fencing: Effectiveness of Legislation and Education

Main Key Informant:
Dr W. Robert Pitt

Background

Many children drown or experience near-drowning in backyard swimming pools and in small kiddie pools (Health Canada, 1997). Children are in greatest danger because they like to play in water, they move quickly, and they can drown in only a few centimetres (1 inch) of water (Health Canada, 1997). In Ontario, 8 to 15 drowning victims die each year in backyard pools. About half of backyard pool victims are young children under 5 years of age (43%), of whom many are mobile toddlers in the 2-to-4-year-old group. Both above-ground and in-ground backyard pools are involved in these incidents (Ontario Drowning Report, 2000). Each year children in Ontario under the age of 5 are treated in hospital emergency rooms following submersion injuries in backyard pools. Those children who survive near-drowning experiences may suffer serious injuries and a variety of long-term disabilities, ranging from moderate to permanent brain damage. Injuries from near-drowning experiences result in severe damage (6% of cases), moderate damage (1% of cases), and measurable neurological deficits (30% of cases; Health Canada, 1997).

Drowning fatalities and near-drowning injuries among young children can be prevented. There are a number of pool safety measures available, including pool alarms, pool covers, and pool fencing. Measures such as alarms and covers are dependent on the human factor for effect – the alarm must be activated or the cover placed every time the pool is to be left unattended (Pitt & Balanda, 1991). This dependency, combined with the fact that toddlers have poorly developed perceptual skills, makes pool fencing the most effective means for preventing drownings and near-drownings in backyard swimming pools. Pool fencing designed to restrict unintended access to swimming pools without reliance on human action (i.e., automatic gate-closer installed) is an effective, passive, environmental intervention to prevent toddler drownings and near-drownings at the pre-event stage as defined by Haddon's (1980) model.

Types of Pool Fences

Isolation fencing is a 4-sided fence enclosing the pool, providing a static physical access barrier between the house and the pool. Three-sided fencing is similar to 4-sided fencing, with the exception that the house door allows direct access to the pool. In this case, the house wall is incorporated as one side of the pool fence. The pool gate, an external gate in a pool fence, with child-resistant latches and automatic closers, provides an entry point to both isolation and 3-sided fencing. Together with the pool fence, the pool gate provides a dynamic physical access barrier to the pool. Perimeter fencing, in contrast, is a fence surrounding the perimeter of the property, primarily intended to prevent trespassing. An unfenced pool refers either to an absence of a pool fence or to an incomplete pool fence not qualifying as 3- or 4-sided (Pitt & Balanda, 1991).

In Australia, drowning continues to be the leading cause of death by injury for children aged 0–4 years (Pitt & Balanda, 1991). Between 1983 and 1987 52% of all drownings of children aged 1–4 years occurred in domestic (backyard) pools and 93% of domestic pool drownings of children aged 0–14 years were drownings of toddlers (1991). Advocacy to promote legislation for isolation fencing around domestic pools resulted from the high incidence of drownings in domestic pools in Australia.

History and Development

In the mid-1970s a series of articles was published within the Australian medical community concerning the drowning and near-drowning rates of young children (Pearn & Nixon, 1977b). These studies "identified an absent or an inadequate fence or gate as a contributing factor in 63% of the cases" (Pearn & Nixon, 1977, cited in Pitt and Balanda, 1991). Although the results of these studies supported the need for effective pool fencing legislation, the government in power at that time failed to take action. In 1986, the issue resurfaced with the publication of Pitt's article (1986) citing the continuing problem of child drowning fatalities and injuries in Brisbane. This publication was followed by another article by Pitt and Balanda (1991) demonstrating the effectiveness of pool fencing in preventing childhood drownings.

Resources

Drowning and Near-Drowning Study in Brisbane, Australia

Pitt and Balanda (1991) conducted a study entitled "Childhood drowning and near-drowning in Brisbane: The contribution of domestic pools." This study sought to "describe the epidemiology of domestic swimming pool drowning and near-drowning in Brisbane and to examine the efficacy of a broad range of preventive options, including pool fences." This study was the first of its kind to properly estimate "the increased risk of drowning and near-drowning associated with an unfenced pool" (Pitt & Balanda, 1991, p. 661).

The Brisbane district represents a large, well-defined urban population with a high rate of pool ownership, and the Mater Children's Hospital holds the largest paediatric emergency department in the state, admitting the majority of childhood immersion injury cases. Drowning and near-drowning data came from the first 5 years (1984–1989) of an ongoing surveillance database enrolling all injury presentations to the Emergency Department of the Mater Children's Hospital.

The study described a case-control study of all children 0–13 years old treated for immersion injury at the Mater Children's Hospital from 1984 to 1989. The population-based control group was identified by administering a telephone survey to a random sample of 1,024 households to assess homeowners with a swimming pool. Two hundred and four households had a swimming pool. Personal interviews were conducted in both the case (100 cases) and the control groups (204 households) to determine pool fencing characteristics (i.e., isolation, 3-sided, or perimeter fencing, and/or presence of self-latching gate).

Analyses were restricted to children who had unintended access to the pool. Perimeter-fenced pools were categorized as unfenced pools for the purposes of this study, as perimeter fencing cannot be considered to provide an effective barrier. "Of 72 children who gained unintended access to a domestic pool, 88.9% were less than 3 years of age and 52.8% were less than 2 years. All 10 of the children who drowned and five who were severely brain damaged (age range, 12–32 months) were in this group" (Pitt & Balanda, 1991, p. 661). No adverse effects recognized were attributable to pool fencing. The statistical analysis concluded that "the risk of a drowning or near-drowning involving unintended access to an unfenced pool is 3.76 times higher than the risk associated with a fenced pool" (Pitt & Balanda, 1991, p. 661).

Implementation

Prior to state legislation in Queensland, limited implementation of pool fencing was in place. Approximately 12 local governments out of 130 required fencing of pools. Where they existed, these laws were variable and lax, requiring only perimeter or three-sided fencing but not isolation fencing (W.R. Pitt, personal communication, April 14, 2000). With a change in government, pool fencing legislation was enacted in 1991.

Standards and Legislation Details

Uniform pool fencing legislation was drafted by a delegation consisting of government officials and members of the medical community. Together, these individuals worked to introduce uniform pool fencing legislation on February 1, 1991, with full implementation by March 1992.

The regulation involving safety requirements on pool fencing was designed by Standards Australia to represent consumer, industry, and medical interests. A committee requiring consensus on safety issues was formed but pool fencing specifications were stalled for many years by pool manufacturers' covert opposition, based on the added cost of a pool fence (W.R. Pitt, personal communication, April 14, 2000). An isolation fence required approximately $4–5K (Australian dollars) for fence installation (Vimpani, 1997). Standards Australia requires that a pool fence should have a minimum clear height of 1.2m from:

- finished ground level;
- any substantially horizontal surface, projections or indents (e.g., tree branches, barbecue stoves); and
- any mesh with opening more than 12mm (AS 1926.1, AS 1926.2, as cited in SPASA, 1998).

A 1.2m fence presents an effective psychological barrier for children attempting to climb a fence (W.R. Pitt, personal communication, April 14, 2000). However, a fence is still ineffective unless it is locked. One critical factor is the presence of a self-latching mechanism or a self-closing gate on the fence, blocking easy access by children. Australian Standards requires that the gate shall close and latch from any position from resting on the latching mechanism to fully open (Pitt & Balanda, 1991).

Queensland legislation, as described in the Local Government Swimming Pool Fencing Amendment Act (1991), requires that all pool fences be erected in compliance with Standards Australia. In addition,

1 for newly constructed swimming pools, a 4-sided fence must be erected to fully enclose the pool; and
2 for pre-legislation swimming pools, 3-sided fencing is allowed, provided that there is no opening in the wall providing access from the building to the pool, or that each opening in the wall is locked (doors) or barred (windows).

The second option was sub-optimal, as it still allowed for unintentional access to the pool through the house. Compulsory isolation fencing was implemented for all new pools.

Public Perception

Uniform pool fencing legislation was actively promoted four to five years prior to its implementation (W.R. Pitt, personal communication, April 14, 2000). The proposed legislation generated great public debate, due both to a poor understanding of the epidemiology and to concerns regarding the erosion of personal freedoms. During this time the issue was highly contentious, involving news headlines, massive public debates, and heated arguments led by educators and behaviourists. Distinguished academics also raised intense criticisms; their main concern was that pool fencing would be incorrectly perceived as a substitute for the parental responsibility of supervising their children. Academics also argued that the fence would delay access by parents to their children in cases of emergency. Moreover, many pool owners were concerned with the aesthetics of their backyard, or were unwilling to pay the extra cost of fence installation. The civil liberty argument led to marches and demonstrations by persons concerned about state intrusion into private property. People felt threatened by the possibility of enforcement officers and aerial surveyors monitoring their private homes.

Despite the controversy and opposition, pool fencing legislation was passed in 1991. Central to the implementation of the legislation in Queensland were 3 critical factors:

1 The government initiative was fully supported by key members of the medical community.

2 The medical community clearly expressed the need for pool fencing to the general public.
3 Collaboration with the Queensland Injury Surveillance Unit provided solid statistical results supporting the legislation and countering arguments raised by academic and public critics (W.R. Pitt, personal communication, April 14, 2000).

During the drafting of the legislation, well-meaning bureaucrats became overzealous and proposed impractical rules that threatened the public credibility of the pool fencing package. For example, pools with an outing to canals were required to erect a fence between the pool and the canal. Barbeque stoves and trees placed near the pool fence had to be dismantled or cut down regardless of whether they provided easy footholds for climbing. The medical community, represented by the interviewee, argued vigorously with the bureaucrats to temper the legislation such that it would be practical for implementation. For example, it was ultimately decided that tree branches, and not the tree, had to be removed. Similarly, barbeque stoves could be retained provided that pool fencing behind the barbeque was raised to 1.8m. In this way, concerns over safety were balanced against the personal rights of a pool owner in his/her backyard. The goal of the legislation was to restrict the access of preschool children to pools, and the rules drafted were sufficient for this purpose.

It was important that both the government and the medical community supported the campaign. Similar legislation passed in New South Wales in 1990, requiring isolation fencing of all new and existing domestic pools, proved to be unsuccessful for political reasons. Though the legislation was supported by 80 per cent of the population, the retroactive element of the new law was met with considerable opposition from a powerful group of pool owners who formed the Pool Fencing Action Group. The minister of local government's subsequent defeat in a state election was partly attributable to the pool fencing law. The new minister was less committed to the issue and supported an amendment of the law requiring only perimeter fencing for existing pools (Vimpani, 1997).

Outcome

There was a high level of awareness following enactment of the legislation, due primarily to the extensive media coverage and in part to the government campaign, which consisted of prime-time television ads and consumer information distribution. Given that there was no enforcement provision within the legislation, implementation relied heavily on the good will of pool owners. The government saw enforcement as a political liability, and was unwilling to take up the task. Once legislation was in place, the public accepted pool fencing as a way of life. Little resistance was encountered, and approximately 80% of pool owners agreed with the legislation. The main problem, however, was the pool gate, and the failure to keep gates closed. Ninety percent of toddlers gain unintended access through a gate left opened, or through a defective latch (W.R. Pitt, personal communication, April 14, 2000). In order to ensure the maximum effectiveness of the fence, pool owners needed to be constantly reminded not to prop open the gate for their own convenience.

Monitoring and Evaluation

The overall success of pool fencing legislation and the public awareness campaign was measured in collaboration with the Queensland Injury Surveillance Unit (QISU). QISU is an ongoing program overseen by Queensland Health to collect injury-related data from hospitals in the South Brisbane District (QISU, 2000). Monitoring and comparing the before and after evidence of drowning rates has reinforced the need for continuing legislation and educational campaigns.

During a time of increased publicity and community awareness, there averaged only 2 drownings per year for the first 2 years (1992 to early 1994), compared to 12 per year previously. It is not possible to determine how much of this reduction was due to the physical barrier itself, and how much to the intense publicity generated by the media prior to legislation. However, from early 1994 to 1997 drowning rates increased again, averaging 11 per year and thus reaching a level similar to the one prior to the legislation and the public awareness campaigns (Pitt & Balanda, 1998). Please refer to Table 1 for details. This increase in drowning rates coincided with the withdrawal of the government-funded public awareness campaign in 1994. Legislation and education is a package: in the absence of a public campaign, compliance levels declined and drowning rates escalated. Continuing health promotion is needed to remind the public of pool safety and compliance issues. Realizing this need, the government has since replenished modest funds (approximately $50K Australian annually) on public awareness campaigns.

TABLE 1:
Drowning Deaths in Queensland

	1987–91 Before legislation	1992–3 Legislation passed	1993–4	1994–5 Campaign withdrawn	1995–6	1996–7
Average number of deaths per year	11.2	2	2	11	12	11

Source: Pitt & Balanda, 1998.

Government Education Campaign

Queensland Health has been collaborating with the local government in 3 main areas (Allen, 1998):

1 A joint marketing campaign focusing on pool owners emphasizing the need for closer supervision of children, maintenance of pool fencing, and for teaching children how to swim.
2 The development of an information package for pool owners which meets an expressed need from both pool owners and individual local government authorities.
3 A renewed link with Laurie Lawrence, a high-profile Olympic swimmer, to conduct the Kids Alive campaign, a program with 5 messages deigned as calls to action for pool owners and parents and caregivers to reduce the level of death and disability as a result of drownings and immersions. The campaign, sponsored by McDonald's, has been successful in educating children and parents about water safety. The aim of the program is Zero Child Deaths by Drowning (http://www.mcdonalds.com.au).

Despite the lack of enforcement, a significant reduction in the number of drownings or near-drownings was achieved through legislation and education. By the late 1990s the rate of drowning or near-drowning had decreased by 50% since the late 1980s. Though the numerical data (refer to Table 1) does not strongly indicate a decline in the number of drowning deaths, it must be noted that pool ownership has more than doubled in the course of 10 years. Prior to 1987, 90% of pool owners had fences, but only 50% were fully compliant with Standards Australia (W.R. Pitt, personal communication, April 14, 2000).

In Ontario, pool fencing regulations are under the jurisdiction of individual cities, where by-laws require building permits for the construction of new pools. However, there is little enforcement of or awareness about the need for the maintenance of pool fences. As demonstrated by the Australian case described here, uniform pool fencing law, when implemented with public awareness campaigns, offers the best strategy in the prevention of toddler drownings.

Prevention of Motor Vehicle and Other Road Vehicle–Related Injuries

For Ontarians of every age, contact with roads is a common if not daily occurrence. Individuals use the roads not only as passengers or drivers in motor vehicles but also as pedestrians, cyclists, and in-line skaters and as participants in sports such as neighbourhood street hockey. Road safety initiatives that address the different ways in which individuals use roads, in ways appropriate for different ages, are vital. Statistics from the Ontario Ministry of Transportation bear out the need for ongoing road safety initiatives: in 1997, more than 85,000 motor vehicle injuries were sustained in Ontario and 38.7% of those injuries were head or neck injuries. The section that follows profiles leading road injury prevention initiatives. These initiatives reflect not only the numerous ways in which individuals use roads but also a variety of approaches to injury prevention on our roadways, including safety enforcement (i.e., red light cameras), road design and engineering (roundabouts and rumble strips), safe road use (i.e., child pedestrian injury prevention), and passenger restraint systems legislation and engineering initiatives (i.e., seat belts and child safety seats).

Best Practices

- Red Light Camera Enforcement
- Roundabouts
- Rumble Strips
- Child Pedestrian Injury Prevention Project (CPIPP)
- RoadWise: A Manitoba Public Insurance Safety Campaign
- SafetyBeltSafe, U.S.A.

Promising Practices

- Retro-Reflective Clothing
- Intelligent Traffic Signals for Pedestrian Detection
- SAFE KIDS Buckle Up: A National SAFE KIDS Campaign Project
- The PARTY Program
- HEROES

BEST PRACTICES

Red Light Camera Enforcement

Main Key Informant:
John Veneziano

Background

The Need for Red Light Cameras

Traffic signals are explicitly designed to control conflicting traffic movements and reduce motor vehicle crashes at intersections. However, the effectiveness of traffic signals is dependent on the level of compliance by motorists with the signals. Enforcement of traffic signal compliance presents 2 major issues: not only is enforcement constrained by limited police resources, it has also become increasingly dangerous for police to pursue violators through urban areas. Red light cameras help to enforce traffic laws by automatically photographing vehicles whose drivers run red lights (Retting, Williams, Farmer, & Feldman, 1999).

Relevance to Neurotrauma

In William Haddon's paper, "Energy Damage and the Ten Countermeasure Strategies," he describes 10 strategies to reduce and prevent injury. Haddon's third strategy for injury prevention is "to prevent the release of the energy" (Haddon, 1973). A driver who decides to run a red light greatly increases the chance of an accident and since red light running usually occurs at high speeds, the release of energy is exceptionally high. Aside from physically restraining a vehicle and its driver from running a red light, there is no possible way to totally eliminate its occurrence. However, it is possible to greatly reduce the incidence of red light running by installing cameras that can produce evidence against drivers, thus deterring offenders who run red lights because they believe they cannot and will not be caught. According to this model, any general deterrent to red light running will reduce its frequency, thus reducing the release of energy, which in turn will finally reduce or prevent injury.

Relevance to Ontario

According to SMARTRISK's 1998 publication, *The Economic Burden of Unintentional Injury in Canada*:

- 2,000 people in Ontario are injured every day, 85 people every hour of every day. Eight Ontarians die daily from these injuries, and over 16,000 are disabled every year. Overall, almost 750,000 Ontarians are injured each year.
- Costs for injuries in 1996 were $2.9 billion – roughly $260 for every citizen on average.
- Implementing a prevention strategy based on buckling up, driving sober, slowing down, and looking first on the roads would result in 900 fewer hospitalizations, over 6,400 fewer injuries treated outside a hospital setting, and over 250 fewer injuries leading to permanent disability, amounting to annual savings of more than $180 million.

The Ontario Ministry of Transportation's Road Safety Annual Report for 1997 indicates that:

- there were a total of 396,704 motor vehicle accidents;
- motor vehicle accidents resulted in 85,527 injuries;
- a total of 7,712 people were admitted to a hospital due to their injuries;
- 2,987 of those people had either head or neck injuries;
- 44.7% of all road accidents occurred at intersections or were inter-section related; and
- there were a total of 5,154 pedestrian accidents at intersections.

Red Light Running Injuries in Ontario

In 1996 there were 44,971 collisions at signallized intersections operated by municipalities in Ontario, accounting for 21% of all motor vehicle collisions in the province. Of these collisions, 17% were the direct result of drivers disobeying a red light. Collisions resulting from red light running are often more severe than other intersection collisions because they typically involve at least one vehicle travelling at high speed (Toronto Council, 1999). It is clear that a reduction in red light running will reduce the number of accident injuries, which will in turn decrease the incidence of neurotrauma.

Red Light Running in the United States

Statistics from the U.S. Department of Transportation show that more than 1 million motor vehicle crashes occur at traffic signals annually, and the number of fatal crashes at traffic signals increased by 24% between 1992 and 1997. During that same period all other fatal crashes increased by only 6%. It is estimated that about 260,000 red light running crashes occur each year in the United States, resulting in 750 fatalities (Retting, Ulmer, & Williams, 1998).

Crashes due to red light running are more likely to cause injury to motorists than any other type of urban crashes. Studies have shown that occupant injuries occurred in 45% of red light running crashes but only in 30% of other urban crash types. Red light running is the most common type of crash, accounting for 22% of all urban crashes and 27% of all injury crashes (Retting, Williams, Preusser, & Weinstein, 1995).

How Red Light Cameras Work

Red light cameras automatically photograph the licence plates of vehicles that drive through a red light. Drivers who enter on yellow and find themselves in the intersection when the light changes to red are not photographed. Only motorists who intentionally disobey a traffic signal after it has turned red are caught by the camera. A red light camera system is connected to the traffic signal system and is triggered only when a vehicle passes through the intersection at a faster speed than a preset minimum speed and at a specified elapsed time after the signal has turned red. The camera records the date, time of day, time elapsed since the signal turned red, and the speed of the vehicle (Retting, Williams, Farmer, & Feldman, 1999a).

History of Red Light Cameras

England, Scotland, Singapore, and Australia have used red light cameras since the 1970s and all have reported large declines in collisions after their installation. In Victoria, Australia, a 32% decrease in right-angle collisions was found at 46 camera-equipped intersections 3 years after installation, which indicates long-term effectiveness (South, Harrison, Portans, & King, 1988).

In the United States, the first red light camera program was implemented in New York City in 1992. Another two dozen municipal red light camera programs were implemented by 1998. In San Francisco, violations declined from 11.1 per 10,000 vehicles to 6.4 after 6 months. In Oxnard, California, a 42% decline in violations was found after 4 months (Retting et al., 1999a).

Occurrence of Red Light Running in a Test City

Red light cameras were used for research purposes in Arlington, Virginia, where more than 30,000 red light violations were recorded over a 3-year period. On average, a red light running occurred every 12 minutes per intersection. This figure increased to every 5 minutes during the peak travel time between 8 and 9 a.m. (Retting et al., 1996).

Resources

The City of Fairfax, Virginia, initially invested approximately $100,000 U.S. to launch the red light camera program. This investment included setting up 3 locations at a cost of about $16,000 each, purchasing 5 additional camera housings to be used as dummy sites, and developing a community outreach campaign. In the beginning, 1 camera was leased for $2,000 per month and rotated around the 3 sites. The lessor was responsible for the servicing and maintenance of the camera and was paid an additional $20.85 for each valid citation issued. After 8 months, 5 additional sites were established at a total cost of $60,000 and a second camera was added into rotation. In October 1999, a third camera was added. The City of Fairfax received $50 in revenue per citation and reached the break-even point about 15 months into the program. As of the end of February 2000, the City of Fairfax had issued over 24,000 citations and collected over $1 million in revenue (J. Veneziano, personal communication, April, 2000).

Study Site

The City of Fairfax, Virginia, has an estimated population of 20,000 and a land area of approximately 6.5 square miles. The city is located in the centre of Fairfax County, which has a population of over 900,000. Both jurisdictions are suburbs of Washington, D.C. The City of Fairfax has 51 signalized intersections within its boundaries and also maintains 3 signals located just outside the city line (J. Veneziano, personal communication, April, 2000).

Three main highways criss-cross the City of Fairfax: Lee Highway and Main Street, both running east-west, and Chain Bridge Road, running north-south. Both Lee Highway and Main Street carry over 40,000 vehicles per day while Chain Bridge Road carries 30,000 to 50,000 vehicles per day. Lee Highway and Main Street parallel Interstate 66, which lies just north of the city line. The interstate carries over 100,000 vehicles per day (J. Veneziano, personal communication, April, 2000).

Implementation

Receiving Approval

In July 1995 a statewide red light camera law took effect in Virginia, permitting municipal governments to establish red light camera programs (Retting et al., 1999b). The approval process included a public hearing and adoption by the city council of a local ordinance. Coordination of the effort involved the police department, public works department, city attorney, courts administration, and district court judges. The process took about a year and a half from the date of the first meeting to the day the program was implemented, July 25, 1997 (J. Veneziano, personal communication, April, 2000).

The Parameters for Red Light Running in the City of Fairfax

A red light running violation occurs when a motorist deliberately enters an intersection after the signal light has turned red. Motorists who inadvertently enter an intersection when the signal light has turned red are not considered red light runners. In the City of Fairfax, a red light violation occurs when a vehicle enters an intersection after a signal has turned red for a minimum of 0.4 seconds and has a measured speed of at least 15 mph. The vehicle must also be travelling straight through the intersection (Retting et al., 1999b).

Choosing the Intersections

Several factors were looked at when selecting the camera sites:

* accident histories
* difficulty of conventional enforcement

- citizen complaints
- traffic volumes
- intersection configuration
- signal operation

Since the City of Fairfax was the first jurisdiction in Virginia to develop a red light camera program, the Department of Public Works decided to start with a small number of camera sites so they could work out any unforeseen problems and assess the workload that would be created (J. Veneziano, personal communication, April, 2000).

Informing the Public

A 30-day warning period in which cameras were used to photograph but not ticket violators preceded actual enforcement. Signs were posted at various locations throughout the city warning motorists of the red light camera program. Postcards were mailed to all city residents announcing the new program. Press releases and media coverage also helped generate awareness of the program (Retting et al., 1999b).

Polling Public Opinion and Awareness

Telephone surveys were administered to a random sample of citizens in order to poll their awareness and opinions of the program approximately 1 month before and 1 year after the program was implemented. For baseline information and for subsequent surveys, 300 responses were collected (Retting et al., 1999b).

Data Collection

Red light violation data were collected at 3 different times for the study: immediately prior to the warning period, 3 months after enforcement, and 1 year after enforcement. Five camera sites were chosen for their histories of red light running crashes. Two noncamera sites were chosen in Fairfax to observe spillover effects, and 2 noncamera control sites were located outside Fairfax to control factors that might affect red light violations, such as weather and travel patterns. The speed limits at all the study sites ranged from 25 to 45 mph (Retting et al., 1999b).

Outcome

Red Light Running Decreases

Red light running violations decreased substantially at all camera and noncamera sites 1 year after implementation. At the 5 camera sites:

- Three months after implementation, red light running violations per 10,000 vehicles were reduced by 7%.
- One year after implementation, red light running violations per 10,000 vehicles were reduced by 44%.

At the two noncamera sites:

- Three months after implementation, red light running violations per 10,000 vehicles were reduced by 14%.
- One year after implementation, red light running violations per 10,000 vehicles were reduced by 34%.

In contrast, at the two noncamera control sites there was virtually no change in violations. Overall, violations decreased 9% after 3 months and 40% after 1 year (Retting et al., 1999b).

Statistically Significant Results

There was no statistically significant difference between the reduction in violation rates at the camera and noncamera sites either 3 months or 1 year after implementation of the red light cameras. There was also no statistically significant difference between the reduction in violation rates at the camera and noncamera sites compared with the control sites 3 months after implementation. However, there was a statistically significant difference between the reduction in violation rates at the camera and noncamera sites compared with the control sites 1 year after implementation of the red light cameras (Retting et al., 1999b).

The Spillover Effect

Red light violations decreased by 14% 3 months after implementation, and by 34% 1 year after implementation at the 2 noncamera sites. This decrease in violations at the noncamera sites is very encouraging, as it indicates that drivers have become more willing and ready to stop for all red lights, not just those equipped with cameras. The spillover effect is very important for cities that may not have the resources to implement a great number of cameras (Retting et al., 1999b).

Public Opinion and Awareness

Only 17% of respondents were aware of the city's plan to use red light running cameras 1 month before enforcement. However, 75% favoured the use of cameras. After 1 year, 89% of respondents were aware of the cameras. Of those that were aware, 84% favoured their use (Retting et al., 1999b).

A large and highly significant reduction in red light violations occurred 1 year after the implementation of the red light camera enforcement program in the City of Fairfax. According to Haddon's (1972) model, this reduction in violations will result in fewer potential accidents, thus reducing the release of energy and ultimately leading to fewer injuries. Given the high number of head and neck injuries sustained in Ontario from motor vehicle accidents, it can confidently be stated that the implementation of red light cameras will help decrease the incidences of neurotrauma in Ontario municipalities.

Roundabouts

Main Key Informants:
Per Garder and Christer Hydén

Background

What Are Roundabouts?

Roundabouts are used moderately throughout Europe and Asia as a form of intersection control. Although roundabouts have been used in other countries for a number of years, they have only recently received attention in North America. Research has proven that roundabouts reduce vehicle conflicts, traffic delays, fuel consumption, air pollution, and construction costs while increasing capacity and aesthetic beauty.

This type of intersection has been successfully used to control traffic speeds and is generally accepted as one of the safest types of intersection design. Unlike traffic circles or circular intersections, which have been proven to have high accident rates, the modern roundabout is designed to reduce speeds and accidents and to manage intersections by accommodating traffic flow in one direction around a central island. It is operated with yield signs at the entry points and gives priority to vehicles within its circuit. Within the roundabout, deflection is used to maintain low speeds, and parking is forbidden. No pedestrian activities are allowed on the central island, and a splitter island is required for pedestrian and vehicle safety.

Relevance to Neurotrauma

Haddon's fourth strategy in injury reduction is "to modify the rate or spatial distribution of release of the energy from its source" (Haddon, 1972). In other words, any reduction in speeds will reduce the severity of injury and the frequency of its occurrence. According to Haddon's model, the reduction of vehicular speeds will decrease their release of energy, thereby preventing and/or reducing unintentional injury. As roundabouts are specifically designed by engineers to reduce speeds, it follows that their implementation will result in a corresponding reduction in unintentional injury.

According to *The Economic Burden of Unintentional Injury in Canada*, a 10% reduction in crashes caused by poor road design and maintenance would result in 380 fewer deaths each year in Ontario (SMARTRISK, 1998a). The implementation of a prevention strategy based on buckling up, driving sober, slowing down, and looking first, would result in 900 fewer hospitalizations, over 6,400 fewer injuries treated outside a hospital setting, and over 250 fewer injuries leading to permanent disability. The net savings to Ontarians would amount to over $180 million annually (SMARTRISK, 1998a).

There were 2,987 cases of head or neck injuries on Ontario highways and roads in 1997. All of the injuries were unintentional and preventable. According to Haddon's (1972) model, a reduction in speed will reduce, if not eliminate, the potential for unintentional injury.

Sites Chosen

This case study examines the implementation and effects of roundabouts in Växjö, Sweden, and Gorham, Maine. These 2 sites are profiled here because they depict the effectiveness of roundabouts in continents with diverse traffic conditions. The Swedish site, Växjö, is highlighted because of the European influence and innovation in roundabouts worldwide. Växjö's citywide roundabout project could be of interest to midsize cities in Ontario that may be considering the implementation of roundabouts. The North American site was chosen for its close proximity and similarity to road and driver conditions in Ontario. The Gorham site provides an excellent example of the potential benefit of replacing a dangerous intersection with a relatively safe one, through the introduction of a roundabout. Overall, both sites demonstrated the versatility and success of roundabouts. The project evaluators for both cities are convinced that the size of a city is not a factor in roundabout effectiveness. They believe that roundabouts are a safer alternative to intersections and are most effective if they are small in size with only 1 lane and a traffic flow of approximately 1,000 vehicles per hour. The success of both projects led the project evaluators to recommend the implementation of roundabouts to replace dangerous intersections with high accident rates in Ontario (P. Garder, personal communication, 2000; C. Hydén, personal communication, 2000).

Växjö, Sweden

Establishing Goals

Since 1986, the Department of Traffic Planning and Engineering (now known as the Department of Technology and Society) at Lund University in Lund, Sweden, has been working with the City of Växjö, Sweden, to develop and test a traffic safety program for the city. Originally, the group was to make a general study of traffic safety in Växjö, but it soon determined that the implementation of roundabouts was the most effective method of improving traffic safety in the city. Växjö was chosen because it was a midsize city of 70,000 inhabitants; the researchers from Lund University did not want a city that was too big or too small. The traffic-planning issues in Växjö were akin to those in other midsize cities in Sweden (C. Hydén, personal communication, 2000). A committee was formed with representatives from Växjö and Lund University's Department of Traffic Planning to ensure that local interests and engineering knowledge were well balanced in the decision-making process. The committee decided on the following traffic safety goals: (1) the number of casualties should decrease continuously, and by at least 50% in 10 years' time; (2) the largest reductions should be for vulnerable road users, and in particular children and older adults; (3) the feelings of unsafety caused by traffic should be reduced as well; and (4) other "social aspects" should be enhanced (Hydén and Várhelyi, 1999).

Roundabouts Are Considered

Researchers from Lund University decided that the speed problem had to be given the highest priority in order to reach the pre-set goals. A traffic program that focused on reducing speeds at intersections would have the greatest probability of increasing safety. Traffic engineers at Lund University were well aware of the speed-reducing effects of roundabouts. Research by Lynam (1987), Davies (1988), Schull and Lange (1990), and Simon (1991) all concluded that small roundabouts significantly increased safety. Van Minnen (1992) found that new roundabouts reduced the total number of accidents by 50% and the number of casualties by 80%. The Norwegian Road Safety Handbook by Elvik, Mysen, & Vaa (1997) listed 5 general reasons why roundabouts improve traffic safety: (1) they reduce the number of conflict points among traffic flows, (2) road users approaching the roundabout have to give way to those in it, (3) all traffic inside the intersection comes from one direction, (4) roundabouts eliminate left turns in front of meeting traffic, and (5) the lateral displacement reduces the speed (Hydén & Várhelyi, 1999).

Assessing the Problem

Members from the Department of Traffic Planning and Engineering at Lund University, led by a professor of traffic engineering, undertook a study of local traffic conditions in the first years of the project. Streets and intersections were classified and extensive traffic counting, speed measurements, and traffic conflict studies were conducted. One year's worth of accidents reported to the health service and the insurance companies were analysed, plus 5 years of accidents reported to the police. Two basic conclusions were reached on the basis of observations of local traffic conditions: (1) the speed limit on the main streets was being exceeded by almost 5 km/h on average, and (2) the most important part of the system is the intersections. This study of accident reports concluded that approximately 75% of unintentional road injuries in Växjö occurred at intersections (Hydén and Várhelyi, 1999).

Secondary Resources

A further study of secondary resources by the research team revealed some general findings concerning speed. Other studies show that a clear positive relationship exists between the speed level and the number of accidents. Research by Salusjärvi (1981); Nilsson (1982); Finch, Kompfner, Lockwood, and Maycock (1994); and Elvik, Mysen, and Vaa (1997) all demonstrated that even small changes in the speed level resulted in significant changes in both the number and seriousness of motor vehicle accidents. Engel and Thomsen (1990) showed that pedestrian safety depends to a large extent on vehicular speeds while Pasanen (1992) showed that the risk of fatal injury for a pedestrian is almost 8 times higher at a collision speed of 50 km/h than at a speed of 30 km/h. Hydén, Odelid, and Várhelyi (1991) concluded from all the preliminary research that speed was the main traffic problem and that measures other than those related to speed would only be fine tuning the system (Hydén and Várhelyi, 1999).

Gorham, Maine

One of the engineers employed by the Maine Department of Transportation had heard of other states having success with roundabouts and thought it would be an appropriate intervention for the Town of Gorham. Research into modern roundabouts in the United States was undertaken and successful implementation of roundabouts in cities such as Montpellier, Vermont (the closest roundabout to Maine), and others in Europe was examined. There are no principal differences between the roundabouts in Europe and those found in the United States. The researchers definitely wanted to differentiate their modern roundabout from a traffic circle, which usually has a high accident rate and low design quality. In response to the belief held by some people that all circular intersections are identical, the researchers emphasized that they were building a modern roundabout that would be designed for safety (P. Garder, personal communication, 2000).

Establishing the Project
In early 1997, the Maine Department of Transportation decided to undertake a project to improve a junction located in the Town of Gorham. The Intersection Improvement Project #FTP675100X in the Town of Gorham studied the intersection of U.S. 202 and State Route 237, which is located about 5 km north of the Gorham town centre and about 13 km northwest of central Portland, the largest city in Maine (Garder, 1998). The major reason for improving this junction was the many complaints from drivers of long delays. The average delay was over 1 minute

during peak hours. The Maine Department of Transportation wanted not only to reduce delay, but also to improve overall safety. Pedestrian safety was a concern because there is a public school nearby (P. Garder, personal communication, 2000).

Traffic Flow
The junction of U.S. 202 and State Route 237 was a 2-way stop controlled intersection; the 2-way stop signs were located on Rt. 237 and augmented by flashing red and yellow lights. The speed limits were 56 km/h on U.S. 202 and 48 km/h on Rt. 237. Rt. 237, which had the stop signs, carried 52% of the daily traffic; 48% of the traffic travelled on U.S. 202, which had the right of way. U.S. 202 is a very busy state highway but Rt. 237 was actually busier at this junction due to heavy use by commuters to and from Portland. The intersection was used by an average of 13,210 vehicles per day (P. Garder, personal communication, 2000).

Other Possibilities
Some thought was initially given to switching the stop signs from Rt. 237 to U.S. 202 but problems were anticipated as drivers do not expect a stop sign on a state highway. The intersection could also have been signalized but this would have required the addition of left-turn lanes, because the right of way was very narrow on the approaches. Installation of signals would also have necessitated the purchasing of property from nearby homeowners and property owners who were very reluctant to sell their land for a signalized intersection. Finally, the intersection was very skewed: there was a 60-degree angle between the roadways. It was agreed that installing signals on such a skewed intersection would be very difficult (P. Garder, personal communication, 2000).

Accident History of the Intersection
The intersection had 18 accidents in the previous 3 years, giving it an accident rate of 1.36 per million entering vehicles. The average accident rate of signalized intersections in Maine is about 0.8. There were 6 injuries and no fatalities at the intersection during those 3 years, giving it an injury accident rate of 0.45. The average injury accident rate of signalized intersections in Maine is 0.25. The conflicts all arose from vehicles having difficulty finding gaps in the traffic and squeezing in when they should not have (Garder, 1998).

Resources

Växjö, Sweden

The City of Växjö paid about 2 million Swedish Kronor ($140,000 U.S.) for the installation of 21 roundabouts. A total of $40,000 U.S. was spent on planning, designing, and other preparations. The cost for the smaller roundabouts was about $2,000–$3,000 U.S. each, while the larger roundabouts cost between $8,000 and $10,000 U.S. apiece. Maintenance costs were about $800 U.S. per roundabout for the 6-month period. The research project was originally funded by the Transport Delegation, now known as the KFB (the Swedish Transportation and Communications Research Board). Further funding was needed during the project; it was supplied by the KFB, as well as the Swedish National Road Administration, the Swedish Association of Local Authorities (SKF), and the National Society for Road Safety (NTF) (C. Hydén, personal communication, 2000).

Gorham, Maine

Engineers from the Maine Department of Transportation designed the Gorham roundabout; the chief engineer approved its design and implementation. Since U.S. 202 is a state highway, the Gorham roundabout was built with substantial federal aid. The total cost of the roundabout was $259,000; construction costs were $169,000, preliminary engineering costs were $40,000, and construction engineering costs were $49,000. Approximately 80% of the costs were covered by federal money, with the remaining 20% paid for with state money. The Town of Gorham was responsible for maintenance costs only. An associate professor of civil engineering at the University of Maine evaluated the roundabout with funding from the Maine Department of Transportation (P. Garder, personal communication, 2000).

Implementation

Växjö, Sweden

The Lund University originally wanted to install 80 roundabouts in the City of Växjö, but city councillors thought that 3 roundabouts would be sufficient for the study. After some discussion, it was decided that 21 junctions would be provided with small temporary roundabouts. The intersections were chosen randomly, though junctions with high traffic volumes were given priority (C. Hydén, personal communication, 2000).

Two different studies
Two different analyses of roundabouts were conducted. The first analysis, a 4-month study, involved a comparison of traffic conditions before the roundabouts were implemented (compiled from analysis of 1 year of accidents reported to the health service and the insurance companies and 5 years of accidents reported to the police) with the results of 4 months of testing (from April to October in 1991) after the roundabouts were introduced. The second analysis was a 4-year evaluation of the long-term impact of 4 remaining roundabouts (2 unchanged and 2 altered). For both studies, the speed of cars was measured with a radar gun on about 100 randomly chosen vehicles per site, and on stretches leading to and from the junction. In total, 600 cars were measured for speed before, and 800 after, the introduction of the roundabouts (Hydén and Várhelyi, 1999). Also, for both studies all the roundabouts were evaluated using speed measurements, conflict studies, and interviews, and video recordings were used for behavioural observations and counting road users at the junctions (C. Hydén, personal communication, 2000).

The 4-month study analysed 21 roundabouts from April to October of 1991. The local Highway Department wanted the roundabouts removed before the winter due to possible problems with snow removal. A total of 16 roundabouts were removed after the first study while 5 remained due to requests from the public and bus companies. Three of those roundabouts remain unchanged while the other 2 have since been rebuilt as permanent structures (C. Hydén, personal communication, 2000). For the 4-month study, police accident reports during the roundabout experiment from April 20 to October 20 of 1991 were compared to the accidents reported during the same time period between the years 1983 and 1990. The traffic conflicts technique, based on the relation between conflicts of a certain severity and accidents, was used to evaluate the safety effects of the roundabout (Hydén, 1987). Interviews were conducted with 157 drivers and 142 bicyclists concerning their opinion of the roundabouts 4 months after implementation (Hydén and Várhelyi, 1999).

In order to investigate the long-term effects 4 years after the initial experiment, police reports of injury accidents for the 3 years before the

roundabouts were implemented (1988–1990) were compared with police reports of injury-related accidents for 3 years after implementation
(1992–1994). Post-implementation results were based on accident measures at all 21 roundabouts for the first 4 months of the intervention, and 4
roundabouts after 4 years of use. Four years later, follow-up interviews
were conducted with 125 road users (25 private car drivers, 26 bicyclists,
26 pedestrians, and 48 professional drivers; Hydén & Várhelyi, 1999).

Gorham, Maine

Construction of the Roundabout
The town council of Gorham approved the project and the contract was
officially signed on April 9, 1997. A pre-construction meeting was held
on April 30th and it was decided that 50 working days would be
allotted for construction. Ground was broken on May 15th and the
roundabout was finished on July 24th (P. Garder, personal communication, 2000). The roundabout was designed to accommodate the largest
tractor-trailer combinations allowed in Maine, as well as any oversized
vehicles travelling along U.S. 202. The design speed, which is the maximum speed at which a driver can travel with reasonable comfort, is the
most important feature of a modern roundabout. Reasonable comfort is
defined as a side-force of around 0.3 g., an acceptable range for design
speeds on a roundabout is between 26 and 37 km/h. The Gorham
roundabout has a design speed of about 29 km/h (Garder, 1998).

Description of the Roundabout
The approach lanes of the Gorham roundabout are 4.5m wide, the exit
lanes are 5.5m wide, and the circulating lane is 5m wide. The central
island has a 7 m diameter and is surrounded by a 21 × 23 m, slightly
oval, truck apron. Any roundabout must be visible to incoming drivers.
The Gorham roundabout has vegetation on the central island and arrow signs facing each approach. The apron is red and lighting illumi-
nates the junction at night. Sight distances for all approaches at the
roundabout are acceptable. Drivers entering the junction can see circulating traffic within the roundabout, as well as traffic entering from the
approach closest to the left (Garder, 1998).

The roundabout has double yield signs at each approach, and yield
lines consisting of 15 cm wide skip stripes. Apart from the arrow signs
on the central island, there are also painted arrows in the circulating
roadway to ensure that all vehicles drive counterclockwise around the
central island. A warning sign with a symbol of a roundabout is located

about 300 m before the roundabout on each approach. At approximately 150 m, another sign is posted with the words "Roundabout Ahead," and a separate yellow speed limit sign recommends a speed of 24 km/h (Garder, 1998).

Public Opinion

A questionnaire was filled out by 68 motorists in the area. Just over 40% knew about the roundabout project before construction started. Of that 40%, roughly 60% were sceptical or opposed to the idea. About 20% were in favour of the project (Garder, 1998). Media support was also very mixed but all parties involved remained faithful to the project (P. Garder, personal communication, 2000).

Outcome

Växjö, Sweden

Speed Reduction

Not surprisingly, the roundabouts reduced speed considerably at the junctions. Four months after implementation, the change in mean speeds was statistically significant ($P < 0.05$) at 7 of the 10 approaches studied. Speeding at these junctions was practically eliminated. There were also speed reductions on the roads between roundabouts. This reduction depended on the distance between the roundabouts. The effect, however, decreased with increasing distance. Where the distance exceeded 300 m, almost no speed reduction was observed. The lateral displacement that the roundabout forces upon the driver has a great effect on the speed of approaching cars to a roundabout. Speed is greatly reduced at even a 2 m deflection. Also of great importance is the fact that speeds did not increase in those parts of the city that were not directly included in the experiment. Moreover, a small, though not statistically significant, decrease of speeds was found. This decrease indicated that drivers did not try to make up for lost time due to the roundabouts (Hydén & Várhelyi, 1999).

Reduction in Injuries

Hydén and Várhelyi (1999) also found that there was almost no difference in the number of accidents between the after and before periods. However, while the total number of serious conflicts did not decrease, they did become less severe. Front-to-front accidents were replaced by small-angle accidents, which are less destructive. The severity of accidents also decreased because the average speed in conflicts decreased from 30.5 km/h to 27.2 km/h. Based on Linderholm's (1992) ratio between serious conflicts and accidents, the total number of expected injury accidents decreased by 44%. Pedestrians experienced an 80% decrease in the total number of expected injury accidents and bicyclists a decrease of 60%, but the number of expected injury accidents for car drivers increased by 12%: an ineffectively designed roundabout actually increased the number of expected injury accidents at the junction by nearly 200% (Hydén and Várhelyi, 1999).

Driver Improvement

Analysis of driver behaviour found that the roundabouts resulted in better interaction between road users at junctions. Drivers' belief that they always have the right of way decreased 4 months after the introduction of the roundabouts. The behaviour of drivers entering from side roads and main roads became almost equal. Consideration for vulnerable road-users from drivers increased, bicyclists were given greater consideration, and pedestrians on zebra crossings were given priority from cars twice as often as before the roundabouts (Hydén and Várhelyi, 1999).

Effective after 4 Years

The 4-year study revealed that the 2 unchanged roundabouts were as effective 4 years later as they were 4 months after their introduction. Though the speed level increased by a few km/h, it was still far below the original speed level and well within the speed limit. The number of injury accidents per year was reduced and the severity of the accidents decreased as well. Unfortunately, one of the rebuilt roundabouts did not fare as well. Though still safer than the pre-roundabout intersection, bicyclist risk increased. The research team believed this increase was due to the fact that the roundabout's inner diameter was increased from an already relatively large 18 m to 24 m. Researchers feel that the most effective roundabouts should be smaller in size and this finding reinforces their opinion (Hydén and Várhelyi, 1999).

Public Opinion

Interviews conducted with 125 citizens for the second study revealed that all road users were satisfied with the roundabouts. Of the people interviewed, 70% felt that safety had improved with the help of the roundabouts and that traffic had become smoother (Hydén & Várhelyi, 1999).

Gorham, Maine

Better Than Traffic Circles

Although 4 accidents were reported in the first 16 months of traffic in the roundabouts, all were minor and caused no injuries. Conversely, there had been 6 police reported accidents per year before the roundabouts were built. The intersection now had an accident rate of 0.62, a considerable improvement over its previous rate of 1.36. Combined damages were estimated at less than $1,500 per accident. Using the British Injury Crash Prediction Model, the roundabout should have 0.55 injury accidents per year. According to this model, there will be 1 serious injury every 13 years and 1 fatality every 422 years. Most injury accidents will be single-vehicle crashes (1 every 4.9 years), approach accidents (1 every 6.5 years), entering/circulating accidents (1 every 14.7 years), and pedestrian accidents (1 every 20.7 years). The average accident rate for older traffic circles in the United States is approximately 2.3, while Maine stands at 3.5, and, as stated, the Gorham roundabout is 0.62, undeniably outperforming traffic circles in terms of accident rates (Garder, 1998).

Reductions in Speed and Delay

The average speed for through traffic on U.S. 202 was reduced to 23 km/h from 56 km/h at the intersection. Using a collision model, the risk of a collision has been reduced by 83%, the risk of an injury by 95%, and the risk of a fatality by 97% (Garder, 1998). The Gorham roundabout slows down all vehicles so that Rt. 237 and U.S. 202 are now equal in terms of priority and delay. The times until gaps are found for traffic from Rt. 237 has been shortened dramatically. The average delay for eastbound, northbound, westbound, and southbound traffic has been reduced to 5.1, 3.2, 7.4, and 2.8 seconds respectively (Garder, 1998).

Increased Pedestrian Safety

Based on his own extensive research, the project evaluator believes that the most important safety characteristics for pedestrians are vehicle speed, vehicle volume, crossing distance, existence of a refuge island, and sight conditions. The Gorham roundabout scores high on all of these measures compared to both pre-intervention scores and to the typical signalized intersection (P. Garder, personal communication, 2000). The prior average speed on the U.S. 202 was 56 km/h, indicating a likelihood of about 1 in 2 that a pedestrian would be killed if involved in an accident with a car. The risk of death at the average speeds in the Gorham roundabout is about 1 in 7 (Teichgraber, 1983). Reaction and braking times are also better at lower speeds, so that the actual collision speed at the Gorham intersection should, therefore, be considerably lower than the average driving speed (Garder, 1998).

Cost Effectiveness

The Gorham roundabout evidence supports the concept that roundabouts save money by increasing an intersection's capacity, making it unnecessary to widen roads between intersections (Ourston, 1993). If the intersection had been signalized, separate left-turn lanes would have had to be provided, and additional right-of-way would have had to be acquired. The Gorham Public Works Director also reported that there were no additional costs for maintenance. Contrary to fears, standard equipment was used for winter maintenance with no problems (Garder, 1998). Directly due to the success of the Gorham roundabout, the Maine Department of Transportation is presently considering the construction of 2 new roundabouts (P. Garder, personal communication, 2000).

Any costs incurred in an intervention of this nature must be weighed against the enormity of potential savings in emotional and health care expenses. Roundabouts effectively reduce speeds on roads where pedestrians and motorists are endangered due to possible high speeds. Almost half of all road accidents in Ontario occur at intersections or are intersection-related. Roundabouts installed in Växjö, Sweden, and Gorham, Maine, reduced speeds and accidents at the intersections in which they were implemented, suggesting that roundabouts are an extremely safe and effective form of intersection design.

Rumblestrips

Main Key Informant:
John J. Hickey, Jr

Background

The Sonic Nap Alert Pattern (SNAP) is an innovative type of rumble strip developed by the Pennsylvania Turnpike Commission in the 1980s to combat the growing number of Drift-off-Road (DOR) accidents. SNAP is a narrow, continuous grooved pattern located just outside the edge line of the pavement. Vehicle tires passing over the pattern produce a rumbling sound and cause the vehicle to vibrate. Drowsy and sleep-deprived drivers cannot predict or prevent when drowsiness sets in; SNAP alerts drivers of their precarious situation. Since the 1950s, highway engineers have tried to reduce DOR accidents by experimenting with different types of shoulder texturing, but with only mixed results. It was not until the late 1980s, when the Pennsylvania Turnpike Commission introduced SNAP, a 7-inch milled continuous shoulder rumble strip, that a definitive design was established. SNAP has become one of the most successful and cost-effective safety innovations in the history of America's highway system (Rumblestrips, 2000). Consideration for its use in Ontario on appropriate highways was recommended by the Research Manager for the Pennsylvania Turnpike (J. Hickey, Jr, personal communication, 2000).

Drift-off-Road Accidents

Drift-off-Road accidents occur when drivers become drowsy or inattentive during driving, carelessly allowing their cars to drift off the road onto medians or into rails, ditches, or oncoming traffic. DOR accidents can also be caused by drivers reaching for things such as cigarettes, lighters, cassette tapes, CDs, cell phones, toll tickets, or children, or reacting to other events while driving. Highway officials recognize DOR accidents as the cause of about a third of all American highway fatalities. Nationwide, DOR accidents are the number one form of all non-alcohol and alcohol-related highway accidents. In 1993, $170 billion U.S. in damages was caused by DOR accidents, and this figure does not include the loss in quality of life for accident victims (Rumblestrips, 2000).

Relevance to Neurotrauma
The ninth injury reduction strategy in Haddon's "Energy Damage and the Ten Countermeasure Strategies" is "to move rapidly in detection and evaluation of damage that has occurred or is occurring, and to counter its continuation and extension" (Haddon, 1972). When a driver becomes drowsy or inattentive and begins to drift off the road, he or she is in the process of being injured. Rumble strips can be used to counter

this process by alerting drivers to their precarious situation, where-upon the driver will move back onto the road and avoid unintentional injury.

Defining the Problem
In 1984, the Pennsylvania Turnpike Commission decided that DOR accidents were a significant safety problem on the PA Turnpike and that a solution was needed. DOR accidents increased from 48% in 1984 to 57% in 1986 on the PA Turnpike. In fact, a study of police accident reports revealed that DOR accidents were the largest contributor to overall accidents on the PA Turnpike (Wood, 1994).

The Pennsylvania Turnpike Commission
Created in 1937 under the offices of the governor to construct a toll superhighway for the state, the Turnpike Commission is currently re-sponsible for the operation and management of the toll road system in Pennsylvania. It is not part of the state's Department of Transportation. The Pennsylvania Turnpike has expanded from its original length of 160 miles to a current length of 506 miles, carrying 114.3 million vehi-cles per year (J. Hickey, Jr, personal communication, 2000).

Initial Development of SNAP

The realization of the scope of DOR accidents provided the impetus for the development of the Sonic Nap Alert Pattern. The SNAP project was led and developed by a bridge engineer (now retired) for the Pennsyl-vania Turnpike Commission, who began by studying accident reports in the hopes of finding possible engineering modifications to improve safety. His initial area of interest was safety near bridges, but the high percentage of DOR accidents could not be ignored. No explanation for these accidents, other than driver inattentiveness and drowsiness, was found. After reviewing police reports, observing the turnpike, and undertaking preliminary research, he made his first sketch of the SNAP concept. Originally, he envisioned SNAP as a narrow, continuous strip of grooves along the right side of the roadway, but the turnpike's bare pavement snowplowing policy eliminated any possibility of raised strips or grooves. A narrow pattern was necessary because mainte-nance vehicles travel the shoulders daily for debris collection and the strip could not encroach on their wheel path. In response to these demands, the bridge engineer sketched a revised design for SNAP that used grooves or indentations instead of raised strips (Wood, 1994). The required testing of this design is discussed below.

Encouraging signs
Other states were also experimenting with different types of shoulder rumble strips as warning devices for drowsy drivers. Many of those experiments involved raised strips or grooves installed across the full width of the highway shoulders, which, as indicated above, the Pennsylvania Turnpike could not adapt due to their service and snowplowing vehicles. However, the California Department of Transportation had installed a rumble strip pattern to reduce DORs on a monotonous road between Las Vegas and Los Angeles with excellent results. CalTrans published a report in 1985 stating that the rumblestrips had reduced DORs by 49% (Chaudoin and Nelson, 1985). Encouraged by those positive results, the Pennsylvania Turnpike Chief Engineer agreed that it was time to proceed with rigorous testing of SNAP and the Pennsylvania Turnpike Commission initiated a full-fledged test of the SNAP design (Wood, 1994).

Resources

Costs for SNAP

Development, research, and evaluation of SNAP were financed entirely by the Pennsylvania Turnpike Commission. The costs for SNAP are now less than $0.30 per 0.305 m of asphalt shoulder. Installation on both shoulders of 1.62 km (1 mile) of highway can be completed in 6 hours for less than $5,000 U.S. Complete installation of SNAP on the entire 815 km PA Turnpike will cost the Pennsylvania Turnpike Commission between $2 and $3 million U.S. (Hickey, Jr, 1997).

Contractors were hired for installation purposes. Trumbull Corporation of Pittsburgh, Pennsylvania provided equipment and conducted initial imprinting trials. Highway Equipment and Supply Company of Harrisburg, Pennsylvania, demonstrated their Bobcat skid-steer loader and planer attachment for field testing. Surface Preparation Technologies Inc. of Mechanicsburg, Pennsylvania, developed and demonstrated a milling machine specifically designed for installation of SNAP; Safety Grooving and Grinding Inc. of Wauseon, Ohio, developed and demonstrated a continuous forward motion grinding system specifically for installation of SNAP (Wood, 1994).

Implementation

Extensive experimentation and evaluation of both preliminary and final designs for SNAP were incorporated into this intervention. Ontario jurisdictions with comparable highways and highway safety issues stand to benefit from these efforts.

Testing at the STAR Facility

In June 1988, testing of SNAP began on a 13-mile portion of abandoned turnpike just east of Breezewood, Pennsylvania, which has been redesignated as a Safety Testing and Research (STAR) facility available for highway testing away from traffic (Wood, 1994). Turnpike engineers tested narrow and recessed SNAP patterns with varying lengths and depths to select an effective design with enough sound and vibration to be perceptible in a truck cab, yet not too severe for cars or motorcycles (Hickey, Jr, 1997). A variety of vehicles, including a turnpike dump truck and motorcycle, were driven at various speeds over 5 different test patterns (Wood, 1994). Drivers were equipped with sound meters held to their ears. The patterns were only required to produce an alerting sound but the tests revealed that they also produced a vibration that could be felt on the steering wheel (Hickey, Jr, 2000).

Final SNAP Pattern Established
After extensive testing, SNAP units with 17.78 × 40.64 cm (7 × 16 in.) indentations, 1 groove per 0.305 m, milled 1.27 cm deep starting 10.16 cm outside the roadway edgeline along the shoulder were found to have the best results. They were also the unanimous choice of the various test drivers due to the sound and vibration they produced. At average highway speeds, the acoustic pitch of 95 cps at 105 kph and associated tactile vibration produced by the vehicle tire drop is sufficient to alert even truck drivers effectively, yet is not too startling for motorcyclists. Maintenance and snowplow vehicles are not affected. Given SNAP's shallow shape and proximity to passing traffic, the grooves remain relatively clear (Hickey, Jr, 1997).

Milling versus Rolling
There were two possible methods for physically implementing SNAP. Milling in SNAP involves the use of a grinding wheel that grinds a

concave shape into the ground; it is done over dry asphalt and material is removed from the ground. Rolling in SNAP is done by pressing in the pattern using a rolling wheel or pad over the wet, hot asphalt. Milling is a simpler process that has no effect on the integrity of the pavement structure. Contractors also prefer to keep the processes of road paving and installation of SNAP separate, and rolling in SNAP was found to interfere with paving a smooth road. It was much more effective and efficient to allow the asphalt to dry, then mill in SNAP. Milled-in rumble strips produce a greater noise and vibration than rolled-in rumble strips (Hickey, Jr, 2000); tests have also shown that rolled-in rumble strips smooth out and lose their shape because this installation process pushes roadway materials out of shape, leaving behind a more flexible asphalt pavement that can recover its shape under traffic pressure. Milled in, the SNAP indentations are not worn or smoothed out after excessive use because material was physically removed, not simply displaced, in the milling process (Hickey, Jr, 1997). Hence, milling in SNAP after repaving and line painting proved to be much more practical and cost effective than the rolled in method (Wood, 1994).

Testing SNAP

Following the positive test results at the STAR facility, the next step was to locate an adequate site on the PA Turnpike for full-scale testing of SNAP under real traffic conditions. Extensive DOR research revealed the turnpike locations with the greatest number of DOR accidents. The westbound lanes between mileposts 82 and 88 had 13 DOR accidents over a 10-month span, yielding an average of 1.3 DOR accidents per month. This 6-mile stretch is mostly a 3% downhill grade with 16 curves of varying degrees (Wood, 1994).

A contractor was hired to install SNAP between mileposts 82 and 88, as well as to repave some shoulder slope improvements and install single-face concrete Jersey Barriers where jagged rock cuts were next to the shoulder. The contractor completed the job in June 1989 and the project underwent evaluation. As of January 1990, there was only 1 reported accident on this highway strip. It could not be determined if the accident was a DOR. There were no reported problems with debris, water, ice, or snow retention in the SNAPs. Given these favourable results, the Pennsylvania Turnpike Commission decided to install SNAP system-wide (Wood, 1994).

Publicity for SNAP

Publicity was generated through state media during the development, testing, and implementation of SNAP due to the great safety implications of the product. The public was well aware of the problems associated with DOR accidents through the national attention they received, such as a report aired on the television show ABC News, "20/20." State media and citizens were very open and enthusiastic to the installation of SNAP, given its potential for reducing DOR accidents (J. Hickey, Jr, personal communication, 2000).

Outcome

The First 5 SNAP Projects

By May 1992 the PA Turnpike had completed 5 repaving projects that included SNAP. A follow-up study in May 1993 of the first 5 completed SNAP projects confirmed the effectiveness of the project (a 70% reduction in DOR accidents) and revealed no noticeable degradation of the SNAP imprints. If SNAP had been scheduled in with normal repaving projects it would have taken nearly 10 years to completely install it on the entire turnpike, so it was decided that the installation would be accelerated by including SNAP in all contracts for roadway resurfacing in 1993 and 1994. New contracts would also be issued specifically to install SNAP on recently paved sections. By the end of 1994, 80% of the turnpike would have SNAP installed. Installation in the remaining sections of the turnpike would take place as those sections were due for their scheduled repaving from 1995 through 1998 (Wood, 1994).

Findings

An average of 41.1 months of accident reports before installation of SNAP were examined and compared to 24.8 months of accident reports after SNAP was introduced, for 53 roadways. These roadways experienced a 60% reduction in DOR accidents. Twenty-five segments were treated with SNAP and RRPM (Recessed Reflective Pavement Markers) without any other pavement or shoulder work. These 25 roadway segments experienced a similar reduction in DOR accidents (63%), suggesting that the other work that was usually performed along with

SNAP treatment did not significantly contribute to the DOR accident reductions (Hickey, Jr, 1997).

The accident rate involving mechanically sound, single vehicles that drove, rather than slid, off the right side of the roadway was reduced from 3.81 accidents per 100MVM (Million Vehicle Miles) before the implementation of SNAP to 1.54 accidents per 100MVM after SNAP was introduced. The total reduction of DOR accidents was 60% over 348 miles (560 km) of roadway, or about 100 fewer accidents per year on the Pennsylvania Turnpike due to SNAP (Hickey, Jr, 1997). As a result of its overwhelming success, SNAP was quickly adopted by the state and installed on all appropriate interstates in Pennsylvania (J. Hickey, Jr, personal communication, 2000).

Accolades for SNAP

In 1994, the International Bridge, Tunnel and Turnpike Association awarded the Pennsylvania Turnpike Commission the IBTTA Innovation Award for their SNAP invention and SNAP is promoted on the Federal Highway Association website as a best practice safety product. SNAP is widely used on many American interstates and 4-lane highways (J. Hickey, Jr, personal communication, 2000).

Child Pedestrian Injury Prevention Project (CPIPP)

Main Key Informants:
Dr Donna Cross, Mark Stevenson, and Margaret Hall

Background

The Child Pedestrian Injury Prevention Project (CPIPP) is a comprehensive pedestrian safety program for school-aged children. It involved a quasi-experimental community intervention trial over a 3-year period in the Perth metropolitan area of Western Australia. The project assessed the effectiveness of combining a school-based pedestrian safety education program with a community-based environmental road safety approach.

In 1995 the pedestrian fatality rate for Western Australian children aged 5 to 9 years was more than double that for Australia as a whole. In fact, pedestrian injury is the leading cause of injury-specific death for this age group not only in Western Australia, but also in other parts of Australia, Canada, and the United States. Those children who survive the collision typically suffer severe neurotrauma; over 80% of critically injured child pedestrians have serious head injuries (Cross, Stevenson, Hall, Burns, Laughlin, Officer, & Howat, 2000).

Child pedestrian injury is a significant public health issue in many of the advanced industrialized nations. Intervention programs such as CPIPP have clear applicability in these jurisdictions, all of which rely heavily on the private automobile for personal transportation. Primary prevention, or avoidance of the pedestrian/motor vehicle collision, involves many factors – child pedestrian behaviour, driver behaviour, road design, and so forth – and there are various opportunities for intervention (Stevenson, Jones, Cross, Howat, & Hall, 1996).

Child Pedestrian Injury Prevention Project

Pedestrian safety is a complex, multifactorial problem calling for intervention on various levels. According to the Haddon (1980) matrix model, the presence of numerous potential risk factors would suggest that intervention strategies be developed on multiple levels (once the hazardous exposures and circumstances are known). The CPIPP was "one of the first major intervention research projects to evaluate the efficacy of a comprehensive school, home, and community education program in association with road environment changes on children's pedestrian-related knowledge and road crossing and playing behaviour" (Cross et al., 2000, p. 179). Planning and design of the CPIPP – which was based in the School of Public Health at Curtin University of Technology in Perth, Australia – began in January 1995. Baseline measures were undertaken in May 1995.

The target population for the intervention was male and female children aged 5 to 9 years. A cohort of children was observed for a period of 3 years, through Years 2, 3, and 4 of their schooling. In all, 2,440 students drawn from 47 schools, a parent/guardian for each student, 106 teachers of these students, and 1,845 community residents were involved in the project. According to a chief investigator of the CPIPP, the 5–9 age group of children was specifically selected on the basis of the existing scientific literature, which suggests that children of this age are most at risk of sustaining a pedestrian injury and that, as a group, they are overrepresented in pedestrian injury statistics (M. Stevenson, personal communication, May 2, 2000).

Goals and Objectives
The long-term goal of the CPIPP is to reduce pedestrian injury rates among children aged 5 to 9 years. However, since it was not feasible to collect injury rate outcome data in this study, the primary aim of the program was to design and evaluate a school- and community-based intervention that would improve children's road-related behaviour and enhance the safety of their road environment (Cross et al., 2000).

Road-related behaviour and safety of the road environment are 2 known risk factors for child pedestrian injury. With this fact in mind, specific intervention objectives were developed on each of these fronts. The behavioural objectives were:

• To increase by 10% the proportion of 5–9-year-old children who practise safe pedestrian behaviour;
• To determine the extent to which 5–9-year-old children perceive themselves as being capable of following safe pedestrian behaviour (self-efficacy);
• To increase by 5% the knowledge level of 5–9-year-old children and their parents regarding pedestrian safety issues;
• To increase by 5% the proportion of parents of 5–9-year-old children who encourage safe pedestrian behaviour through verbal instructions and modelling; and
• To increase by 40% parental knowledge of the limitations of perceptual skills among 5–9-year-old-children.

With respect to the environmental objectives, the aim was to modify positively the physical environmental risk factors for child pedestrian injury. More specifically, the desired modifications targeted:

• the speed of vehicular traffic;
• traffic flow; and
• the volume of traffic.

Furthermore, an implicit objective of the CPIPP was to contribute to the growing body of health promotion research on the prevention of pedestrian injuries in children (Australian Injury Prevention Database website: http://www.spmed.uq.edu/au/aipd).

Stakeholders

As is generally true of community-based research projects, many stakeholders were involved with the CPIPP. According to a chief investigator of the project, the key stakeholders included: Main Roads Western Australia; the Traffic Board of Western Australia; RoadWise, an educational road safety organization; the Western Australia Department of Transport; the Western Australia Police Department; the Education Department of Western Australia; school principals and teachers; parents; and Perth community residents (M. Stevenson, personal communication, May 2, 2000).

At the time of development and implementation of the CPIPP, Main Roads Western Australia and the Traffic Board of Western Australia were very interested in being involved in providing schools, teachers, and parents with up-to-date road safety materials. Previously these groups had experienced some difficulty trying to involve schools in road safety issue and to evaluate their efforts. Moreover, many of the programs offered tended to be categorical rather than comprehensive (M. Hall, personal communication, May 5, 2000).

School principals and teachers expressed concern about always having to take on new road safety programs, which meant additional demands on resources (time and money). The CPIPP research team, however, was "able to facilitate and coordinate these activities" (M. Hall, personal communication, May 5, 2000). The project's plans both to train teachers to implement the new curriculum and to pay for replacement teachers during the training sessions were well received by school officials as they posed no additional burden upon educational resources.

In post-program surveys, the teachers reported tremendous satisfaction with the project. The curriculum materials were well organized and easy to follow. School officials were pleased that the outcomes were positive in terms of changes in student behaviour. High praise was also given to the communication links established with the parents of the children and to the fact that support systems were put in place to allow the intervention programs to continue past the life of the program (M. Hall, personal communication, May 5, 2000). In fact, the pedestrian safety curriculum materials developed by CPIPP have been incorporated into a comprehensive Kindergarten – Year 10 road safety education program and disseminated statewide (Cross et al., 2000).

Resources

In this section, the theoretical model underlying the CPIPP is described, as is the project's sources of funding.

Model

When developing the model for the CPIPP, members of the research team were keenly aware of the fact that inadequate program planning is to blame for much of the ineffectiveness of prior health promotion and injury prevention interventions. In a journal article written about the project, the investigators note that "increasing attention has been given to the use of recognized planning models to enhance the quality of injury control interventions. A significant proportion of programs, however, are developed with relatively little consideration given to planning frameworks or theoretical models" (Howat, Jones, Hall, Cross, & Stevenson, 1997, p. 282).

The CPIPP was based on a modified version of the PRECEDE-PROCEED model (Green & Kreuter, 1991), an increasingly popular health promotion planning framework. According to CPIPP investigators, "the value of the model is that it forces the planner to assess thoroughly the factors associated with the problem that is the focus of concern. A series of diagnoses precedes the development of the interventions, their implementation, and evaluation" (Howat et al., 1997, p. 283). The model devised for the CPIPP consists of 6 phases or steps:

1 Epidemiological Factors Assessment: identify the epidemiological details of the problem and characteristics of the groups at risk.
2 Social Factors Assessment: identify the specific problems of the communities to be studied.
3 Behavioural and Environmental Factors Assessment: identify behavioural and environmental factors causally associated with child pedestrian injuries and then develop objectives for each identified risk factor.
4 Contributing Factors Assessment: identify and then classify as predisposing, enabling, or reinforcing the contributing factors for each behavioural and environmental risk factor identified in Step 3.
5 Intervention Strategy Selection: develop strategy objectives in rela-

tion to the identified risk factors and then select intervention strategies to address these strategy objectives.
6 Evaluation: plan the evaluation of the intervention trial with respect to process, impact, and outcome.

A total of 13 main strategy objectives were developed to inform the CPIPP interventions (see Howat et al., 1997). The school-based interventions targeted students, parents, and teachers; the community-based interventions included media outreach, a community advisory group, and the Safe Routes to School program.

The CPIPP investigators believe that there were many advantages to using the PRECEDE-PROCEED model as part of the planning of the Project. For instance, the model forced the development of clear, measurable goals and objectives; indeed, it provided a useful checklist specifying the 6 main steps to be considered during program planning (see above). In addition to facilitating the planning process, the model proved helpful both with ongoing monitoring and periodic implementation reviews. In the words of the researchers, "the ultimate benefit of the model is that appropriate interventions are likely to result and the likelihood of a rigorous evaluation design is enhanced" (Howat et al., 1997, p. 286).

Funding

The CPIPP was funded by a health promotion research grant awarded to the Centre for Health Promotion Research, School of Public Health at Curtin University by the Western Australia Health Promotion Foundation (Healthway). This grant, for the 3-year period 1995–1997, was for $226,369 (Australian dollars).

Owing to the high costs associated with the evaluation of the project, especially the environmental intervention, more funds were needed. Additional funding support for the evaluation was provided by the Traffic Board of Western Australia and Main Roads Western Australia.

Office equipment and work space for project staff were supplied by the Centre for Health Promotion Research at Curtin University of Technology.

Implementation

The Child Pedestrian Injury Prevention Project was a quasi-experimental trial with 2 intervention groups and a comparison group. The project employed a multifaceted approach with both behavioural and environmental interventions. Three communities in the Perth metropolitan area were assigned to one of the intervention conditions: Intervention Group 1 (the high intervention group) received both a community/environmental road safety intervention and a school-based pedestrian safety education program; Intervention Group 2 (the moderate intervention group) received only the school-based pedestrian safety education program; and the Comparison Group received no road safety intervention whatsoever.

Listed below are the specific intervention strategies employed in the respective intervention groups. The school-based educational interventions were:

- development of road safety curriculum materials for student activities;
- road safety training for teachers; and
- ongoing teacher support.

The community-based environmental interventions included the following:

- establishment of a Community Road Safety Advisory Committee;
- development of a community action project;
- organization of awareness-raising activities through the media, local shopping centres, competitions, a Road Safety Carnival, and the distribution of stickers;
- development of a sponsorship kit and community action manual;
- implementation of the Safe Routes to School program, with strategies including travel surveys, road safety policy development, identifying and marking safe routes for walking to school; and
- implementation of engineering/environmental changes to reduce road safety hazards and to test 40 km/h speed zones.

Both the school-based and community-based interventions were implemented over a 3-year period (1995–1997).

Effective Practices

The decision to provide teacher training as well as paid teacher relief was cited by a CPIPP program director as a critical factor in the success of the school-based safety education intervention (M. Hall, personal communication, May 5, 2000). As indicated above, in the past, teachers were somewhat reluctant to commit to road safety initiatives: there were too many programs and very little coordination among them, resulting in great demands placed on the teachers' time with little support to assist them. The CPIPP team maintained regular contact with the teachers in the intervention trial and provided significant follow-up support. In addition, the teachers greatly appreciated the fact that the curriculum materials in the CPIPP road safety program were developed on the basis of a rigorous formative evaluation, which included focus group meetings with both teachers and parents as well as pilot testing of the curriculum with the teachers (M. Hall, personal communication, May 5, 2000).

With respect to the community-based environmental trial, the factor that proved most effective in implementing the intervention was the formation of the Community Road Safety Advisory Committee. The committee was formed to develop intervention strategies and to facilitate the various community-based activities associated with the interventions. Membership of the committee included the following: a city councillor, a traffic engineer, 2 advocates for road safety, a police officer, 2 community residents, a representative from Main Roads Western Australia, and 2 CPIPP research team members (Stevenson, Iredell, Howat, Cross, & Hall, 1999). According to a CPIPP project director, the role of the Community Road Safety Advisory Committee was critical in that it served to link together the parents, the schools, and the community with the researchers at Curtin University. For instance, the committee initiated the development and dissemination of 2 road safety resources for local community groups and organized a community-wide sticker distribution campaign promoting the message Safe Drivers Save Lives (Stevenson et al., 1996).

One factor that greatly facilitated the operation of the CPIPP was the voluntary assistance of students in the School of Public Health at Curtin University. Given the laborious nature and extensive range of the data collection involved, the comprehensive evaluation plan (especially for the environmental interventions) would not have been feasible had it not been for the student volunteers (M. Hall, personal communication, May 5, 2000).

Decision Making and Planning

Investigators and staff on the CPIPP received advice and direction from the Project Advisory Committee. The membership of this committee was broad-based and consisted of key representatives from the community (e.g., parents, teachers, residents), government (e.g., police, traffic engineers, Education Department officials), and academia (e.g., CPIPP investigators). The committee met twice during the first year of the project and on an annual basis thereafter to monitor the progress of the project. For instance, all curriculum materials were reviewed by the committee in order to provide feedback to the CPIPP investigators.

To deal with the ongoing management of the CPIPP, a Project Management Committee was formed. This committee was comprised of the three Chief Investigators, two project directors, and other select staff members. The Management Committee met on a fortnightly basis over the 3-year period in order to review the progress of the project and to strike subcommittees as necessary.

Outcome

This section presents a description of the evaluation of the CPIPP, followed by an overview of the various methods of dissemination of information.

Evaluation

The evaluation component of the CPIPP was incredibly extensive. The evaluation plan included formative, process, and summative research efforts. The elements of the evaluation are listed below.

1 Formative Evaluation:
   – exhaustive literature review;
   – review of available resources;
   – focus group meetings with parents, teachers, and local public administrators; and
   – pilot testing of curriculum materials with teachers.
2 Process Evaluation:
   – awareness of the project and its components by students, teachers, parents, and community residents;
   – participation rates in the project;
   – attitudes towards the project;
   – teachers' perceptions of the usefulness of the teacher training, follow-up support, and educational materials;

- curriculum implementation rates;
- assessment of the quality of selected intervention components; and
- media coverage of local traffic safety issues.

3 Summative Evaluation:
- students' pedestrian safety-related knowledge, attitudes, behavioural intentions, and skills;
- students' self-reported pedestrian behaviours and self-reported injuries;
- teachers' pedestrian safety-related knowledge, attitudes, and behavioural intentions regarding use of the program with their students;
- teachers' self-reported pedestrian behaviours;
- parents' pedestrian safety-related knowledge, attitudes, and behavioural intentions regarding use of the program with their children;
- parents' self-reported pedestrian behaviours;
- local community ordinances;
- community members' awareness and perceived effects of the program;
- Community Road Safety Advisory Committee members' perceptions about the committee and its effects;
- reduction in traffic speed and volumes; and
- cost effectiveness of the intervention strategies.

As noted above, no data on actual injury rates were collected during the course of the CPIPP. Given that the long-term goal was to reduce the incidence of pedestrian injury among children, this is an obvious weakness of the project, especially with respect to the evaluation of the outcome of the interventions (M. Stevenson, personal communication, May 2, 2000). It was known from the outset, however, that the collection of injury outcome data would not be possible (owing to limited funding) so analyses that this data would have allowed were never included as part of the evaluation plan.

In terms of the available data, the results observed were encouraging. Children in the high and moderate intervention groups were significantly more likely to cross the road with adult supervision than were those in the comparison group. Similarly, those children who received the educational intervention (i.e., the road safety program) were significantly more likely to play away from the road than were those children who did not receive the intervention. There were no significant differences between the intervention and comparison groups on the measures of children's pedestrian safety knowledge, possibly owing to methodological limitations with the instrumentation (see Cross et al., 2000).

Regarding the community/environmental interventions, the results were equally positive. Greater road safety activity was observed in the high intervention group, which was the only group to receive the environmental interventions. More specifically, "the level of community/environmental activity evident in intervention group 1 was 2.3 times greater and 5 times greater when compared with intervention group 2 and the comparison group, respectively" (Stevenson et al., 1999, p. 29). The findings also indicated a significant reduction in the volume of traffic on local access roads in the high intervention group, but not in the other 2 groups. Based on the results of prior research, the observed 9% reduction in volume could lead to a reduction in the incidence of childhood pedestrian injury by up to 18%. Moreover, this reduction in traffic volume on local streets did not result in an increased speed of traffic on those streets, which is a common undesired consequence of reducing volumes (Stevenson et al., 1999).

The CPIPP is "one of the first school- and community-based programs to show that it may be possible to decelerate the relative increase of pedestrian-related risk taking in children" (Cross et al., 2000, p. 180). The various environmental interventions contributed to significant reductions in the road-related risk factors. Taken together, then, the findings of the CPIPP suggest that a combination of community/environmental interventions and road safety education programs are likely to reduce the rate of childhood pedestrian injury. These results have important implications for future childhood neurotrauma prevention initiatives.

As for limitations of the project, both contact persons cited concerns with the outcome measures. Since it was not possible to collect actual injury rates, the impact evaluation of the CPIPP was restricted to assessing the effect of the interventions on knowledge and behaviours (M. Stevenson, personal communication, May 2, 2000). The reliability of these outcome measures was also questioned. Although there was observational and interview validation of a sub-sample of students, the evaluation of the behavioural findings was based on the self-report data of young children, which is not always reliable (M. Hall, personal communication, May 5, 2000).

Dissemination of Information

The investigators involved with the CPIPP have published a sequence of academic papers in peer-reviewed scholarly journals detailing the development, implementation, and evaluation of the project and a Final Report on the project was published in 1998. There have also been numerous presentations at various national and international conferences as well as at state and local road safety group meetings.

Key findings from the project were also disseminated to stakeholders and residents at a full-day seminar at a local auditorium. Project staff were involved in writing articles about the project for local newspapers and consented to many media requests for interviews. Information on the project is also available via the Internet on the Centre for Health Promotion Research website (http://www.curtin.edu.au/curtin/dept/health).

RoadWise: A Manitoba Public Insurance Safety Campaign

Main Key Informant:
Dennis Bell

Background

In industrialized countries and increasingly in developing countries, motorized vehicles represent a leading cause of injury and death. Indeed, the International Federation of Red Cross and Red Crescent societies noted, in its 1998 World Disasters Report, that, by 2020, road crashes will be the third largest killer in the world. Alarming statistics for automobile-related injury, however, go largely unnoticed by the general public, and the epidemic scope of the problem does not make the headlines of newspapers. In Canada, road safety concerns all of us at every stage of our lives as passengers, as pedestrians, as users of the road, and as drivers on the road. The road represents a very proximal danger to nearly all Canadians. As the only insurance company for drivers in Manitoba, Canada, Manitoba Public Insurance (MPI) saw a need to increase public awareness and to reduce the incidence and

TABLE 1. Neurotrauma claim trends (Source MPI, December 1999)

Type of claim	1994	1995	1996	1997	1998
Chronic pain	7	202	275	141	125
Brain damage	67	61	29	36	35
Quadriplegic	3	4	3	4	1
Paraplegic	4	7	1	4	1
Whiplash	9,925	9,193	7,820	6,538	6,977
Total	10,006	9,467	8,128	6,723	7,139

severity of motorized vehicle injuries, not only as a way to deduct from the bottom line, but also as a way to promote social good. It was in response to this realization that MPI conceived of its RoadWise campaign in 1993.

The RoadWise program is an ongoing campaign launched in 1996 after 3 years of development. The campaign targets all Manitoban drivers and pedestrians and, in 1999, reached 98 communities throughout the province, including aboriginal and Hutterite communities and youth at-risk. Neurotrauma injury incidence in this Canadian province is shown in Table 1.

MPI considers the RoadWise campaign social marketing – where a social agenda is harnessed to a business strategy. This social marketing strategy fits MPI, a monopoly insurance provider that is both a financial institution and a not-for-profit organization. The RoadWise campaign enables MPI to make better use of its charitable and philanthropic activities and allows the insurer to take a leadership role in road safety with benefits for both the public and the corporation.

History and Development

MPI is empowered to introduce, establish, supervise, finance, and promote research or education related to safety and the reduction of risk in respect to any branch or class of insurance in which the corporation is engaged. The mission of MPI is "to protect Manitobans from the human and economic cost of automobile accidents" (MPI, December 1999). The goal of the RoadWise program is to create a social agenda for change in the way people drive in Manitoba. This campaign began as an awareness program and has developed into program delivery with 8 prevention strategies:

1 Children's Traffic Club

The Children's Traffic Club was developed in 1999 as a state-of-the-art modular educational program in conjunction with Manitoba Education. Over the next 3 years, this program will expand to be fully integrated with the existing curriculum and will reach 210,000 students annually. The program is based on an evaluated model developed in Scotland over 5 years and provides a structured way to introduce road safety concepts directly into the classroom. These safety concepts progress in sophistication from pre-school through to grade 9. The concepts are target-group appropriate and focus on the way each grade level is most likely to use the road (i.e., as passenger, as pedestrian, as cyclists, as drivers). The program is seen as a natural training program for the Driver Education program that follows.

2 Enhanced Driver Education

Since 1987, MPI has managed a High School Driver Education Program. The program provides 25 hours of in-class training and 16 hours of in-car training from road safety professionals using a curriculum that is constantly tested against the best practices of other jurisdictions. In the past, MPI paid one half of every student's tuition; the tuition has now been lowered to further encourage enrolment. In 1999, the program will have reached 70% of eligible new 16-year-old drivers in the province. MPI is conducting a longitudinal study of the driving performance of its driver education graduates compared to non-program users. The program seeks to combat driver over-confidence, a sometimes dangerous result of driver education, by emphasizing attitude and awareness along with driving skills. The measuring tools for evaluation are still in the development stage, but will utilize the most current concepts generated on the issue, particularly those advocated by Transport Canada and the University of Sussex. Furthermore, an exhaustive analysis of accident records will be conducted. As a result, the evaluation will include measures of proclivity to risk-taking behaviour, among other attitudinal measures.

3 High-Risk Driver Campaign

In an additional attempt to reach young drivers, a television ad campaign using innovative commercials addressed drinking and driving, seat belt use, peer pressure and other issues. These ads were first launched in 1996 and utilized an episodic approach in which each of the 4 ads depicted a different result of a driver's carelessness. The advertisements won a number of international marketing awards and produced a 90% recognition rate amongst the target population. Furthermore, this ad campaign produced the largest increase in self-reported behaviour change from baseline than any other MPI media-based awareness campaign. Each year, the campaign has changed in an effort to remain fresh; the current ads no longer utilize the episodic approach but deal with risk-taking behaviours in a stand-alone approach.

4 Drinking and Driving (RoadWatch)

In a provincewide initiative between MPI and police agencies, the RoadWatch program increased the level of roadside enforcement for drinking and driving. Statistics gathered during this program show that impaired driving has decreased from previous annual rates. Also, a tracking survey done in Brandon, Manitoba, shows that 73% of the respondents indicated that they believed the chance of a drunk driver being stopped at a checkpoint had increased, and this was a significant gain over the 54% of respondents who reported so at the beginning of the campaign.

5 Occupant Restraints

Click In to Win is an innovative program developed for the RoadWise Campaign. This program uses an incentive-based approach by offering seat-belt users the opportunity to win one of 16 27-inch colour televisions if they are confirmed by law enforcement to have been wearing a seat belt when stopped at a safety checkpoint. Transport Canada reported an increase in seat-belt use in the province after the program had run. Also, the rate of response for the program increased in its second year.

Misuse of child restraint systems is more common than one might expect. Several recent studies report misuse rates between 62.9% and 79.5% (c.f. Eby & Kostniuk, 1999). In order to combat this problem, MPI and the Winnipeg Fire Department began a program that allows parents to bring child car seats into fire stations around the city and have the seat and installation inspected free of charge. Plans are underway to extend the program to rural parts of Manitoba.

6 Speeding

This campaign utilized television and billboards to call attention to the consequences of a speeding collision to drivers. The campaign was augmented by increased police surveillance of speed limits. While pre-campaign measures have been amassed, final statistics are still not available due to a lag in the time between the gathering of the statistics and their release by the provincial government. Year-on-year trends, however suggest that the ads are playing a role in reducing speeding on Manitoba roads.

7 Motorcycle Safety

This educational campaign included direct mailings to motorcyclists, and placing billboards targeting other drivers. The goals were to provide information about safety practices and equipment to motorcyclists, and to increase driver awareness of motorcycles during the summer months.

8 Senior Road User Safety

An Ontario study has shown that, on the basis of kilometres driven, older drivers are involved in approximately the same number of collisions as 16–24-year-old drivers. Furthermore, seniors who are involved in an accident are more likely to die from their injuries or take longer to recover. The Older and Wiser Driver booklet was produced to address this issue. The 25-page booklet addresses safe driving from an older person's perspective and provides tools for self-rating driving capability along with other information geared towards the mature driver. The booklet has only recently been developed so evaluation of its effectiveness is not available at this time.

The RoadWise program addresses both the event and pre-event phases of injury as defined by Haddon (1980). For example, the pre-event phase, the period in which the interplay of factors determines if an injury event will occur, is addressed by programs that develop skilled and unimpaired drivers, such as the high school driver education program and RoadWatch. Programs that address the event phase include the High-Risk Driver Campaign, Click In to Win, and child safety seat inspections. These programs affect the time of crisis (the event phase) by influencing the degree of injury that will occur. Aspects of host, agent, and environment, the factors defined by Haddon as coming together during the pre-event and event phases, are also addressed by the RoadWise campaign, to different degrees for each component. Similarly, Table 2 depicts how each program fits into the three Es of injury prevention and the evaluation component of the programs.

TABLE 2.   Effectiveness of the RoadWise Program

RoadWise component	Education	Engineering/ environment	Enactment or enforcement	Evaluation*
Traffic club	✓			*
High school driver's ed.	✓			✓
High-risk driver campaign	✓			*
RoadWatch	✓		✓	✓
Click in to win	✓		✓	✓
Child car seat inspections	✓	✓	✓	*
Speeding campaign	✓		✓	*
Motorcycle safety	✓			*
Older & wiser driver	✓			*

*The effectiveness of media and direct educational campaigns for the RoadWise program have been assessed through surveys and self-reported changes in driving behaviour. Checked rows indicate specific assessment of the intervention.

As stated earlier, the impetus for this program came in 1993. After an extensive review of past interventions both within and outside Manitoba, MPI felt that a new program must address or incorporate the following conclusions:

- an integrated approach which simultaneously addresses as many elements of the system simultaneously as possible is more likely to succeed;
- the magnitude and cost of the problem must be recognized and put on the public policy agenda;
- cooperation and collaborative effort on the part of many partners is essential;
- sufficient resources and multiple interventions over an extended time period are required to sustain a critical mass of awareness across the community; and
- the development of intervention must be guided by a systems approach to the problem.

MPI developed a number of objectives and goals for the Road Safety division of MPI and for the RoadWise program. As part of an overall corporate plan to provide innovative and effective driver safety programs, the Objective for Road Safety was: "To expand their driver safety program and include a strategy of life-long learning for Manitobans. It will start at the pre-school level and continue throughout adulthood."

Goals connected to this objective were threefold:

1 to seek the cooperation of the Manitoba Department of Education to introduce driver safety teaching models into the public school curriculum;
2 to expand the number of community-based partnerships; and
3 to consult with industry experts to create a suitable driver safety index whereby MPI can measure the comparative safety of Manitoba drivers against other North American jurisdictions.

The immediate objectives of the RoadWise initiative were:

• to increase public awareness of the major causes of collisions other than speeding and drinking and driving by more than 3% from the baseline awareness of 58%; and
• to achieve an expected improvement in attitudinal and behavioural changes by at least 6% among the monitoring public with respect to bad driving habits.

The ultimate objectives of the initiative were:

• to reduce the number and severity of traffic crashes resulting from unsafe driver actions by 3% in 5 years; and
• to protect the public from the effects of motor vehicle-related losses.

Stakeholders and Collaborators
Stakeholders in the development of RoadWise were primarily police agencies and a division of Driver Vehicle Licensing. Subsequent supporters included agencies such as the Selective Traffic Enforcement Committee (STEC), and policy analysis and other government agencies such as Highways, Health, and Justice. Later collaborators included the Addiction Foundation of Manitoba, the Canadian Automobile Association (CAA), and IM-PACT. MPI sees the program as a collaborative effort, but mass advertising and educational campaigns are largely MPI's responsibilities. MPI utilizes their already good relationship with

policing agencies to coordinate programs and time campaigns based on trends in data. Fundamentally, the programs are an MPI initiative.

MPI found increasing support over time as they were able to demonstrate the effectiveness of the programs. The corporation was assisted in this endeavour by its strong relationship with police, medical, and professional agencies.

Resources

Road Safety became a strategic corporate goal for MPI in 1993. As such, Road Safety was established as a formal department. The corporation devoted considerable financial resources and corporate effort to the department, and is continuing to do so. Recently, the structure was reorganized such that mass media campaigns and advertising are carried out through a separate department, leaving Road Safety free to concentrate on program design and analysis. This restructuring is in keeping with Road Safety's new focus on public responsibility, in addition to public awareness.

Implementation

The most effective strategy as perceived by MPI has been the use of media; however, the department feels that this medium has achieved as much as it can in terms of raising public awareness of Road Safety issues and of the RoadWise campaign. Future strategies will engage in more direct contact with the target population, or in a personal presence in communities.

Each program under the RoadWise campaign is data driven and targets a particular demographic (i.e., the road-user population that commits a given offensive behaviour and the incidence rate) for which an initiative can be built and evaluated. This use of data to develop programs for specific target groups builds diversity into the RoadWise program and accounts for its seamless approach to every age group and provincewide reach.

From the outset, MPI provided its new department with ample funding for media campaigns and program development. The availability of financial resources was a great help to implementation. One barrier to the implementation of the campaign was that it dealt with public awareness of an issue that was not new or fresh. The need to reinvent the problem in an attention-grabbing way posed a challenge for the program developers. Also, the difficulty in accessing timely statistics on injuries and accidents (these statistics are released quite slowly from the government) proved a hindrance in some evaluation areas, although ongoing customer consultation (through comment cards) helped provide a basis for feedback and redevelopment. Another difficulty for MPI is reaching beyond the education component to the engineering and enforcement components of a model injury prevention program.

As a Crown corporation, MPI is invested in and accountable to bureaucratic political processes that deal with road safety; there is, however, substantial autonomy for development of programs within MPI. Partners in decision making may include the Manitoba Road Safety Coordinating Committee (MRSCC) and the Police Advisory Council (PAC). Also, MPI always uses a collaborative approach in the development of programs with government and non-government stakeholders. When collaborating, MPI develops an agreement that establishes clear terms of reference for each group and sets out roles and responsibilities. In the event of disputes, this document is called on to assist in resolution. In most cases, MPI takes primary responsibility for a given campaign.

Outcome

MPI notes that an unexpected outcome of the program was the wide acceptance of the RoadWise logo and concept by the public and especially by young people. This brand awareness provides immediate recognition of RoadWise campaigns and creates an immediate context for any RoadWise endeavour. Essentially, people know who they are and why they are there.

Evaluation

The RoadWise Public Awareness campaigns have a clear evaluation framework in place. The framework comprises an ecological study, in which pre-and post-measures form the bases for evaluation. The framework also includes other evaluation designs described in the Table 1 of the *ONF Guide to Program Design and Evaluation Planning*; for example, archival data. The RoadWise evaluation framework includes clear and measurable goals, specific evaluation criteria, and a plan for integration of the findings. The evaluative criteria include a public awareness index, self-reported changes in attitudes and driving habits, changes in the perceived level of risk associated with the collision contributory factors addressed in the campaign, changes in police reported at-fault accident contributory factors, changes in annual MPI claims data, and cost benefit analyses of the media campaigns. Data sources include tracking telephone surveys, claims data, and other statistical data.

Program Successes

The program has been successful in meeting 2 of its 3 major goals: 1) acquiring the cooperation of the Manitoba Department of Education and 2) expanding the number of community-based partnerships (e.g., the Child Car Seat Inspection Program). The program has not yet been able to develop a Driver Safety Index that is useful and valid both within and outside Manitoba. While a number of factors might contribute to the reduction in casualty crash involvement since the program's inception in 1996, it is likely that the program played some role in producing the concurrent self-reported changes in attitude towards safety in general as well as self-reported changes in driving behaviour.

Ongoing Development

RoadWise's success in meeting its initial goals has in essence challenged the developers to show greater innovation and creativity in order to meet raised expectations. The next step in the campaign will be to move away from public awareness and towards public accountability. Furthermore, the restructuring of the Road Safety department has helped to define the role of Road Safety more clearly as being development and analysis oriented and not media centred.

This program is intended to be an ongoing and evolving program. As such, the results of the evaluation will be used to assess the program and to make changes accordingly. One such avenue for redevelopment is through dissemination of the program results to stakeholders through regular meetings and annual reports. This sharing of information provides opportunity for further collaboration. Furthermore, because Manitoba has a small population, the relevant collaborators are generally well known and identifiable within the injury prevention community, allowing for both formal and informal connections.

While the roots of the RoadWise campaign lie in public education, the developers have made efforts to touch on the engineering and enforcement aspects which are so necessary to effective injury pre-vention. For example, the campaign enabled engineering issues to be addressed with its child safety seat campaign, and funded overtime for police checkpoints for impaired drivers. This effort to span the hallmarks of good injury prevention programs is to the credit of RoadWise.

Also worthy of attention is that each RoadWise component program is data-driven in terms of development and implementation, and in-cludes an evaluative component designed by MPI's strategic research services. The results are then reinvested into the program. In this way, the program is able to evolve. Having achieved increased public aware-ness of Road Safety issues, RoadWise is now moving towards public action and accountability as a goal. Finally, the program is also unique because it knits together a complete list of road safety issues and covers the lifespan in its reach.

SafetyBeltSafe U.S.A.

Main Key Informant:
Stephanie M. Tombrello, LCSW

Background

SafetyBeltSafe U.S.A. is a non-profit organization dedicated to child passenger safety in motor vehicles. The agency states that its mission is to "help reduce the number of serious and fatal traffic injuries suffered by children by promoting the correct and consistent use of safety seats and safety belts." SafetyBeltSafe U.S.A. maintains relationships with the Society for Automotive Engineers and automobile manufacturers and is known for its up-to-date technical materials.

Consumers

While the organization sees parents as the ultimate target group for their efforts, their consumers are primarily information and service providers who disseminate SafetyBeltSafe U.S.A.'s materials. The ef-forts of the organization are thus multiplied without the need for unsustainable staffing levels. Parents, however, are also direct recipients of SafetyBeltSafe U.S.A.'s services. The organization maintains a website and 2 toll-free phone lines as a direct contact to parents. These measures also suggest that the potential reach of the organization is worldwide.

Collaborators

SafetyBeltSafe U.S.A. is described by its executive director as a diverse group with numerous partnerships, affiliates, and members. Included in its collaborative profile are ongoing relationships with the local and international corporate world. For example, current projects include partnerships with Nissan North America, American Honda, Allstate Insurance Company, and Toyota Motor Sales, U.S.A., among others. Although it is available to carry out private contracts, the agency will not enter an exclusive relationship with any one corporation. Since its inception, the organization has worked with all law enforcement agencies in the country.

History and Development

SafetyBeltSafe U.S.A. was founded 20 years ago with an initial mandate to serve Los Angeles County in California. The impetus for the founding of the organization occurred in 1980 when the current executive director of SafetyBeltSafe U.S.A. attended a state conference on child passenger safety issues. At this conference, discussion among individuals of various professional backgrounds from Los Angeles County highlighted the need for an organization dedicated to child passenger safety within the county. In response, the organization was initially founded as a grassroots intervention under a different name. When the organization began to achieve national recognition, its current title was adopted in order to reflect the national span of the organization.

SafetyBeltSafe U.S.A. runs a number of initiatives that address child passenger safety. The organization's available services include the following programs:

1 Safe Ride Helpline
The Safe Ride Helpline provides telephone counselling to parents who need help choosing or correctly installing safety seats. The helpline is also an important resource to provide technical consultation and materials review for professionals and advocates. A further resource to

callers is the SafetyBeltSafe U.S.A. website (http://www.carseat.org), which also provides email links to the organization for online inquiries.

2 Training

SafetyBeltSafe U.S.A. provides training for advocates, law enforcement officers, safety and health care professionals, educators, social service providers, and staff of child restraint distribution programs. The organization has provided more than 200 8-hour workshops since 1980 and in doing so has provided training to more than 6,000 advocates and professionals. The organization also provides special technical seminars as well as a 4-day training program for national certification. Indeed, before a national program existed, SafetyBeltSafe U.S.A. developed a statewide program to certify Child Passenger Safety Specialists under a grant from the California Office of Traffic Safety (Tombrello, 1996).

3 Public Awareness Campaigns

SafetyBeltSafe U.S.A. continually generates press releases, public service announcements, and posters. The organization fosters long-term relationships with mass media personnel including reporters, columnists, and feature writers. In the first 5 months of 1999, SafetyBeltSafe U.S.A. was able to verify 20 instances of media coverage.

4 Publications and Technical Resources

SafetyBeltSafe U.S.A. publishes a bimonthly newsletter, brochures, reference guides, and technical updates. The organization's website contains a technical update area that has up-to-date information on over 50 topic areas related to child passenger safety. Also, the site provides information needed by parents to purchase the best seat for their child, their vehicle, and their needs in a step-by-step format. Organization staff hold technical teleconferences for Californians bimonthly, participate in bimonthly program teleconferences in California, and are active in materials review both directly and through the California materials review committee. Automatic Updating is a service available to SafetyBeltSafe U.S.A. members; whenever the recall/replacement part list is updated, a packet of revised or new materials is sent on to these subscribers.

The initiatives of SafetyBeltSafe U.S.A. target both the pre-event and event phase of an injury-inducing incident as described by Haddon

(1980). Furthermore, the efforts of the organization cover the 3 major areas of injury prevention: education, engineering, and enactment. The following section describes the current initiatives of SafetyBeltSafe U.S.A. and how they address these 3 areas.

In 1998 SafetyBeltSafe U.S.A. created a 3-year plan of action specific to the State of California that included 39 objectives with the goal of expanding the Child Passenger Safety Net. A large portion of the goals involved education. While safety seat use is legislated throughout North America and compliance is good, rates of safety seat misuse are extraordinarily high. For this reason, education about proper use is an essential component of injury prevention work in this area. SafetyBeltSafe U.S.A. employs a multilateral approach to education through methods that include training, workshops, contests, media blitzes, safety seat checkups, and helpline responders.

SafetyBeltSafe U.S.A. is also committed to expanding enactment and enforcement of child safety regulations. Within its 3-year plan, at least 5 of the objectives deal directly with this aspect of prevention. The methods include: the issuance of safety belt citations and well-publicized enforcement saturation operations by an enforcement agency (Los Angeles Sheriffs Department); safety seat checkups to help caregivers comply with legislation; education of law enforcement agencies; recognition to officers who write citations for child restraint violations; and collaboration with Judicial Council. SafetyBeltSafe U.S.A. actively consults on legislative/regulatory initiatives at the state and federal levels.

Finally, SafetyBeltSafe U.S.A. addresses engineering aspects in the plan through its effort to develop a standardized data collection protocol for safety seat checkups and a methodology to rank various types of misuses. Information collected in this standardized way may help support 2 objectives: the development of intuitive child restraint systems that are difficult to misuse and the legislation of independent attachment systems for safety seats in motor vehicles.

Resources

Aside from a small endowment fund, SafetyBeltSafe U.S.A. does not have permanent funding. Instead, the organization has sought grants, memberships, and donations to cover administrative costs and has funded initiatives through diverse means. In some cases, the agency obtains government funding for California-specific initiatives; in others, it relies on its fundraising expertise. One example is the franchising of a program developed by SafetyBeltSafe U.S.A. called Family Safety in the Car. The program licensees and their instructors must be trained in child passenger safety and follow the prescribed program in its entirety since it involves providing services for courts and evaluating safety seats. Under this arrangement, SafetyBeltSafe U.S.A. earns $1 from licensee costs for every student enrolled in the program. Fines levied upon violators of child restraint and safety belt laws represent an additional source of program funding. Finally, the organization sells the data they collect as another way to support their initiatives.

Implementation

SafetyBeltSafe U.S.A. routinely collaborates with other stakeholders such as agencies and professionals in the field. Many of the initiatives of the organization involve law enforcement, health, and social agencies. Also, the organization collaborates with the Society of Automotive Engineers, manufacturers, and legislators.

Effective Practices

The organization recognizes the need to make its message relevant to the target population, and that this need is best accomplished by understanding and respecting the unique and variable composition of that group. Accordingly, SafetyBeltSafe U.S.A. has programs that target the diverse population of California. For example, the organization provides both an English- and a Spanish-language hotline in recognition of this diversity. At least one brochure is available in a dozen languages. SafetyBeltSafe U.S.A. also recognizes that prevention of injuries relies on a number of interrelated aspects, such as good design and societal values, and for this reason attempts to engage as many agencies as possible in safety initiatives. Cultural sensitivity has been a component of the hundreds of Educator Workshops held for at least the past 15 years.

Decision Making and Planning

SafetyBeltSafe U.S.A. maintains both a board of directors and an advisory board. Decision making is generally the responsibility of the approximately 15 paid staff members under the general guidelines of the elected Board of Directors that meets monthly. Others involved in planning include trained volunteers, part-time helpers, program consultants, and bilingual resource personnel. Most initiatives for the organization are based on contracts that have specific outlines and objectives. The specificity of this arrangement generally obviates the need for dispute resolution mechanisms within the organization. In its 20-year history, 1 member has resigned as a result of a disagreement over a position taken by the organization (S. Tombrello, personal communication, May 4, 2000).

Outcome

Ongoing Evaluation

While SafetyBeltSafe U.S.A. continually compiles data, especially through the Family Safety in the Car, Helpline, and Safety Seat Checkup services, staff is cautious in claims for direct effects on specific behaviour measured. Understanding the nature of data analysis, and often lacking funding for specific research, they are hesitant to apply this data as an evaluative measure because its collection is not subject to proper scientific controls. Nevertheless, the score card has shown that careful, though limited, data analysis has been borne out by other research in the field. Data collection through Family Safety in the Car has been controlled carefully and has proved a useful resource since more than 30,000 violators/students have participated in the program. Evaluations submitted at each Educator Workshop by students and at safety seat checkups by families are carefully reviewed. The organization does employ other approaches to evaluation, such as program monitoring, client satisfaction, and outcome/impact evaluation, which are discussed in Chapter 3 of the *ONF Guide to Program Design and Evaluation Planning*.

Expanding the Child Passenger Safety Net

A report on the first year of the 3-year plan indicates that program objectives that targeted levels of safety seat usage for infants and toddlers have been surpassed and that misuse levels are lower than the targeted reduction. The improvement in U.S. rates of child safety seats is a marked success, and other indicators suggest that overall, the plan is progressing well. Furthermore, objectives regarding education and enforcement have been met by the organization. A revised usage survey tool has been developed and implemented, and final evaluation will be made after one more year.

Other Successes

Safety Seat Voucher Program
From 1994 to 1996, SafetyBeltSafe U.S.A. piloted an education and safety seat voucher distribution program to low-income clients in Los Angeles County (Tombrello, 1997). SafetyBeltSafe U.S.A. was designated by the Los Angeles County Department of Health Services to establish the program, which would be funded by fines collected for violations of the safety seat law. This program, which covered 88 cities in the county, overcame challenges such as the lack of problem awareness in the target populations (in some communities, child passenger restraint was not seen as an important issue), and resulted in 1,289 individuals being educated about child passenger safety. Nine hundred and five of the participants received a voucher for $35 towards the purchase of a child safety seat and 73% of the vouchers were redeemed. Also, 161 participants returned for a safety seat checkup and errors were generally minor (a $10 grocery voucher was offered as an incentive for the checkup). Based on the success of this pilot project, the Los Angeles Department of Health Services expanded the program and hired SafetyBeltSafe U.S.A. as a technical and program consultant.

Legislative and Regulatory Efforts

SafetyBeltSafe U.S.A. has had a number of successes in the area of legislation and regulation since its inception in 1980. These successes include:

- petitioning of the National Highway Traffic Safety Administration to require shoulder belts in the rear seats of all post-1989 passenger vehicles;
- assisting the California Senate Transportation committee in writing the 1983 child restraint law;
- discovery of a counterfeit, illegally imported car seat in the late 1980s and then working with the LAPD and City Attorney in the investigation which led to confiscation of thousands of dangerous products and a subsequent public awareness campaign;
- passage of the 1984 national law earmarking funds for child passen-

ger safety efforts in every state, leading to attending the bill signing in the White House Rose Garden as a guest of the congressman who carried the legislation; and
• petitioning the Federal Aviation Administration to protect children under age 2 by requiring that they be properly restrained on aircraft. This effort has been ongoing since 1982; a current rule-making process has been underway since June 1999.

Dissemination

SafetyBeltSafe U.S.A. utilizes a variety of methods to distribute information to stakeholders. The most commonly used methods include the organization's website, helplines, media, pamphlets, and follow-up information packages to callers.

SafetyBeltSafe U.S.A. has run a number of initiatives (not all described in this profile) that incorporate both education and enactment. While data is routinely collected by the agency, it prefers not to place a great deal of emphasis on data due to the lack of controls and related perceptions of methodological weaknesses. The agency does monitor the effectiveness of its programs, however, and should not be faulted for not drawing direct causal relationships between observational data on safety seat use and its programs. The observations required by the state are of a general geographical area. It is unknown if those being observed were directly affected by the SafetyBeltSafe U.S.A. program.

PROMISING PRACTICES

Retro-Reflective Clothing

Main Key Informant:
Viola Hoo

Background

Night-time and low-visibility hours on roads can be hazardous for professionals, workers, and pedestrians who are on or near the road, but unseen by approaching motorists (3M Canada Company, n.d.-a). Due to reduced visibility, the risk of pedestrian injuries increases during twilight and night hours. This increased risk is only moderate for children, since they generally are not walking during the night hours. Nonetheless, "more than half of all pedestrian deaths and injuries occur when pedestrians cross or enter streets" (National Safety Council 1994 as cited in Luoma, Schumann, & Traube, 1995, p. 378). Prevention of pedestrian injuries during the night hours has been approached in a number of different ways, including increased street lighting and the use of retro-reflective (commonly referred to as reflective) clothing. Increased street lighting has proven to be expensive, and thus may not be practical in rural areas. Retro-reflective clothing appears to be an inexpensive and feasible alternative.

Retro-reflective Material

"Retro-reflection occurs when surfaces retain a portion of the directed light to its source" (3M Canada Company, n.d.-b). Retro-reflective materials appear brightest to observers located near the light source, such as a driver and the headlights of his or her vehicle. This is true for drivers at any angle, which makes retro-reflective surfaces excellent for night visibility (3M Canada Company, n.d.-c).

It is possible to buy both retro-reflective clothing and retro-reflective material, which can subsequently be attached to any article of clothing. Retro-reflective material is lightweight, flexible, and comfortable to wear. It is easily sewn, ironed, or stuck onto uniforms, jackets, vests, sportswear, footwear, and accessories (3M Canada Company, n.d.-a).

Research studies have shown that retro-reflective markings on clothing increase the distance at which pedestrians remain visible at night. Although the majority of studies to date have been conducted in laboratory settings, Luoma, Schumann, and Traube (1995) replicated the main features of an earlier laboratory study by Owens, Francis, and Leibowitz (1989) in a field study.

Effects of Retro-reflector Positioning on Night-time
Recognition of Pedestrians

The study was conducted in a predominantly dark road environment where over half of the encounters included a pedestrian crossing. It investigated the potential effects of retro-reflector positioning on recognition of night-time pedestrians (Luoma et al., 1995). Four retro-reflector configurations were tested: 1) no retro-reflectors on the pedestrian, 2) retro-reflectors on the torso, 3) retro-reflectors on the wrists and ankles, and 4) retro-reflectors on the major joints.

Participants
Thirty-two paid subjects participated in the study. Sixteen subjects were between the ages of 20 and 28, and 16 were between the ages of 60 and 77. There were 8 females and 8 males in each group. Subjects performed a recognition task while seated in the front and rear passenger's seats of a car driven on a dark road with low-beam lamps illuminated (Luoma et al., 1995). The subjects were asked to press a hand-held response button whenever they recognized a pedestrian on or alongside the road ahead of the subject vehicle. They were told not to respond to anything else on the road. A timer was connected to each subject's response button.

Resources

Manufacturers like 3M Canada Company produce reflective products. These materials are sold in roll goods, which are then sold to either converters or garment manufacturers. Converters take the manufacturer's product and make it into a saleable item such as a sticker or an armband (V. Hoo, personal communication, February 29, 2000). Converters also have the capability of screen printing or die-cutting reflective materials (V. Hoo, personal communication, February 29, 2000).

Implementation

The Luoma et al. (1995) study was conducted on rural roadway sections with only sparse traffic. Along the route, 9 locations were chosen for the experimental sites where the subject vehicle encountered a pedestrian. In addition to the pedestrian targets the route included retro-reflective traffic signs, roadside reflector posts, and other types of retro-reflective markings. As well, there were a number of distractions, including:

- 4 encounters with traffic cones;
- 3 encounters with a bicycle; and
- 2 encounters with a barricade with retro-reflector stripes.

The experiment was conducted at least 50 minutes after sunset and it lasted for approximately 45 minutes. It was conducted only on nights without active precipitation or water on the road surface, and in locations free of lighting from buildings, and free of other traffic.

Outcome

The findings of the Luoma et al. (1995) study determined wrists and ankles configuration, as well as the major joints configuration, lead to significantly longer recognition distances than when the markings are attached to the torso. "This was the case whether a pedestrian was approaching the vehicle (156–169 m vs. 96 m) or a pedestrian was crossing the road (241–249 m vs. 136 m)" (Luoma et al., 1995, pp. 380–381).

"When the retro-reflective markings were attached to pedestrians, the crossing condition yielded 42–53% longer recognition distances than the approaching condition. When a pedestrian had no retro-reflectors, the recognition distance in the crossing condition was 13% shorter than in the approaching condition" (Luoma et al., 1995, p. 380). The effect of the walking direction indicates that pedestrians with retro-reflective markings are more visible when they are crossing the road. This result is significant as most pedestrian accidents occur when pedestrians cross or enter the road (Luoma et al., 1995, p. 381).

The findings also revealed that the older subjects in this study needed shorter distances (i.e., to be closer) to recognize a pedestrian. "The magnitude of this difference was even larger when pedestrians were approaching the vehicle, which is a more demanding condition because of less movement, than when they were crossing the road" (Luoma et al., 1995, p. 381).

Retro-reflective clothing has the potential to reduce the risk of injury to pedestrians during the night-time and low visibility hours. The results of Luoma et al. (1995) study measuring the recognition distance of subjects in response to retro-reflector positioning on pedestrians look promising. Further work needs to be done, however, to determine whether or not the use of retro-reflective clothing actually reduces the number of injuries and fatalities among pedestrians.

Intelligent Traffic Signals for Pedestrian Detection

Main Key Informant:
Dr Oliver M.J. Carsten

Background

Statistics from the United States indicate that pedestrians are involved in a high percentage of fatal motor vehicle crashes (Sarkar, Nederveen, & Pols, 1997). In Canada, deaths relating to pedestrian injury account for the second highest incidence of deaths due to road traffic accidents in the under-20 age category (Health Canada, 1997). Because brain and spinal cord injuries are a common result of motor vehicle crashes (SMARTRISK, 1998a), increased safety for pedestrians, who are the most vulnerable group of road users, should be addressed. Current signalized crossings cater to vehicle demand, thus resulting in several problems for pedestrians. In most countries, the following problems for pedestrians are commonly found at the typical signalized crossing (Carsten, Sherborne, & Rothengatter, 1998):

- pedestrians should push a button to indicate their intention to cross, however, they frequently do not;
- time provided for crossings are inadequate; and
- signal response to pedestrian demand is inadequate; the pedestrian stage is available only at particular points in the signal cycle.

After observing microwave vehicle detectors at a tradeshow, the principal investigator of the Vulnerable Road User Traffic Observation and Optimization (VRU-TOO) project believed that these devices, if converted to pedestrian detectors, had the potential to ameliorate pedestrian problems. Consequently he approached the manufacturer of the vehicle detectors and presented them with the idea. Fixed on top of traffic signals, the detector registers the approach of a pedestrian and can be employed at signalized crossings to:

- replace normal push-button mechanisms;
- activate the pedestrian stage earlier;
- extend the pedestrian stage for late arrivals; and
- extend the pedestrian stage for a large number of detections.

The VRU-TOO project was part of a transport research project funded by the European Commission, Dedicated Road Infrastructure of Vehicle Safety in Europe (DRIVE II). There was an open call for proposals and the VRU-TOO research team bid for the task in the area of systems for vulnerable road users. The project ran from 1992 to 1995 as part of the European Community DRIVE II Programme. The research team was an international consortium created for the implementation of this project, and consisted of members from the following institutions: the Institute for Transport Studies, University of Leeds; West Yorkshire Highways Engineering and Technical Services; the Traffic Research Centre, University of Groningen; the Department of Traffic Planning and Engineering, Lund Institute of Technology; FCTUC, University of Coimbra; FEUP-DEC, University of Porto; and TRENDS (Transport Environment Development Systems), Athens.

The VRU-TOO system for pedestrian detection was outfitted in 3 cities, Leeds, England; Porto, Portugal; and Elefsina, Greece. Consortium members for the project made individual arrangements with their respective city councils for the implementation of the detectors.

Objectives

Recognizing that signalized crossings had to be more responsive to the needs of pedestrians without negatively affecting vehicle traffic, the project implementations had the following goals:

- to reduce pedestrian wait time;
- to increase pedestrian comfort and safety; and

- to accomplish the above objectives with minimal negative effects in vehicle traffic queues, delays, and capacity.

Configuration of the VRU-TOO system was tailored to the national regulations of each country, to the particular signal system of each site, to the layout of each junction, and to the observed flows of pedestrian and vehicular traffic.

Resources

Detection Unit

The microwave detector is based upon the Doppler radar principle. The mixing of reflected energy at 2 points in the receiver enables the detector to differentiate between retreating and approaching targets. Detection frequencies of 10.5 or 24 GHz were used and resulted in an adjustable detection range of 8 to 25 m. Careful positioning and angling of the detection unit prevented vehicles from being detected over pedestrians. The ability to adjust the signal timing at a crossing enables conditions of the intersection to be taken into account; for example, the signals can be set to run at fixed intervals during times of day with high traffic volume or they can be adjusted to take into consideration the size of pedestrian demand.

Implementation of the system added approximately 20% to the cost of building a new traffic signal (O.M.J. Carsten, personal communication, April 20, 2000). The system can also be affixed to existing traffic signals.

Evaluation

The safety, comfort, and behaviour of pedestrians and the effect of the VRU-TOO system on vehicle traffic were assessed before and after the implementation of the detection units. Counts of pedestrian-to-vehicle conflicts, as described by Hydén (1987), were used as the primary indicator of pedestrian safety. Other criteria for pedestrian safety included the following:

- percentage of pedestrians violating a red light;
- number of encounters between pedestrians and vehicles; and
- normative pedestrian behaviour (including approach to the curb,

head movements made to observe traffic, and use of the crossing facility).

Pedestrian comfort was monitored by:

- expected delay time (i.e., the time between arrival at the crossing and the onset of the pedestrian green);
- realized wait time (i.e., the time between arrival and departure);
- the percentage of pedestrians who experienced long wait times (10, 20, or 30 seconds);
- the percentage of pedestrians arriving on green; and
- the percentage of pedestrians who started and completed their crossing on green.

Conflict observations were also conducted. Pedestrian behaviour and interactions with vehicles were evaluated by video analysis.

Implementation

The research team included professionals from the fields of electronics, highway engineering, traffic psychology, and traffic safety. Necessary permission for implementation was sought with the appropriate ministries, highway authorities, and so forth. Members of the consortium were involved in discussions of how to implement the system, while exact signal timing was decided by the traffic control or traffic management unit of the individual city concerned. Negotiation of the exact nature of manipulations was a process of give and take with traffic authorities.

One obstacle to the wide-scale implementation of this detection unit was the lack of an industrial stakeholder involved in the manufacture of whole signal systems (O.M.J. Carsten, personal communication, April 20, 2000).

Outcome

The number of observed pedestrian-to-vehicle conflicts in Leeds and Elefsina was reduced, indicating increased pedestrian safety. Unsafe red light violations also declined in Leeds. A decrease in expected delays and a reduction in long wait times were exhibited at most sites, indicating improved pedestrian comfort. As well, the proportion of pedestrians beginning and completing their crossing on a green light increased in all 3 countries. No major side effects on vehicle traffic were noted as a result of the implementation of pedestrian detectors. For a more detailed description of results, please see Carsten et al. (1998).

The results of the study were generally positive. They varied, however, among sites. Characteristics of the sites and manipulation of the detectors also varied. While the use of pedestrian detectors can help decrease conflicts and reduce injuries, further research is warranted to determine the most effective methods of implementing these devices and to measure long-term effects while controlling for confounding variables. To date, it has been determined that signals can provide pedestrian stages as they are needed, activate the green for pedestrians more promptly, extend the pedestrian stage for late arrivals, and account for pedestrian demand at intersections. Moreover, these detectors can be adjusted to the conditions of individual signalized intersections. Currently, the timing of traffic signals is established in favour of motor vehicles. The detection system described has the potential to compensate for the neglected needs of pedestrians.

SAFE KIDS Buckle Up: A National SAFE KIDS Campaign Project

Main Key Informant:
Camilla Taft

Background

In response to recommendations made in the 1995 Blue Ribbon Panel on Child Restraint and Vehicle Compatibility report, the U.S. National SAFE KIDS Campaign (NSKC) began a pilot initiative at O'Donnell Pontiac–GMC in Ellicot City, Maryland, to gauge feasibility of a dealer-based car seat safety program. The organization collected surveys of Car Seat Check Up attendees, new car owners, and dealership employees as well as focus group data from 7 sessions that measured general awareness of child passenger safety and effectiveness of safety messages.

Based on findings from the pilot phase, SAFE KIDS approached General Motors as a potential partner for SAFE KIDS BUCKLE UP (SKBU). In 1997, SAFE KIDS and General Motors (GM) launched SKBU. This nationwide initiative is just one of many SAFE KIDS projects; for information about other National SAFE KIDS Campaign initiatives, please visit their website at http://www.safekids.org.

History and Development

The Blue Ribbon Panel (whose report inspired the creation of SKBU) recommended automobile dealers as a primary conduit for passenger safety information. Accordingly, the SKBU program targets parents and caregivers through GM dealerships in the United States. GM vehicle owners, however, are not the only intended recipients of the campaign efforts.

The National SAFE KIDS Campaign is the combined effort of more than 280 SAFE KIDS Coalitions comprised of a cross-section of community leadership:

- law enforcement officers;
- firefighters and paramedics;
- medical and health professionals;
- educators;
- parents and volunteers;
- business leaders;
- public policy makers; and
- kids.

These coalitions are involved in bringing the SKBU program to their communities. SKBU also involves other health and education partners. The Campaign enlisted OB-GYNs, family physicians, paediatricians, emergency physicians, community health centres, children's hospitals, and Head Start workers as conduits of information and asked them to encourage referral of parents to checkup events.

As recommended in Chapter 2 of the ONF's *Guide to Program Design and Evaluation Planning* (1999), SAFE KIDS developed a number of objectives and goals for the SKBU program. Originally, the program had 4 goals:

1 to answer the Blue Ribbon Panel's call to action;
2 to provide GM dealership employees with basic child passenger

safety education through workshops conducted by trained specialists;

3 to give parents and caregivers hands-on instruction about proper car seat use; and
4 to deliver free educational materials to the public via a toll-free number.

In 1998–1999 additional goals included:

5 to intensify media coverage to increase public outreach; and
6 to conduct original nationwide research to determine precisely how car seats are being misused.

The SKBU program addresses both the host and environment aspects of injury at the event phase as defined by Haddon (1980). Much of the SKBU program is aimed at education and awareness and accomplished through advertising, reading materials, and education partners. The other aim of the program is to change the environment of the injury event phase in 3 ways:

1 by reducing child safety seat misuse;
2 by distributing car seats to needy families; and
3 by providing recall information.

Stakeholders and Collaborators

Stakeholders in the development of SKBU were primarily SAFE KIDS coalitions, GM, and GM dealerships. As noted earlier, these coalitions represent a cross-section of community leaders and the grassroots reach of the campaign. Other partner organizations include:

• the American Academy of Family Physicians;
• the American Academy of Pediatrics;
• the American College of Emergency Physicians;
• the American College of Obstetricians and Gynecologists;
• the National Association of Children's Hospitals and Related Institutions;
• the National Association of Community Health Centers; and
• the National Head Start Association.

The reach of the campaign to minority communities has been facilitated since 1999 by the partnership between SAFE KIDS, GM, the National Association for the Advancement of Colored People (NAACP), and the National Council of La Raza (NCLR) in a related child safety seat distribution program (discussed further below).

Resources

GM entered into a 5-year $10.6 million partnership with SAFE KIDS to promote correct car seat and safety belt usage. As of July 1999, the program costs have been $7.2 million. Almost $2 million of this total has been awarded directly to the coalitions as grants to support the program initiatives: Check Ups, training sessions, and workshops.

Implementation

The SKBU program was launched with a high-profile media campaign on August 28, 1997. The campaign reinforced its media efforts by offering a toll-free number for complimentary child passenger safety educational materials. SAFE KIDS continues to promote its materials through venues such as magazines and television. The campaign developed a variety of media and educational materials that were tested with target audiences to ensure effectiveness.

GM dealers and management were reached through targeted mailings that provided child passenger safety data, local coalition contact information, and a toll-free number for questions. Dealers continue to learn about SKBU through corporate publications and the campaign's newsletter.

From the original pilot project at one dealership, the program has expanded to include more than 2,250 GM dealerships in the United States (SKBU, May, 2000). In partnership with state and local SAFE KIDS coalitions, these dealerships host Car Seat Check Ups and provide educational materials for customers. Also, more than 1,630 dealership staff members have been trained in child passenger safety.

Other national partners and their local affiliates in the health and education fields help to increase the span of SKBU educational materials, as well as to provide referrals to Car Seat Check Ups.

The Car Seat Check Ups initiative has expanded with the donation by Chevrolet of 51 Venture vans to be used as mobile fitting stations. These vans allow coalitions to take child passenger safety "to the streets," reaching more kids and caregivers who need this information in the community. They also enhance the program's visibility, especially where there is not enough room at a particular dealership to house an event. The vans come fully equipped with the makings of a Car Seat Check Up including signage, tents, and a starting supply of car seats.

Along with brochures, advertising, and Check Ups, the SKBU program developed a video that demonstrates effective child restraints for infants, toddlers, children, and youths as well as providing information about safest practices for child passengers.

In May 1998, GM, the United Auto Workers Union (UAW), SAFE KIDS, the NCLR, and the NAACP came together to distribute child safety seats to needy families in the United States as part of America's Promise (a set of 5 basic promises made to every child in America). GM and the UAW committed $5 million over 3 years to the project. SAFE KIDS coalitions provided training to NCLR affiliates and NAACP branches in 9 cities. The representatives then trained and educated families on proper usage of car seats before distributing free car seats (Cruz & Mickalide, 2000). This initiative extended the range of SKBU to minority and underserved communities.

Outcome

As of February 2000, SKBU reports the following numbers:

Initiative	Total
GM dealer Check Up events	1,550
Check Up attendees	118,456
Seats checked	46,190
Misuse rate	89%
Recalled seats	5,401
New safety seats given away	11,005
Educational workshops	418
Dealer staff trained	1,602

Source: *On the Move*, February, 2000.

Initially the program set 4 goals, and then expanded those goals to 6. Each goal has been fulfilled, including the completion of a study of child safety seat misuse in February 1999 that sets out recommendations for experts, the media, government, and car seat manufacturers.

Evaluation

The SKBU program has surpassed each of its goals. The number of dealership staff trained and the number of car seats inspected is more than double the original goal, and calls to the toll-free number are greater than 7 times the predicted 10,000 calls. More than 2 million brochures have been distributed and more than 5,600 car seats have been given to needy families. Furthermore, through the related America's Promise car seat distribution program, over 13,000 new car seats have been distributed to needy families in minority communities.

Program Successes

Safe Kids has documented 26 children whose lives may have been saved as a direct result of their car seats being adjusted at SKBU Check Up events. The SKBU program received the 1999 Allstate National Safety Award out of 500 entries. This award carries a $25,000 grant from the Allstate Foundation.

Ongoing Development

Regrettably, in materials reviewed for this report no mention was made of plans for evaluation of the impact of SKBU upon rates or severity of injury in car seat users. The campaign will however continue its education initiative by expanding its dealership partnership base through continuing coalition grant support, as well as by maintaining partnerships with health and education providers. SAFE KIDS will also continue to participate in Child Passenger Safety Week each year to take advantage of one time of the year when much of the media and public are focused on transporting children safely. Finally, the America's Promise program will continue to advance its achievements and partnerships.

The PARTY Program
Sunnybrook and Women's College Health Sciences Centre, Toronto, Canada

Main Key Informants:
Joanne Banfield, RN, and Sheila Mongeon

Background

Every week dozens of high school students from across the Greater Toronto Area make their way to Sunnybrook and Women's College Health Sciences Centre (SWCHSC) to attend PARTY, which is the acronym for the teen-focused program Prevent Alcohol and Risk-related Trauma in Youth. PARTY is a day-long (8:45 a.m. to 3 p.m.) program that follows the course of a typical trauma case from occurrence through transport, treatment, rehabilitation, and community reintegration. The program is offered Tuesdays and Fridays during the school year at this location, and the applicability of the program to other jurisdictions is now well documented, with over 40 PARTY programs spread across Canada.

The PARTY program was initially conceived in 1985 by an Emergency Room nurse at SWCHSC. Several youths in her neighbourhood had expressed a desire to visit the trauma centre where she worked to see first hand where people involved in motor vehicle collisions were taken for treatment. The students believed that this type of experience would help them in their desire to discourage drinking and driving in their community. The ER nurse agreed that this idea might prove effective and, with an eye towards increasing risk awareness and preventing injury, began to consider a program that would bring in entire classes of teenagers to participate in guided tours of the ER and recovery units. The planning took place through 1985 and the inaugural PARTY program was delivered in January 1986 at SWCHSC.

Today, there are 44 PARTY programs operating in Canada (including SWCHSC) as well as a single U.S. program in Minnesota. While all of these programs are similar in nature, only recently has there been an attempt to monitor and standardize the operation of each individual program. At the present time, the PARTY name is trade-marked in Canada and is being trade-marked in the United States. Also, a set of national standards has been developed under the coordination of the SMARTRISK Foundation, which acts as the PARTY program national secretariat.

At SWCHSC, PARTY operates out of the Office for Injury Prevention. The manager of trauma injury prevention coordinates all aspects of the program, which continues to increase in popularity with each passing year. In fact, it is impossible to meet the current demand from school boards wanting their students to participate. To date, over 20,000 teens have participated at this site alone.

Consumers

The target population of the PARTY program is male and female high school students aged 16 and over (i.e., Grade 11 through Grade 13/OAC), drawn from a 300 km radius around Toronto. On a typical program day, a high school class of approximately 30–35 students accompanied by an adult leader (usually a teacher) will attend. The initial decision to target this specific age group was made in view of the fact that these students would be of legal driving age in the Province of Ontario (J. Banfield, personal communication, March 20, 2000).

More recently, however, the program has been made available to Grade 10 students (i.e., 15 year olds). This change was made for 2 reasons. First, the elimination of Grade 13/OAC after the 2000–2001 school year will significantly reduce the current target audience. Second, available evidence suggests that youth are becoming involved in high-risk activities at younger ages so it was considered prudent to begin targeting youth in advance of attaining legal driving age. Motor vehicle collisions involving teens, which are the leading cause of serious head and spinal cord injury for this age group, are both predictable and preventable and thus a major concern for neurotrauma prevention initiatives (J. Banfield, personal communication, March 20, 2000).

Goals and Objectives

The PARTY program's mission statement is "to promote injury prevention through reality education, enabling youth to recognize risk and make informed choices about activities and behaviours." This strategy is consistent with Haddon's (1980) theory of injury prevention at the primary level, which is to prevent the occurrence of the hazard in the first place (i.e., the pre-event phase), and emphasizes the importance of making self-interested choices regarding risk-taking behaviour. The specific goals and objectives of the program are listed below.

1 To reduce the incidence of risk-related trauma in youth:

- provide youth with positive alternatives and strategies to encourage smart choices;
- expose youth to the potential social and physical limitations that can result from traumatic injury, using reality education; and
- encourage youth to directly apply strategies learned at PARTY.

2 To empower youth to recognize risk and make informed, safe choices:

- identify potentially dangerous situations and behaviours through personal testimony, videos, slides, and active participation.

3 To increase awareness of personal responsibility for choices:

- encourage youth to examine their attitudes, decisions, and actions.

4 To increase knowledge of the impact of serious injury on quality of life:

- encourage youth to think about potential loss of independence, friends, self-esteem, and control of their bodies as a result of injury.

5 To promote injury prevention initiatives:

- demonstrate PARTY program's active participation in promotion of injury prevention initiatives at a local, provincial, national, and international level.

Implicit in these objectives is the important contribution the program makes as part of the growing community effort to reduce preventable injuries owing to alcohol and risk-related activities (PARTY Program, 1999).

Resources

This section of the report presents a discussion of the model underlying the PARTY program as well as its sources of funding.

Model

Strictly speaking, the PARTY program is not based upon a specific injury prevention model or program. Rather, development of the program was founded upon "the belief that in order to improve and better understand adolescent health, sectors of education, government, health care, and community services need to focus on eliminating the barriers that prevent youth from making informed choices" (PARTY Program, 1999). At the time of development, there were few, if any, programs of its kind in operation; indeed, pre- and post-testing conducted in area schools indicated a pressing need for this type of injury prevention program. This indication was further supported by the teen trauma statistics at SWCHSC.

The principle underlying the design/format of the PARTY program is the value of reality education. That is, the typical classroom lecture format is avoided as much as possible in order to involve the participants more directly and more completely in the actual experience of injury and recovery. The program day is organized such that the group is walked along the common course of injury and treatment of someone who has been involved in a motor vehicle crash or other trauma. Teaching techniques include:

- simulated trauma resuscitation;
- slide presentations;
- interaction with flight paramedics and trauma nurses;
- question-and-answer periods with health care professionals such as physicians, nurses, and social workers;
- tours of the Trauma Room, Critical Care Unit, and Neuro-Intensive Care Unit; and
- personal contact with injury survivors at the Toronto Rehabilitation Institute (Lyndhurst Site), a local spinal cord rehabilitation centre.

Topics discussed throughout the course of the day include: the effect of alcohol/drugs on decision making, judgment, concentration, and coordination; basic anatomy, physiology, and the mechanics of injury; the nature of injuries that can be repaired and those that cannot; and the effect of traumatic injury on families, friends, and future plans.

Very few significant (i.e., structural) changes have been made to the program since its inception in 1986. In recognition of the fact that other risks in addition to alcohol consumption contribute to injury among teens, a minor name change occurred in 1988 in which the words "risk related" were added (the PARTY acronym initially stood for Prevent Alcohol-Related Trauma in Youth). Over the years, the degree of hands-on or personal experience with the aftermath of major trauma has been enhanced. For example, participants now actually handle various pieces of medical equipment, perhaps a catheter or a halo vest, while a member of the PARTY Team explains the function of the item. Also, the amount of time spent in direct contact with injury survivors has been increased. It is believed that these changes, though minor, are important with respect to the ongoing effort to personalize the program.

Funding

The PARTY program initially received one-time seed funding from the Ontario Ministry of Health in 1985 to develop the program. Following the development phase, ongoing operating funding was applied for and received through the Emergency Health Services Branch of the Ministry of Health. Until 1998 an annual application was made for continued funding. Regular stable funding is now maintained by the Ministry of Health as part of its annual base operating grant to SWCHSC. Since this funding has remained at the same level for many years, however, the program regularly exceeds its budget and relies on SWCHSC to cover the cost over-runs. Office space and equipment is provided on-site by SWCHSC.

In 1998 the Office for Injury Prevention at SWCHSC received funding from the Ontario Neurotrauma Foundation ($80,000 over 2 years) to investigate the potential effectiveness of a Junior High PARTY Program. The objectives of this study were twofold: to determine the prevalence of risk-taking behaviour in youths aged 12–14 and to conduct a needs assessment with regard to developing a large-scale prevention program targeting this age group. This research resulted in the adaptation of the existing PARTY program for the junior high school population. At the present time, the Junior High PARTY Program is operating in 5 Toronto-area schools in a pilot study. A request for funding ($60,000/year for 3 years) has been submitted to the Ontario Neurotrauma Foundation to conduct an extensive evaluation study and to expand the program across the province.

Although there is no cost for attending the PARTY program (other than that for transportation to SWCHSC), a $100 deposit is required for each class to reserve a specific date. This deposit is returned to the school after the visit; however, approximately half of the time the deposit is donated to the program. Also, on many occasions, participating classes have undertaken their own fundraising efforts to assist the program in covering its expenses.

Implementation

The PARTY program employs a multidisciplinary approach to risk awareness and injury prevention. Indeed, the program could not succeed without the collective contributions of educators (teachers, principals, Board of Education officials), the Toronto Rehabilitation Institute, Lyndhurst (physical/occupational therapists, injury survivors), and

SWCHSC (trauma nurses, paramedics, physicians). Each of these collaborators is committed to expanding the foundation of injury prevention. For example, as Canada's largest trauma centre, injury prevention is a significant component of SWCHSC's mandate. The president/chief executive officer of SWCHSC welcomes any opportunity to become involved with new prevention initiatives and is fully supportive of the operation and continued development of the PARTY program.

Effective Practices

The original ideas of both bringing students on guided tours of the ER and critical care units and having them meet actual injury survivors have proven to be key to the success of the PARTY program. According to the program manager, it is these 2 aspects of the program that have the greatest and most enduring impact on the students. While many concepts are discussed and a great deal of information is passed along during the course of the day, it is always the true stories and the one-on-one experiences that the students report as their lasting memories of their visit.

The PARTY program makes allowances for cultural differences and all team members are sensitive to diversity issues that may arise during the course of the day. For example, donating blood and receiving a blood transfusion may be common medical practices, but they are not accepted by Jehovah's Witnesses. Cultural differences such as these rarely pose problems; rather, these sorts of issues are usually raised by the students themselves for further discussion.

When a problem does arise, it is viewed as an opportunity to improve the implementation of the program. For instance, a nurse new to the PARTY team had been choosing inappropriate injury survivors to speak with the students (e.g., a patient with a traumatic head injury) and teachers had made mention of this on the evaluation forms. This feedback precipitated the development of implementation guidelines and teaching packages for the nurse tour guides. Each group (nurses, paramedics, social workers, etc.) is now trained in the effective delivery of the program and receives a set of guidelines and protocol to follow.

A short video was developed for use in cases where a class is unable to participate in the PARTY program. While the video cannot replace a visit to PARTY, it can introduce some of the important concepts covered in the program and has proven useful in stimulating classroom discussion about risk awareness and injury prevention. A manual and discussion guide is available to assist the teacher or other first-time presenter. A new video is being planned in which the activities portrayed by the teens in the docudrama will better reflect both the interests (e.g., extreme sports, raves) and the problems (e.g., suicide, designer drugs) of today's youth. The feasibility of developing a PARTY program website is also being pursued.

The interests and activities of teens are diverse and constantly changing. In order to stay current, the program is flexible in terms of meeting the evolving needs of its target audience. For example, issues such as youth violence, raves, and the use of new designer drugs (e.g., Ecstasy) have been added to the slide presentation and are now raised in the group discussion periods. According to the program manager, the success of the PARTY program is due, in large part, to the fact that "it is highly targeted. It's a program for teens and about teens ... We don't talk about seniors' issues" (J. Banfield, personal communication, March 20, 2000).

Decision Making and Planning

The PARTY program has an Advisory Committee, which meets regularly on a quarterly basis. The mandate of the committee is to review the operation of the program and to engage in short- and long-term planning. The committee, which is chaired by the PARTY program manager, is comprised of 8–10 individuals involved with the program, including representation from nurses, the SWCHSC Foundation, Lyndhurst, and the Head of the Trauma Department at SWCHSC.

All decisions are made on the basis of consensus. The program manager describes the nature of the relationship among the committee members as harmonious and respectful. One contentious issue that arose early in the history of the program illustrates how such cases are handled. When those developing the program were searching for potential funding, an offer of sponsorship was received from a beer company. The program was in serious need of additional funding and there was considerable debate over this offer. The committee ultimately reached the decision, however, that such a relationship would be inappropriate given the age of the participants in the program. It has now been written into the mandate of the PARTY program that no funding is to be accepted from alcohol-related companies or the pharmaceutical industry.

Outcome

In this section, the evaluation of the PARTY program is described, followed by an overview of the methods of dissemination of information.

Evaluation

All participants are given a PARTY Program Follow-Up Form to complete during the week following their visit. Essentially, this brief form inquires about: a) participants' feelings about SWCHSC and Lyndhurst; b) whether their visit will have any effect on their activities and lifestyle; and c) the most-liked and least-liked aspects of the program. Finally, participants are asked whether they recall what the acronym PARTY stands for. The adult leader (again, typically a teacher) is encouraged to complete a Follow-Up Form as well.

Over the years, provincial officials from both the Ministry of Health and the Ministry of Education have attended the PARTY program and provided written comments and suggestions. All of this feedback is carefully considered and constructive criticism is passed along to the PARTY team.

Other, more scientific methods of evaluation have also been employed. For instance, a long-term outcome study of the PARTY program was undertaken in 1993. This type of evaluation is referred to as summative evaluation, as its primary objective is to summarize the impact or performance of the program (ONF, 1999). The major research question is: Do those students who have attended the PARTY program have different rates of driving-related offences and injuries compared to a control group of students who have not attended the program? The evaluation is being conducted in conjunction with researchers at SWCHSC and the University of Toronto, with assistance from officials with the Ministry of Health and the Ministry of Transportation.

The study group will consist of consenting PARTY program participants who have provided both their Ontario health card number and driver's licence number. The control group, matched for age and geographical location, will be obtained anonymously through Ministry of Health and Ministry of Transportation databases. Students entering the study at onset will be tracked for a maximum of 10 years, whereas those entering at a later phase in the study will be tracked for a minimum of 5 years. Statistical analyses will be performed to investigate differences in the injury and incident records of the 2 groups, as well to examine potential age and gender differences. Results will not become available until 2004.

The PARTY Team at the Ottawa General Hospital has recently completed a short-term evaluation of its program (Nuth, Mongeon, Currie, & Curran, 1999). The objective of this summative evaluation (ONF, 1999) was to determine the impact of the PARTY program on injury prevention knowledge, attitudes, and behaviours at 6 months after completion of the program. To measure these outcome variables, the researchers utilized the Spinal Cord Assessment of Risk Inventory (SCARI), a 32-item self-report measure with sound psychometric properties (Currie, DeGagne, Cwinn, Mongeon, & Seymour, 1995).

A convenience sample of 257 Ottawa-area high school students was drawn for the purposes of the evaluation. The students completed the SCARI immediately prior to beginning the PARTY program and then again 6 weeks later. The final sample consisted of 203 students (52% female; mean age = 16.5 years). The results indicated a significant improvement in the level of injury prevention awareness after having visited PARTY; in fact, scores improved on 3 of the 5 SCARI sub-scales. The students demonstrated greater knowledge of head and spinal cord injury risk factors, more positive general attitudes towards safe behaviours, and more positive attitudes specifically regarding helmet use. There was no statistically significant change in frequency of reported helmet use or level of high-risk behaviours reported (Nuth et al., 1999).

Dissemination of Information

Until 1998, annual reports were prepared for the Ontario Ministry of Health detailing the operation and budget of the PARTY program. These reports are no longer required, following the Ministry's decision to make permanent the program's funding through the annual base operating grant to SWCHSC.

With regard to other stakeholders, Board of Education officials and school principals receive copies of *In Their Own Words*, a compilation of students' comments on their visit to PARTY as culled from the Follow-Up evaluation forms completed during the previous year. The comments quoted below reflect the considerable impact the program has had on participants:

It made me realize how one little mistake can affect you for the rest of your life.

I really respect and admire the people at Lyndhurst Rehabilitation
Institute for their bravery and I thank them for speaking to us because it
has made an impact on me.

A learning experience that scared me out of my wits!

(Source: *In Their Own Words*)

Finally, there is also outreach to the community through the media.
For instance, an article describing the PARTY program ran in the March
2000 edition of the SWCHSC newsletter. Many similar pieces have
appeared in various newspapers and national magazines over the years.
The Ottawa PARTY program was featured in a detailed profile on the
CBC Evening News in April 2000. An interesting and promising possi-
bility for the future involves a partnership with YTV (Youth Television
Network). Information on the PARTY program is also available via the
Internet on the SWCHSC website (http://www.sunnybrook.on.ca/serv-
ices/injury).

HEROES

Main Key Informant:
Kim Diamond

Background

Toronto-based SMARTRISK's HEROES program is a mobile stage production whose objective is to introduce young people to the notion of
"smart" risk-taking behaviour and to empower them to make simple
decisions that will significantly reduce their risk of injury. The program
consists an hour-long presentation that includes high-tech audio-visual
components, injury-survivor testimonials, a local student presenter, a
question-and-answer period, and suggestions for future courses of strategic action. All components of the presentation are designed to provide knowledge as a tool for minimizing the chance and severity of
youth injury. While studies have been conducted to measure audience
responses to and recall of the central messages of the show, linking
these evaluations to injury rate outcomes has not been attempted.

Instead, HEROES aims to serve an important role in initiating other injury prevention activities within a community, as well as to express an unmistakable, but affirming, message to youth.

History and Development

The SMARTRISK Foundation is a non-profit organization founded by a Toronto-based paediatric heart transplant surgeon who became active in injury prevention after becoming aware that unintentional injuries to youth provided the majority of organs donated for transplant. The accounting firm PriceWaterhouseCoopers, although no longer a corporate partner, extended temporary support through provision of office space, equipment, and expert advice. The organization's original name, the Canadian Injury Prevention Foundation, was changed to SMARTRISK in 1995 to better articulate its objectives. The flagship program, HEROES, was developed in 1992 in an effort to encourage sensible risk-taking behaviour among youth. Other SMARTRISK programs include:

- the Stupid Line Public Service Announcement Campaign;
- SMARTRISK On-line Services and the Canadian Children's Safety Network; and
- the SMARTRISK Ambassador Program (with the Canadian Forces Snowbirds and two high-profile Canadian astronauts).

Consumers

The HEROES program is intended for a grade 9–12 audience, although local feeder schools (grades 7–8) are sometimes invited to attend. SMARTRISK identifies motor vehicle crashes as the leading cause of injury for this population. Falls, drowning, burns, sports injuries, firearms-related incidents, and suicide attempts are also named as significant to the group. In 1998, over 600,000 students across Canada have been participants in the program (SMARTRISK, 1998b). It is projected that this number will reach 800,000 by the end of 2000 (K. Diamond, personal communication, May 3, 2000).

Focus upon this population is determined by evidence that unintentional injury accounts for more deaths among youth than all other causes combined, and that as many as 90% of these injuries are predictable and thus preventable (SMARTRISK, n.d.). SMARTRISK's (1998a) recent publication, *The Economic Burden of Unintentional Injury in Canada*, indicates that serious injury to the head and the spinal column are prevalent (ranked first and second in most categories) outcomes of motor vehicle crashes and falls. These are the leading injury scenarios for the target population, and are thus a major concern for neurotrauma prevention.

Strategy

HEROES, developed between 1990 and 1992, was based on a model for a touring injury prevention presentation originally designed by the University of Alberta Hospital (K. Diamond, personal communication, May 3, 2000). An important modification of this template was the shift towards offering constructive and safe options rather than simply a long list of "don'ts." The strategy underlying HEROES addresses both primary and secondary prevention of injury. Consumers are encouraged to make self-interested choices as to their risk-taking behaviour. The 5 key messages of the program promote these choices: Buckle Up; Drive Sober; Look First; Wear the Gear; Get Trained. By emphasizing both pre-event (e.g., proper training) and event phase (e.g., protective equipment) measures, HEROES aims to reduce both the incidence and the severity of unintentional injury outcomes.

HEROES is designed to reduce/prevent injury by addressing the unique needs of youth. A central assumption is that risk taking helps to make life enjoyable, and that this enjoyment can be preserved while issues of safety awareness are promoted. Through an upbeat, attention-grabbing presentation (including, for example, rock music) it aims to negate the association of "safety" with "boring." Also, by emphasizing positive choices and courses of action, it avoids being overly prohibitive or "preachy" and so makes the most out of teenagers' concern over being independent and in control. Addressing teens "in their own language," so to speak, reflects the program's twofold objective of promoting a message of agency without alienating its audience or appearing staid.

Objectives

HEROES is intended to initiate interest in injury prevention that will continue after the conclusion of the event and provides suggestions as to how this might be accomplished. SMARTRISK On-line Services, for example, is cited as a resource that allows interested parties to share resources and strategies among each other and with specialists across Canada.

Additionally it is believed that youth, as the target audience for the promotion of informed risk-taking behaviours, have the potential to begin a social movement and mobilize public opinion in the interests of unintentional injury prevention. The fitness and environmental movements are described as instances in which increasing public demand has turned an existing issue into an everyday concern. It is hoped that HEROES can help to make "injury prevention the next hot issue on the Canadian social agenda," and that this will result in appropriate preventative legislative developments (SMARTRISK, n.d.).

Resources

Key to understanding HEROES' strategy is the underlying assumption that it is unrealistic to expect people, particularly youth, to cease risk-taking behaviours altogether. The concept of The Stupid Line (i.e., a certain amount of risk is adequately safe; another is stupid) is employed to suggest active choice making, individual empowerment, and taking responsibility for one's own health through rational risk calculation, in different situations (SMARTRISK, 1998d).

Collaboration

Clear consideration of the developmental issue of adolescent independence and the challenges of presenting a message of caution to this group, of the fiscal and emotional costs of injury, and of the value of making injury prevention a topical social and legislative concern may be taken to reflect a degree of multidisciplinary perspectives within the HEROES agenda. Also, by being given an opportunity to hear from and interact with an injury survivor, teens are confronted with a potential outcome of poorly planned risk taking as a reality rather than an abstraction. The value of this portion of the presentation has been confirmed in a study investigating student responses to the event (see below).

Additionally, HEROES has worked with community organizations and safety coalitions, such as Mothers Against Drunk Driving and Ontario Students Against Impaired Driving.

Funding

A portion of HEROES' expenses is paid by the program itself. The HEROES mobile stage show is available to requesting parties for a fee of $2,500 for a single day, $1,500 for each subsequent day, and $400 for an evening presentation to parents. The following public and private interests provide major external funding for the HEROES program:

- Royal & SunAlliance;
- Ford Canada and the Ford network of Dealers;
- Parks Canada;
- Harvey's Youth Foundation; and
- Canadian Pacific.

Implementation

A definite asset to the HEROES program is the extensive assistance provided by SMARTRISK to parties interested in arranging a show. SMARTRISK provides a comprehensive guide to hosting the event, including a media kit to promote it and an outline of what arrangements can or must be made to guarantee the best possible experience. Noteworthy among these are suggestions as to how and where to advertise the event, how to approach potential supporters, and encouragement to follow up on the presentation with related activities and/or make HEROES a centrepiece for other injury prevention awareness activities. SMARTRISK's support, together with the fact that HEROES travels to the audience, makes the program highly replicable and easy to distribute.

Feedback

Ongoing evaluation of the HEROES prevention strategy is accomplished through distribution of a questionnaire to be completed by the event host. This questionnaire solicits general information about participation and promotion, details of other activities initiated in conjunction with the HEROES show, and feedback from stakeholders. Changes made to the format as a result of this participation include updating the music to match audience tastes and tailoring the background images to reflect injury scenarios that typify a given community.

Additionally, the firm Smaller World Communications (SWC) was commissioned by SMARTRISK in 1997 to conduct a survey of high school students who had been audience members for the HEROES show. Parties seeking support for injury prevention initiatives should note that the Ontario Neurotrauma Foundation (1999) publication, *Guide to Program Design and Evaluation Planning for Ontario Neurotrauma Foundation Project Applicants: Rehabilitation and Prevention*, emphasizes the importance of, and provides a comprehensive framework for, proper evaluation planning. The purpose of this study was to measure changes in "knowledge, attitudes and behavioural intentions, find out what students thought about the HEROES presentation, and obtain students' recommendations for improving the presentation" (SMARTRISK, 1998c, p. 70). The full study was conducted in 1998–1999. The most effective aspect of the show, as determined by student rating, was the talk by the injury survivor. In terms of changes to the strategy, the study made the following recommendations:

• Emphasize that schools should plan follow-up activities such as discussions after the show.
• Incorporate more injury survivors and/or examples of unintentional injuries.
• Consider removing the student presenter from the show (SMARTRISK, 1998c, p. 71)

Outcome

The SWC evaluation provided additional feedback as to the success of the HEROES prevention strategy. The major findings were that 1 month after seeing HEROES, student recall of the 5 key messages was generally not good, but that awareness that injury is the leading cause of death among youth rose. More significant positive changes were found in students' knowledge and beliefs than were found in their behavioural intentions. The greatest positive changes were seen in beliefs that injuries could be prevented, "that you can do things to prevent being injured," and "their behavioural intentions to make sure the area is safe before doing an activity" (SMARTRISK, 1998c, p. 71). Regrettably, the study makes no recommendations as to how or whether problems of message recall and/or changes in behavioural intent ought to be addressed by SMARTRISK.

Notwithstanding, the literature includes numerous outstanding reviews of the HEROES program from important stakeholders such as students and educators. Perhaps the most validating of these for the program's organizers comes from an eleventh grade Toronto student:

> The HEROES program is different ... we've learned that smart risk taking isn't just a one-time decision, it's a lifestyle.
>
> (SMARTRISK, n.d.)

Prevention of Sports, Playground, and Recreation-Related Injuries

Traumatic injuries sustained during recreational and sporting activities occur throughout the lifespan. These injuries mean loss of life, or quality of life, for a larger number of people than might immediately be expected; SMARTRISK (1998) advises that recreational injuries contribute significantly to the 13.2% of injury-related deaths and the 26.6% of hospitalizations in Canada that cannot be accounted for by the more obvious causes. Neurotrauma prevention interests should take note that, in this category, damage to the head, brain, and spinal cord represents 26% of deaths and 54.9% of hospitalizations.

The types of initiatives taken to reduce the frequency and severity of sports, playground, and other recreational injuries are also diverse. In this section, 2 outstanding interventions are profiled. In the case of Victoria, Australia, impressive gains in bicycle helmet wearing, and corollary reductions in head injuries to cyclists, were realized through a combination of legislative and educational measures. Similarly, in northern Ontario, a program utilizing police officers for a directed law enforcement and safety education effort has been instrumental in a substantial and progressive reduction in the rate of snowmobiling injuries.

Additionally, 3 promising interventions are profiled. In recognition of the seriousness of recurrent concussions in athletes, an innovative university-based study aims to better understand patterns of concussion recovery and to develop guidelines for safely returning to play after the fact. Fair-Play Rules in Youth Ice Hockey illustrates that encouraging injury reductions can be affected through simple rule changes in organized children's hockey. In the United States, a nationwide plan for reducing playground injuries in children lays out guidelines for improving the safety of these environments through better supervision, design, and maintenance.

Naturally, the injuries addressed in this section represent only a small proportion of the types of trauma sustained in the sports and recreational contexts. Conspicuous by its absence, for example, is a prevention strategy effectively addressing the substantial risk associated with recreational diving from heights, a leading cause of death, paralysis, and other injury. The profiles in this section are meant as guidelines for efforts to continue this important work. There is much to be accomplished.

BEST PRACTICES

- Bicycle Helmets: Educational and Legislative Intervention to increase Use in Victoria, Australia
- Snowmobile Trail Officer Patrol Program (STOP)

PROMISING PRACTICES

- The Varsity Athlete Concussion Research Project
- Fair-Play Rules in Youth Ice Hockey
- The National Action Plan for the Prevention of Playground Injuries

BEST PRACTICES

Bicycle Helmets: Educational and Legislative Interventions to Increase Use in Victoria, Australia

Main Key Informant:
Max H. Cameron

Background

Bicycle riding is chosen by millions of people worldwide for exercise, recreation, or transportation purposes. An unfortunate by-product of this popularity is the significant toll of human suffering and strain to social resources that result from bicycle-related injuries and fatalities each year. Studies conducted in Canada suggest that this toll can be substantially reduced if policy makers and other interested parties direct efforts towards lessening the frequency and severity of bicycle-related unintentional injuries (SMARTRISK, 1998; Morris, Trimble and Fendley, 1994). Rates vary among communities and nations, but some studies estimate that close to 1,000 deaths and more than a half million emergency room visits occur annually in the United States alone as a result of bicycling injuries (Centers for Disease Control and Prevention [CDC], 1995). Head injuries account for the majority of the most severe of these cases, suggesting that bicycle helmets represent an important measure for injury-prevention interests.

Coleman, Munro, Nicholl, Harper, Kent, and Wild (1996) describe a 3-point test for assessing the real value of any injury prevention intervention/strategy. These authors indicate that evaluations can be centred upon questions of "efficacy, effectiveness and implementation, all of which conditions have to be satisfied for the effectiveness of an intervention to be confirmed" (p. 59). In the case of bicycle helmets, efficacy and effectiveness have been proven in laboratory tests of helmet design and performance in simulated situations and in studies of real-world cycling unintentional injuries (Thompson, Rivara, & Thompson, 1999). Indeed, although it is true that they represent only an event-phase strategy (i.e., they can reduce the severity but not the occurrence of cycling mishaps), the studies mentioned above clearly establish the protective potential of helmets. The issue, then, is not whether bicycle helmets could be useful, but rather which practices should be considered exemplary in increasing their use. In the terms set out by Coleman et al. (1996), the issue is one of implementation.

Implementation strategies for increasing bicycle helmet use have tended to fall under the general categories of education (disseminating information to increase awareness of the benefits of helmets) or legislation (enacting laws to mandate their use for a given population). While instances of success for each of these approaches have been documented (Rivara, Thompson, Thompson, Rogers, Alexander, Felix, & Bergman, 1994 [education]), many studies and reviews suggest that the most positive results may be best realized by combining both approaches in an intervention (Rivara, 1995). The success of an integrated approach is well illustrated in the case of Victoria, Australia's efforts to increase bicycle helmet use between 1980 and 1990.

On July 1, 1990, Victoria, Australia, enacted legislation requiring the use of a safety-approved bicycle helmet for all cyclists (unless exempted) in the state. The government bodies and officials most immediately responsible for this legislation were the Victorian Road Traffic Authority, the minister for transport, and the minister for police and emergency services. This initiative is noteworthy by virtue of the fact that it represents the first of its kind, anywhere in the world. Helmet-wearing rates jumped dramatically immediately thereafter, from 31% in March 1990 to 75% in March 1991, and increased again to about 83% for all age groups in the city of Melbourne by mid-1992 (Henderson, 1995). Moreover, increased wearing rates have been associated with a 70% reduction in serious head injuries to cyclists over the 2 years following the introduction of the legislation.

Multifaceted Implementation

Even this very broad description of helmet-use trends would seem to indicate the importance of legislation to intervention planners. Yet, while legislation alone has shown significant improvements in some instances, the outstanding results in Victoria are in part related to the fact that its law came on the heels of a longer-term effort to promote bicycle helmets through other channels. It should be noted that in the decade preceding the legislation, during which these activities peaked, helmet use in Victoria increased from about 5% to the 31% mentioned above. The effort comprised:

- research into the efficacy and effectiveness of various helmet designs and the subsequent development of an Australian Standard for the manufacture and sale of protective bicycle helmets;
- strategy planning;
- school-based education;
- mass media–based awareness raising;
- publicly funded discount schemes to minimize helmet cost as a barrier to their purchase; and
- consultation and feedback from experts, stakeholders, and other concerned parties.

Collaboration

Public and private interests supported the initiative. The Victorian Road Traffic Authority established the Bicycle Helmet Promotion Task Force, a group whose membership included "all the interested organizations in the state, including doctors, manufacturers, retailers, cycling and motoring organizations, the police, the Education Department, the State Bicycle Committee, the Australian Brain Foundation and the media" (Wood & Milne, 1998). An evolution of an existing helmet education and advocacy group, the Task Force was responsible for analysis of available information and development and promotion of helmet-related activities.

Collaboration with the Education Department and schools was an important aspect of the promotional effort. A bicycle-safety module (Bike-Ed) was developed in 1980 for distribution in public schools. In 1983 the Department demanded that a helmet be worn by any student participating in public school cycling activities.

Consumers

While helmet safety education efforts were directed at Victorians generally, and while the current legislation is virtually universal, it should be noted that special attention was focused upon children and adolescents. This focus was largely accomplished by wide dissemination through both the school system and youth-geared mass media. The Victoria program's targeting of children and youth, and efforts to reduce helmet costs, should be seen as great strengths of the intervention strategy. Research conducted in Australia and elsewhere has suggested that the cost of helmets can present a barrier, particularly among low-income families and/or families with more than 1 child. A major report, for example, notes a study in Barrie, Canada, in which observed helmet-use among primary-school children jumped from 0% to 22% after the implementation of a significant helmet subsidy, compared to no observed change with education alone (cited in CDC, 1995).

The same report also suggests focusing upon children under the age of 15, because they are more likely than adults to be bicycle riders, and to sustain bicycle-related head injuries, but generally have lower helmet-wearing rates. Furthermore, becoming accustomed to using a helmet while young increases the likelihood that this behaviour will be maintained into adulthood. Related to this likelihood is the possibility of eventually increasing use among adolescents, a persistently hard to reach group, by reducing the threat of social stigma and peer derision associated with looking foolish or appearing unduly cautious while wearing a helmet.

Resources

As described above, this program profited from the involvement of a wide range of injury-prevention interests: cyclists and cycling groups, other road users, various branches and levels of government, community groups, mass media partnerships, medical facilities, injury-prevention consumers, and consumers and manufacturers of helmets as well as researchers and coordinators. The contributors had an impact in a variety of ways, including:

- provision of funding;
- assisting in distribution of promotional materials and other information;
- providing feedback and voicing concerns;
- participating in law enforcement; and
- participating in ongoing evaluation and planning.

Additionally, the promotional campaign, begun in the 1980s, benefited from the creation of a "helmet-friendly" public climate in previous decades. During the 1960s and 1970s, legislation requiring the use of motorcycle helmets, seat belts, and child restraints was introduced, as were random breath tests for blood-alcohol and engine restrictions for inexperienced motorcyclists (HEA, 1996). Early research into prevention of head trauma in bicyclists could therefore profit from what had previously been learned through studying motorcycle injuries (Wood & Milne, 1988). In the late 1970s consumer demand for effective and comfortable bicycle helmets contributed to the implementation of an Australian Standard; in 1990, that standard was amended in response to demand for lighter, cooler helmets. Previously, discomfort had been a major impediment to increasing helmet use.

Implementation

The educational phase can thus be understood as growing out of, establishing, and drawing upon a diverse base of expert and community support, and building on earlier injury prevention initiatives. Moreover, it set the stage for across-the-board helmet legislation. An important contribution of this period was an Inquiry into Child Pedestrian and Bicycle Safety by the Social Development Committee of the Victorian Parliament. The first report of this committee included the recommendation that a comprehensive strategy, including cyclist and community participation, be outlined for the enactment of mandatory helmet wearing as soon as possible (Cameron et al., 1994). The current law, the Road Safety Bicycle Helmets Regulations 1990, is a direct result of this report.

Another resource crucial to the success of the Victoria intervention, and its present selection as an exemplary practice, has been evaluation of its implementation. VIC ROADS (the state Roads Corporation of Victoria) and the Monash University Accident Research Centre (MUARC) both conducted a series of observational studies examining helmet-wearing rates. MUARC has also examined changes in bicycle use and has made use of data from hospitals and insurance claims to analyse changes in head injuries and deaths among Victoria cyclists since 1981. These data have been the basis for evaluations of the law and for the identification and analysis of positive and/or negative trends and they contribute to a wider understanding of successful injury-prevention approaches. Given the interdisciplinary nature of the stakeholders and collaborators in this case, these assessments can be of great value to other interested parties from a similarly broad range of disciplines.

Effective Practices

It might be suggested that the single most effective practice indicated in the case of bicycle helmets is the simple fact of legislation, immediately after which the overall percentage of helmet wearing more than doubled. Other factors contributing to the successful implementation of the Victoria bicycle helmet efforts stem from its integration of the legislative and the educational approach. Notable among these are:

- frequent evaluation of the effectiveness of both phases;
- cultivation of partnerships representing a wide range of concerned public and private interests and contributions;
- rebate schemes, which helped to increase the knowledge, use, ownership and general acceptance of helmets, pre-law;
- dissemination through schools, which provided access to important young consumers;
- the breadth of persons and scenarios covered by the legislation, which prevented ambiguity and encouraged adults to act as role models; and
- gentle enforcement: while penalties increased following legislation, they were seldom severe and thus may have minimized hostility.

Persons concerned that any legislation demanding the use of safety equipment would be seen as inherently heavy-handed would do well to consider this example.

Outcome

Cameron et al. (1994, p. 330) articulate an organizing principle of the integrated approach: "If the community understands the benefit of a safety measure, and a reasonable proportion has already been persuaded to adopt it voluntarily, then considerably increased use can be achieved through a law, even with relatively moderate levels of enforcement." The combination of approaches has proven highly effective in increasing bicycle helmet use. Over time, they have worked to produce a culture of safety and, for the most part, voluntary compliance. This conclusion is supported by the findings of the observational, hospital, and insurance claim data mentioned above.

Evaluation

Injury prevention interests in Victoria, Australia, observed an increase in bicycle helmet use from less than 5% in 1980 to about 83% in 1992. At the same time, a 70% reduction in deaths or hospitalizations due to serious head injuries to cyclists was reported. Although it is difficult to prove a direct relationship between these initiatives and changes in the behaviour of people, evaluation studies suggest a significant reduction in serious head injuries among cyclists. Several factors may be taken as reasonable evidence of their impact:

- There was a gradual increase in helmet use, and a corresponding decrease in head injury, during each year of the promotion.
- Each time a helmet rebate scheme was launched consumer interest and response was strong, suggesting a desire to participate.
- Making helmets mandatory for all cyclists was associated with a jump, from 31% to 75%, in overall wearing rates.

These outcomes reflect reliable scientifically gathered data collected in field studies and from insurance claims, hospital admissions, and emergency room records, over nearly two decades, in Victoria.

Shortcomings

Injury statistics indicate that the risk of sustaining severe injury while cycling is greater for males than for females (SMARTRISK, 1998). In 1993, of the 102 cyclists aged 5–16 killed or severely injured in New South Wales, Australia, 85 were male (Henderson, 1995). Despite this incidence, the literature reviewed in preparation for this evaluation made no mention of a strategy to target males. The absence of such a focus was addressed by a senior research fellow with the MUARC who provides road safety strategic advice to Australian state governments and internationally (New Zealand, South Africa), who argued that while this discrepancy is a serious matter, it would be difficult to justify a strategy that accepted the exclusion of females (M. Cameron, personal communication, April 27, 2000).

Another, unforeseen, challenge has been the fact that cycling exposure in Victoria dropped considerably following legislation. Although a greater and growing percentage of cyclists are wearing helmets, the number of people cycling has, unfortunately, decreased. In terms of cost analyses, it would be prudent to consider balancing lost quality of life and health benefits of cycling against gains realized through helmet use.

A significant and lingering problem is that, despite substantial gains in helmet use in general, rates remain substantially lower for teenagers than for other age groups. Although teen helmet use rates certainly improved, this improvement coincided with a substantial decrease in bicycle use among this group. Developmental concerns over independence and social image make youth difficult to reach and generally more prone to risk-taking behaviour. Finch, Ferla, Chin, Maloney, and Abeysiri (1997) have addressed this problem in a review of teenagers' attitudes towards bicycle helmets. The study, commissioned by VIC ROADS, made a number of recommendations:

- Future educational efforts should emphasize the importance of helmets in all cycling scenarios, not only those in which danger is obvious.
- Youth are more likely to wear helmets they help to choose. Lighter, stylish, and well-ventilated helmets should therefore be emphasized.
- The perception that fines are rarely imposed and low should be addressed.
- Continued efforts in adult-targeted education schemes will be beneficial, as parents may encourage their children to wear helmets.

The fact that this study has been conducted should be taken as demonstrative of a commitment to addressing the discrepancy in wearing rates and continued interest in the intervention generally.

A final concern is the voice of dissent coming from persons who oppose helmet legislation on the grounds that it increases the burden of responsibility for cyclists without addressing the role played by (far less vulnerable) cars in cyclist injuries (HEA, 1996, p. 28). While this line of reasoning may be valid, it seems less convincing in the case of the Victoria initiative, which coincided with drunk-driving and other driver-focused campaigns, that probably made roads safer for cyclists. Nonetheless, the argument may profitably call the attention of injury prevention programs to the value of alternative or complementary strategies such as traffic calming, physically separating non-motorized traffic, or reducing aggressive driving, in the interests of all road users.

These considerations aside, impressive gains in bicycle helmet use, and reductions in head injury, have been realized in conjunction with Victoria's collaborative initiative. As one of the more successful interventions of its kind, it is widely disseminated and cited in academic and government publications as an exemplar. Many of these publications can be obtained through the Monash University Accident Research Centre website.

Snowmobile Trail Officer Patrol Program (STOP)

Main Key Informant:
Lynn Beach, Provincial Snowmobile and STOP Coordinator, OPP

Background

Like most motorized vehicles, snowmobiles pose an injury risk to riders. To date, many snowmobile-related injuries have been examined and studies have identified "alcohol use, night time driving, speed and driver errors as factors associated with snowmobile related injuries" (Rowe, Therrien, Bretzlaff, Sahai, Nagarajan, & Bota, 1996). Males from 18 to 35 years of age are the highest risk group for snowmobile-related injury and fatalities. Furthermore, approximately 20% of snowmobile-related injuries occur to the brain and spinal cord (L. Beach, personal communication, March 28, 2000).

During the winter season, Sudbury, a north-eastern Ontario city, sees its snowmobile population double as a result of recreational snowmobile tourism. In the 1999–2000 season alone, 360,000 snowmobilers registered their snowmobiles in the Ontario area (L. Beach, personal communi-cation, May, 2000). Unfortunately, this popular winter sport is the leading cause of winter drowning and is a major cause of injury (Rowe, Johnson, Milner, & Bota 1992; 1994). As a popular venue for snowmobiling, northern Ontario has significantly higher snowmobile-related hospital admission rates than the rest of Ontario (Rowe et al., 1996). Moreover, approximately 20% of snowmobile-related injuries occur to the brain and spinal cord (L. Beach, personal communication, April, 2000).

Sudbury politicians, aware of increased revenue from tourists, encouraged snowmobile tourism and supported development of more snowmobile trails. Sudbury OPP and regional police officers, however, struggled with the lack of enforcement to ensure safety for the increased number of riders during the height of the tourist season. These concerns led to the development of a number of initiatives, including the Snowmobile Trail Officer Patrol Program (STOP).

Injury Prevention Strategies Employed

Many strategies have been employed in the Sudbury area to prevent snowmobile-related injuries from occurring. These prevention strategies are aimed at Haddon's (1972) pre-event stage of prevention:

- development of a task force on snowmobile safety;
- public service announcements over the past 3 years regarding snowmobile safety;
- legislative changes such as the introduction of a universal by-law regarding snowmobile safety; and
- increased local police surveillance and training of snowmobile officers (the Snowmobile Trail Officer Patrol program).

As a result of the increased rate of snowmobile ridership in Sudbury during the winter seasons and the risk of disabling neurotrauma-related injuries, a Snowmobile Trail Officer Patrol program was initiated in the 1992/1993 winter season as a pilot project in Sudbury, Ontario. In this community-based policing program instituted to prevent snowmobile-related death and hospitalization (Rowe et al., 1996), community volunteers are trained to become snowmobile trail officers (special constables) to assist law enforcement on snowmobile trails. The STOP officers patrol trails, ticket snowmobile violations, and issue warnings to riders. Other duties for STOP officers and police officers include providing educational seminars and driver training programs for snowmobile riders.

History and Development

The original developers of the STOP project, a police officer, a police sergeant, and two snowmobile club members, arranged a community meeting to address the issues of increased riders and limited law enforcement resources. People from trauma units, snowmobile clubs, police departments, political offices, and First Nations' territory attended. The police sergeant requested the meeting after the January 1993 fatalities from snowmobile unintentional injuries in Sudbury totalled 6 people. Statistics indicated that fatality rates would increase in February and March of that same year (L. Beach, personal communication, March, 2000). The lack of resources preventing law enforcement officers from patrolling the trails and ensuring that safe driving practices were being followed was highlighted at this meeting, and STOP was conceived as a way of supplementing the available resources.

Resources

Support for the STOP initiative was multifaceted.

* the local MPP from the Ministry of Northern Developments and Mines provided initial financial support;
* a retired OPP commissioner supported the initiative verbally;
* the Sudbury Regional Police and Ontario Provincial Police each provided 1 officer to help plan meetings, develop policies, and train volunteers; and
* the original 2 snowmobile club members from the Sudbury Trail Plan Association volunteered time to support the project.

Funding

A combination of funds and support from the provincial/local government, police agencies, and committed volunteers help maintain the STOP program. Funding and support from the Ministry of the Solicitor General created the new OPP position of Provincial Snowmobile & STOP Coordinator. Ontario's current coordinator plans and visits international committees and promotes the STOP program to other towns in Ontario and across Canada. Funding and support from various other organizations contribute to the STOP program safety message. The major funding comes from the Ontario Federation of Snowmobile Clubs. That organization also has a provincial coordinator who works alongside the police provincial coordinator. Some examples of corporate and provincial sponsors include: Bombardier-SkiDoo, Mustang Ice Rider/ Survival Wear, Ontario Snowmobile Safety Committee, Kimpex Action, Cantel/AT&T, Canadian Tire Corporation, Produmax, Labatt's, and the Ontario Ministry of Transportation. Local sponsors include small businesses and local Canadian Tire and Tim Horton's stores (Beach and Robinson, 1998/99).

Resources Needed

An increase in Ministry of Transportation and other government financial support is needed to improve research and data collection concerning safety issues and injuries related to snowmobiling. Given the high rate of ridership in Sudbury and the rest of the province during the winter season and the seriousness of injuries that can result from this popular winter sport, the Ministry of Transport should prioritize snowmobile safety (L. Beach, personal communication, March, 2000).

Implementation

At the onset of the project, the OPP sergeant and the regional police officer trained community volunteers. The trained volunteers, named special constables, learned laws and safety measures needed for riders in the region of Sudbury. Training entailed evaluations, written exams, and trail rides with both civilians and the police.

Awareness of the new program was heightened through information events at public schools and at community meetings. Other educational methods include distributing safety brochures, posters, and videos from the International Snowmobile Manufacturers Association (ISMA) to advertise safety measures and reinforce laws. The media, including local newspapers, radio, and television, is also used to spread the STOP program and safety issues to a larger audience.

Currently, 30 OPP officers and 70 STOP volunteers patrol and enforce safety laws on the snowmobile trails in the Province of Ontario. A STOP officer's job description now incorporates police involvement with the STOP program. Education and enforcement must go together, according to a police sergeant: "The community will not tolerate drinking and riding anymore, not just the police" (L. Beach, personal communication, March 28, 2000).

Driver Training and Educational Programs

Further safety legislation includes licensing. In Ontario, people under 16 years of age must have a snowmobile licence to ride trails with snowmobiles. People over the age of 16 who have a valid driver's licence are not required by law to have a snowmobile licence.

The Ontario Federation of Snowmobile Clubs Driver Training program enables 12–16-year-old riders to obtain a licence. This full-day course teaches laws, safety, courtesy, and fatality statistics. Recently, the program was adapted to include parents for half of a day of training. Unique to this program is a collaborative, volunteer community approach that combines the efforts of police officers, youth, parents, and the community in order to increase the commitment to snowmobile safety.

Target Population

The program targets the highest risk population (males between 18 and 35 years of age) of snowmobile riders. It also targets local snowmobile riders because the majority of injuries and fatalities occur within the local population. The STOP program would like more funding to offset the cost of audience-drawing strategies such as racing videos and endorsements by snowmobile racing celebrities to enhance and promote safety strategies.

Considerations

Weather, time, and funding are all factors that require consideration when implementing the STOP program. Police officers must adjust their rigid schedules to incorporate flexible patrol hours, which are often determined by the amount of snow on the trails. Advanced planning requires that the STOP officers and police have time to prepare and deliver education and driver training programs early in the fall. Once the snow falls and trails open, riders focus on riding rather than learning new skills and training.

The provincial coordinator(s) adjusts the STOP program according to the results of surveys and statistical analysis regarding trends. For example, research indicates that the high-risk group, males between the ages of 18 and 35, sustain fewer injuries and fatalities when travelling with female companions. With the assistance of additional funds, opportunities for promotion of family snowmobile riding as a preventative measure can be implemented (L. Beach, personal communication, March, 2000).

Decision Making

Community involvement is pursued in the decision-making process. The community perspective helps direct changes to the program that reflect specific environmental and community needs. For instance, communities comprised largely of farmland require safety strategies that consider electric and barbed wire fences. Final decisions and plans are implemented by the provincial coordinator(s) and the provincial STOP officer and must meet the high standards expected by the Ministry of the Solicitor General and the 5 partnering police agencies.

A 3-person discipline committee in each area resolves disputes and policy conflicts at a local level. If a conflict persists, the provincial coordinator(s) suggests strategies to facilitate reaching a resolution. Inquiries, made by phone and email, provide information and feedback from the provincial coordinator(s) (L. Beach, personal communication, March, 2000). To further facilitate communication processes and the implementation of the program, the provincial coordinator provides updates to the OPP superintendent and the OPP Deputy Commissioner, prepares an annual report, and delivers the report to corporate sponsors (L. Beach, personal communication, March, 2000).

Outcome

One demonstration of the program's effectiveness is noted by STOP officers who report positive relationships between riders and officers. All data collected from STOP Officers are measured and compared with fatality statistics for the season. Data include the number of charges laid, hours on patrol, special functions attended, number of collisions, on or off trail location, number of warnings issued, and the number of reporting notices issued (L. Beach, personal communication, March 28, 2000). Other measures of effectiveness include compliance and acceptance of the law by the community, recognition of dangers from riders, and feedback from the STOP officers. Positive, unexpected results include out-of-province interest in the STOP program, STOP officer rescue aid, a focus on injury prevention rather than crime prevention, and the fostering of police partnerships with civilians.

Efficacy Studies

Funded by the Ministry of Health Trauma Network, a study entitled *The effect of a community-based police surveillance program on snowmobile injuries and deaths* (Rowe et al., 1996) examines effectiveness of the STOP program in preventing deaths and hospitalization related to snowmobile trauma in Sudbury, Ontario.

Study Design

Hospital records from the General Hospital in Sudbury, coroner's reports, and emergency room surveillance data were collected on snow-mobile admissions and deaths in Sudbury for the 1990–1995 snowmobile seasons. The study compared the data of the pre-STOP seasons (1990–1992) with that of the post-STOP seasons (1993–1995). Cases were included if trauma had resulted in serious injury following a snowmobile crash; non-trauma-related injury and fatality were excluded. Only snowmobile injuries sustained within the region were included.

Demographic (e.g., age, gender), event (e.g., riding status, time of day), and outcome (e.g., severity of injury, length of hospitalization) data was collected. To insure reliability, a second reviewer examined a subset of randomly selected charts. Disagreements were resolved by consensus.

Results

The injured populations and circumstances were similar between the pre- and post-STOP seasons. Data was statistically analysed using 2-tailed t-tests for continuous data and chi-square and/or odds ratios for ordinal data with significant results (p < .05; Rowe et al., 1996).

According to the Rowe et al. (1996) study, significant findings included lower injuries and fewer admissions to hospital, with the result of significant economic savings following the STOP intervention. Admissions to hospital were reduced by 45%. The estimated savings in acute emergency department and hospital costs are $218,870 over the study period, or $72,960 per year. Please see Rowe et al. (1996) for details regarding how acute care, in-patient costs, and earning data were estimated.

Alternate explanations for the results were addressed, and the authors of this study provided plausible explanations for confounding factors. Importantly, this region was unique in demonstrating a decreased snowmobile death and injury pattern. The study thus demonstrates that "snowmobile injuries and deaths can be significantly reduced through targeted surveillance and public education, centred on alcohol awareness and safety" (Rowe et al., 1996). The majority of snowmobile injuries and fatalities are associated with a number of modifiable risk factors. Hence, to be effective as a prevention strategy, a multifaceted approach involving a coordinated multilevel, community-based perspective is necessary.

PROMISING PRACTICES

The Varsity Athlete Concussion Research Project

A University of Toronto and Toronto Rehabilitation Institute Collaboration

Main Key Informant:
Vicki L. Kristman

Background

Concussion in sport is an ongoing, serious challenge for society; difficult questions, such as when is it safe to return to play, if ever, beleaguer coaches, players, and sports medicine personnel. With professional athletes, such as Eric Lindros, sidelined by concussion, the issues about recovery from concussion have become increasingly publicized.

Although often considered an innocuous injury, concussion is, by consensus definition, a mild traumatic brain injury (MTBI); it involves a traumatically induced alteration of consciousness that does not necessarily involve a loss of consciousness (Kelly, Nichols, Filley, Lillehei, Rubenstein, & Kleinschmidt-Demasters, 1991; Kelly, 1999; Esselman & Uomoto, 1995; American Academy of Neurology, 1997; c.f., Barth, 1989). Symptoms of concussion may include concentration and other cognitive problems, as well as headache, dizziness, loss of coordination or balance, and irritability. The consequences of sustaining multiple concussions (Collins, Lovell, & McKeag, 1999) or of returning to play too soon after a single concussion (Collins et al., 1999) can be severe and irreversible.

Concussion Diagnosis and Recovery

Unfortunately, there is a lack of consensus regarding when it is appropriate for an athlete to return to play following a concussion, partially because of inadequate methods for diagnosing concussion and determining when symptoms of concussion have fully resolved. Moreover, concussions in sport often go undiagnosed for a variety of reasons (e.g., athletes who do not want to risk loss of playing time do not report symptoms). These issues require our serious attention.

One of the difficulties in investigating issues concerning diagnosis and recovery from MTBI is that there is typically no information about pre-morbid functioning: in order to determine whether subtle problems in functioning are due to concussion, one has to infer what pre-injury functioning was like for a given individual.

U of T/Toronto Rehab Program

In order to obviate this problem, the University of Toronto (U of T)/ Toronto Rehabilitation Institute (Toronto Rehab) program of research utilized a collection of pre- and post-injury data from a group of individuals at risk for concussion through sport, thereby providing the opportunity to assess recovery patterns of cognitive functioning and to make comparisons to pre-injury functioning. In order to determine when symptoms are fully resolved, this program of research employs neuropsychological testing as the "gold standard" for diagnosis of concussion and for determining when symptoms of concussion have resolved.

The program includes the following research objectives:

- to validate a protocol for the assessment of post-concussive deficits;
- to empirically validate return-to-play guidelines;
- to better understand the pattern of recovery from concussion in previously concussed individuals;
- to examine the rate of cognitive and emotional recovery from concussion; and
- to elucidate factors that contribute to protracted recovery from concussion.

In addition, a long-term clinical objective is the baseline neuropsychological testing of all athletes at risk for concussion in order to allow for a more conclusive diagnosis of concussion in athletes who sustain a blow to the head.

Resources

The research team includes two professors from the Faculty of Physical Education and Health, University of Toronto, and their colleagues at Toronto Rehab. Other co-investigators include a doctoral candidate in Psychology at York University, a psychometrist at Toronto Rehab, the professor and chair of neurosurgery at the University of Toronto, the head of neuroradiology research in the Department of Medical Imaging,

University of Toronto, and a University of Toronto doctoral candidate in epidemiology. These individuals provide expertise in the medical management of concussion, neuropsychological diagnosis, neuropsychological testing (which includes testing of cognition and emotion), experimental design, and statistical analysis. Materials for pilot testing have been provided by the Neurology Service of the Toronto Rehabilitation Institute. The Faculty of Physical Education and Health at the University of Toronto has provided administrative, coaching, and infrastructure support. The research team is currently seeking funding for this long-term project from several sources.

Implementation

The multidisciplinary research group has just completed the first year of the study. During that time, the research design was finalized and baseline data collection was begun on varsity athletes deemed at risk for concussion. Such athletes (i.e., football, rugby, ice hockey, basketball, lacrosse, volleyball, field hockey, and soccer players) were given a battery of neuropsychological and psychological tests to establish a baseline measure of cognitive (i.e., coordination, speed, concentration, and memory) and emotional functioning. Once a baseline is established, if an athlete experiences a concussion, he or she will be retested immediately and then at regular intervals until recovery is complete (defined as a return to normal medical and cognitive status or "baseline" functioning). Three groups of volunteer athletes will be studied: 1) concussed athletes (determined on site by therapists and team physicians using the U of T Sideline Concussion Checklist), 2) knee-injured athletes (as an injury control group), and 3) a non-injured varsity control.

Outcome

This prospective study will reveal incidence and prevalence rates of concussion in varsity athletes at risk for concussion. It will provide objective guidelines for identifying concussion in the sport context so that diagnosis need not rely on athlete report of symptoms. Also, return-to-play guidelines, based on empirical evidence from neuropsychological testing, will be developed.

The program of research will have theoretical and widespread practical importance for scientists, practitioners, and policy makers who seek to understand and intervene in the concussion recovery process.

Findings from this study on athletes will help to determine a rate of cognitive and emotional recovery following MTBI that can then be used as a model of uncomplicated recovery for the general population. Because MTBI also occurs in the workplace, at home, and as a result of motor vehicle or bicycling unintentional injuries, the conclusions and recommendations gleaned from this research will benefit a much wider population than high-performance athletes.

Fair-Play Rules in Youth Ice Hockey

Main Key Informant:
Dr William O. Roberts

Background

Falls and sports-related injuries have been found to be the primary causes of hospital stays and emergency department visits in U.S. children, and therefore account for a considerable amount of health care costs (Brust, Roberts, & Leonard, 1995). A Canadian study of cervical spine injuries in ice hockey found an increase from 1 injury per year from 1976 to 1979 to 13 injuries per year from 1982 to 1986, with 64% of all injuries occurring in male players aged 11 to 20 (Brust et al., 1995). A push or body check from behind, resulting in head-first collision into the boards, was found to be the most common cause of spinal cord injuries (Brust et al., 1995). A number of studies reveal that body checking and illegal play account for a large proportion of ice hockey injuries (Brust, Leonard, Pheley & Roberts; and Stuart, Smith, Nieva & Rock, 1995).

Youth ice hockey is relatively free of injury in age groups under 11, where intentional body contact is prohibited (Brust et al., 1995 in Roberts, Brust, Leonard, & Herbert, 1996). However, as players progress through each age category, injuries have been seen to climb (Brust et al., 1995), as risk of injury increases due to high-speed collisions (Roberts et al., 1996). In Ontario, body checking is introduced at the peewee level where players are 11 and 12 years of age. Incorporating concepts of fair play and sportsmanship into the scoring of ice hockey seasons or tournaments provides a means of controlling increasing violence in ice hockey (Vaz, 1982).

Resources

A review of various applications of good conduct reward systems promoting fair play showed that there are greater decreases in the number of penalties incurred as more points are awarded for acceptable behaviour and as the pre-established penalty threshold for fair-play points awarded is lowered (Marcotte & Simard, 1993). The following rules for promoting fair play can be used:

- points can be added to season or tournament point totals for staying under a pre-established limit of team penalties per game;
- points can be deducted for exceeding a pre-established limit of team penalties per game;
- individuals exceeding a preset number of penalties per game can be suspended from the following game; and
- suspensions can be applied to a coach of a team that is regularly penalized for illegal play.

One study (Roberts et al., 1996) compared the occurrence of injuries in a Junior Gold tournament of players aged 17 to 19 playing under fair-play rules and regular rules. The round-robin portion was played with fair-play rules while the championship round was played with regular rules. While fair-play rules were not used in the championship games, the policy of a game suspension for more than 5 individual penalties incurred in a single game remained in effect. Points for fair play in the Junior Gold Tournament round-robin games were awarded as follows:

- wins garner 13 points, ties 7 points, and losses 0 points;
- +1 point for each period won;
- +1 point for highest total shots on goal;
- +1 point for a shutout;
- for a win, a maximum score of 19 and a minimum score of 12 was set; and
- for a loss, a maximum score of 4 and a minimum score of −2 was set.

Implementation

In establishing a fair-play system, the greatest difficulty has been keeping the reward simple and easy to administer (Roberts et al., 1996).

Outcome

There was an approximately twofold increase in penalties assessed and injuries experienced in championship games where regular rules were used, compared to round-robin games where fair-play rules were used (Roberts et al., 1996). Injury rates were reported per 1,000 athletic exposures and describe the risk of injury to which an athlete is exposed during participation in a game or practice. In games where fair-play rules were implemented, injuries occurred at a rate of 26.4 per 1,000 athletic exposures; the injury rate in the championship games in which regular rules were used was 135.5. Comparing notable injuries, i.e., concussion, facial laceration, or injury of moderate or greater severity, the injury rate during the use of fair-play rules was 5.7 per athletic exposure, versus 27.6 during the use of regular rules. While playing under regular rules, the number of penalties, as well as the rate of penalties assigned, almost doubled per game (7.1 versus 13 penalties per game), as compared to games played under fair-play rules. It was also observed that competing teams were generally assigned bonus points during fair play, while they were above the pre-established limit of penalties required to receive bonus points during regular games.

The fair-play concept can reduce both injury and penalty rates in ice hockey and thus should be given consideration. It has been suggested that the concept may also be applied to other contact sports for the reduction of injuries and rule infractions.

The National Action Plan for the Prevention of Playground Injuries

The University of Northern Iowa, Cedar Falls

Main Key Informant:
Dr Donna Thompson

Background

For most children, playgrounds are a major place for both play and educational activities. Each year thousands of children in Canada sustain injuries in childcare, school, and park playgrounds. These injuries range from abrasions and cuts to broken limbs and concussions and even death. While children should be challenged and allowed to test their limits during outdoor play, a lot can be done to prevent or reduce injuries.

The National Program for Playground Safety (NPPS)

The National Program for Playground Safety (NPPS) was created in October 1995 to help communities across the United States examine issues surrounding playground safety. The National Action Plan for the Prevention of Playground Injuries is one of the first steps towards helping to prevent many needless injuries. The purpose of the National Action Plan is to provide a blueprint of action steps to be taken to develop safe playgrounds. It is designed to be used by parents, teachers, recreation and park personnel, caretakers of children, and other concerned adults.

Goals

The National Action Plan is divided into 4 sections. Each section features 1 major goal and outlines actions to be taken to achieve that goal at national, state, and local levels.

1 Goal: Provide proper supervision on playgrounds

- Action 1: Appraise current supervision plans.
- Action 2: Specify the supervision methods to be used.
- Action 3: Enhance supervision practices.

Children need the guidance of adults to help them make appropriate choices about safe play equipment, behaviour, and activity. Research has shown that in the school setting where active supervision takes place, playground injuries can be reduced significantly.

2 Goal: Design age-appropriate playgrounds

- Action 1: Assess the age-appropriate design of playgrounds.
- Action 2: Choose age-appropriate equipment.

- Action 3: Advocate for all playgrounds being designed age appropriately.

There should be separate play areas for younger children (under age 5) and older children. "When there are not separate areas for children, the probability that young children (children under age 5) will access equipment that is too large for their physical, emotional, social, and intellectual development is significantly increased. In turn, this can increase the exposure to injury" (Hudson, Mack & Thompson, 2000, p. 8).

3 Goal: Provide proper fall surfacing under and around playground equipment

- Action 1: Evaluate current surfacing situations.
- Action 2: Select proper surfacing under and around equipment.
- Action 3: Improve surfacing for the future.

"Falls to surfaces are cited as a contributing factor in 70% of the playground injury data" (Hudson et al., 2000, p. 8). "Thus, proper surfacing under and around the playground equipment is a crucial element in providing a safe play environment" (Hudson et al., 2000, p. 8).

4 Goal: Properly maintain equipment on playgrounds

- Action 1: Review maintenance policies and procedures.
- Action 2: Improve maintenance practices.

Playground equipment needs to be checked for rust, splinters, protruding bolts, missing or broken parts, and gaps (which could entrap the head of a child). Older equipment and equipment made from wood and metal (as opposed to plastic) appear to have the most maintenance problems. "Without routine inspection and repair, any equipment will fall into disrepair and thus pose a hazard to children using the equipment" (Hudson et al., 2000, p. 8).

Each of these goals interact with one another in creating a safe play environment.

The National Action Plan emphasizes that in order "to be successful, playground safety has to be a partnership among local, state, and national levels" (Thompson & Hudson, 2000).

Resources

Collaborators

The National Plan for the Prevention of Playground Injuries was co-authored by members of the Faculty of the School of Health, Physical Education, and Leisure Services at the University of Northern Iowa, Cedar Falls, Iowa.

Funding

Funding for the National Action Plan for the Prevention of Playground Injuries was provided through a grant from the Centers for Disease Control and Prevention in Atlanta, Georgia.

Implementation

The action steps were evaluated informally via attitude surveys conducted at conferences and over the telephone. A more formal evaluation is to be completed in 2001 (D. Thompson, personal communication, May 17, 2000).

Outcome

The NPPS has disseminated over 20,000 copies of the National Action Plan for the Prevention of Playground Injuries to parents, teachers, administrators at childcare centres, schools, recreation centres, governors, senators, and others at conferences (D. Thompson, personal communication, May 17, 2000).

Each year, children are unintentionally injured in playgrounds. The action steps look promising, as they serve as a valuable resource for parents, playground safety specialists, educators, recreation and park personnel, caretakers of children, and other concerned adults. The guidelines, however, need to be formally evaluated to determine the extent of their effectiveness in preventing injuries amongst children in playgrounds.

Prevention of Farm-Related and Occupational Injuries

The workplace is a potentially hazardous environment. Both farmers and small business owners often lack the extensive resources of big businesses to implement formal health and safety policies and procedures. In addition, farms and other small businesses are difficult areas to legislate (Kelsey, 1994).

In Canada, tractor rollovers are the leading cause of fatal injury as well as a cause of injuries that result in hospitalization (CAISP, 1999, p. 5). The ROPS Rebate Scheme, an Australian program, is profiled as a best practice as it incorporates information and awareness programs, education, and regulation to equip tractors with rollover protective structures as a preventative measure at the event phase of Haddon's (1972) matrix.

Two other promising programs are profiled: North American Guidelines for Children's Agricultural Tasks (NAGCAT) and Farm Response. NAGCAT provides a list of general guidelines indicating appropriate work for children in the field of agriculture. Farm Response is a program aimed at training farm workers and family members to respond appropriately in the event phase of a farm-related accident. Neither of these programs has been evaluated to date.

Every year, Canadians are injured as a result of a fall in the workplace. "Fall related injury accounted for 17 percent of work-related injuries and 12 per cent of fatalities in the workplace. Falls were also found to be the second highest cause of work-related deaths" (SMARTRISK, 1999, p. 9). They are a leading cause of serious head and spinal cord injury and, as such, are a concern for neurotrama prevention initiatives. Therefore, the Small Business Falls Prevention Project is profiled as a promising program. This project emphasizes injury prevention at both the pre-event and event phase of Haddon's (1980) model.

All workplaces have hazards. The aim, therefore, is to reduce the risks associated with those hazards. By emphasizing proper training (i.e., pre-event phase) along with the use of protective equipment (i.e., event phase), all of the prevention strategies profiled in this section aim to reduce the incidence and the severity of unintentional injury outcomes on both the farm and in the small business workplace.

Best Practices

* Tractor Rollover Protective Structure (ROPS) Rebate Scheme 1997/98

Promising Practices

* Small Business Falls Prevention Project
* North American Guidelines for Children's Agricultural Tasks (NAGCAT)
* Farm Response Program

BEST PRACTICES

Tractor Rollover Protective Structure (ROPS) Rebate Scheme 1997/98

Main Key Informant:
Dr Lesley M. Day

Background

Farm machinery–related injuries are significant from a medical perspective as they commonly lead to fractures of the limbs, head and spinal cord injuries, major lacerations, and crush injuries (CAISP, 1999). When machinery-related injuries are divided by machinery type, tractors are the leading cause of hospitalized farm machinery injuries for both children and adults. From 1990 through 1996, 133 children (aged 0–14) and 471 adults (aged 15–59) were hospitalized as a result of tractor-related injuries (CAISP, 1999). The average length of stay in hospital for treatment of these injuries is 2–5 days (CAISP, 1999).

In addition to being responsible for a number of disabling injuries, tractors account for a large proportion (47.5%) of fatalities in the farm workplace (CAISP, 1997, Figure 3.1). "Various forms of tractor rollover and run over are the leading causes of death among Canadian farmers and their families" (CAISP, 1997, Figure 5.1.1). From 1991 through 1995, 109 fatalities involving tractor rollovers in Canada were reported (CAISP, 1997, Figure 5.1.4).

Tractor Rollover Protective Structures (ROPS)

Tractor rollover protective structures, with seat-belt use, are designed to protect tractor operators in case of an accidental overturn. There are 2 types of ROPS for use on agricultural tractors: 2-post and 4-post structures. Safety cabs (rollover protective enclosures) may be constructed with either design. The tractor operator is protected because the ROPS is engineered to prevent a collapse of the structure in the critical zone, or the operator's station. "The effectiveness of rollover protective structures in preventing death in the event of a tractor rollover has been demonstrated in Sweden, Great Britain and Norway" (Springfeldt, 1993 cited in Day & Rechnitzer, 1999, p. 13; Thelin, 1990).

Tractor Rollover Protective Structure (ROPS) Rebate Scheme

In 1985, regulations were introduced in the state of Victoria, Australia, requiring ROPS on tractors manufactured or imported as of July 1981, and/or ROPS to be fitted where practicable to all tractors used by employees (WorkCover Authority cited in Day & Rechnitzer, 1999). The passing of these regulations, together with the number of tractor rollover incidents in work-related deaths in Victoria and the demonstrated effectiveness of rollover protective structures, encouraged 2 organizations to increase the level of ROPS fitment to tractors (Day & Rechnitzer, 1999).

The Health and Safety Organization (HSO) and, later, the Victorian WorkCover Authority (VWA), set out to increase the level of ROPS fitment to tractors by running the 1987, 1990, and 1994 ROPS rebate schemes. These schemes encouraged farmers to purchase and fit their tractors with ROPS. For each ROPS purchase and fitment farmers would receive a financial rebate, which served as an incentive.

However, as the 1985 regulations did not extend to include pre-1981 machines, a number of tractors, especially older ones, were not fitted with ROPS. In 1996, there were an estimated 17,420 tractors without ROPS in the state of Victoria (Day & Rechnitzer, 1999). These tractors were considered a hazard to farmers.

The 1997/98 ROPS rebate scheme was created to facilitate the fitment of ROPS to all previously unprotected tractors, with some limited exemptions. The approach included information and awareness programs, education, and regulation. This program addressed the event phase of Haddon's 1980 model by encouraging farmers to take the precautionary measure of fitting their tractors with ROPS in order to reduce the risk of fatality and the risk and severity of unintentional injury should a tractor rollover occur.

History and Development of the Tractor ROPS Rebate Scheme 1997/98

The success of the tractor ROPS rebate scheme 1997/98 was due to a combination of factors, including previous rebate schemes, the development of partnerships, and state regulation.

Previous Rebate Schemes

The 1987, 1990, and 1994 rebate schemes each included various promotional activities and a financial rebate for ROPS fitment. In 1987 the Department of Labour launched a Tractor Safety Awareness Campaign, which ran for 2 months and resulted in the issue of 389 rebates. In 1990 the Health and Safety Organization ran a further campaign for 10 months that produced 1,436 rebates. The HSO ran a similar campaign in 1994 for 7 months, resulting in 1,116 rebates.

Development of Partnerships

"In Victoria there has been a long history of concern by government and individuals regarding tractor rollover deaths that preceded the introduction in 1985 of the regulations requiring ROPS on all post-1981 tractors" (Day & Rechnitzer, 1999, p. 21). This concern, along with the development and implementation of the 1987, 1990, and 1994 ROPS rebate schemes, created the necessary partnerships between the Victorian WorkCover Authority, the Victorian Farmers Federation (VFF), and the Farm Machinery Dealers Association (FMDA).

Regulation

In 1996 the Victorian Farmers Federation (VFF) passed a resolution at their annual conference that "no tractor should be permitted to be operated after January 1, 1998, on any farm in Victoria unless it is fitted with a ROPS or a similar structure having the same effectiveness" (Farmsafe Victoria Meeting Notes, September 1996 cited in Day & Rechnitzer, 1999, p. 21). This was a monumental move; previously the VFF had strongly opposed legislation requiring that all tractors be fitted with ROPS.

ROPS Rebate Scheme 1997/98

The timing of the 1997/98 rebate scheme was perfect. The earlier rebate schemes had served as pilot studies, strong partnerships had developed with key organizations, and the VFF supported the fitment of ROPS to all tractors.

The 1997/98 scheme was funded by the VWA and administered under contract by the VFF. A steering committee was established to advise on the implementation and administration of the scheme. Membership in the steering committee included members of the VFF, VWA, and FMDA. Proposed regulatory amendments, publicity and education, and an incentive in the form of a rebate were the main components of the 1997/98 scheme (Day & Rechnitzer, 1999). The goal of the scheme was to facilitate the fitment of ROPS to previously unprotected tractors, via a rebate of $150 for each pre-1981 tractor fitted with ROPS meeting the specifications of Australian Standard #1636. The fitment had to be carried out by a member of the FMDA or a qualified engineer or mechanic. Tractor owners could fit the ROPS themselves on the condition that a signed indemnity form was provided with the application (Day & Rechnitzer, 1999).

The scheme was launched in April 1997, in Lardner, Victoria. The public relations section of the VWA was responsible for publicity, including a series of television advertisements, press releases, and articles in the print media. The VWA conducted a mail-out to a commercially available list of 39,990 farmers. The mail-out consisted of an application form for the ROPS rebate and supporting material. In addition, tractor rollover incidents and the rebate scheme were the main focus of VWA displays at agricultural shows and field days from the launch until August 1998. The VFF also provided publicity in its material to members. As well, the VWA and the VFF conducted 4 tractor and ROPS information sessions for orchardists (individuals who work in orchards) to assist this group in responding to the scheme and impending regulatory amendments (Day & Rechnitzer, 1999).

This scheme was very successful, with an average of 146 rebate applications received by the VFF each week for the 20-month duration. Before the 1997/98 ROPS rebate scheme, the number of operational tractors in Victoria without ROPS was estimated at 17,420; after completion of the program there were an estimated 5,291 operational tractors without ROPS. "The scheme reduced unprotected tractors by 70%" (Day & Rechnitzer, 1999, p. 25).

Resources

Funds for the Tractor ROPS Rebate Scheme 1997/98 were provided by the Victorian WorkCover Authority, participating farmers, and the Victorian Farmers Federation. The VWA allocated part of their annual state budget as funding for the program. This funding covered costs for the rebates ($2,000,000 AU), advertising ($229,000 AU), administration contract ($40,000 AU), rebate application forms ($15,932 AU), and the list purchase and mailing ($30,465 AU). The most significant contributors were the participating farmers who purchased the ROPS and paid for installation ($5,561,947 AU). The VFF provided in-kind staff time, "significant but not quantifiable" (Day & Rechnitzer, 1999, p. 25).

Although there was sufficient funding for the program, some farmers felt that the rebate could have been larger. Farmers were expected to pay for the ROPS (on average about $500 AU), plus the fitment of the ROPS to their tractor ($100 AU), minus the rebate of $150 AU (E. Young, personal communication, April 4, 2000). Therefore, the total cost to the farmer was approximately $450 AU for each tractor (E. Young, personal communication, April 4, 2000).

Implementation

Effective Practices

The success of the ROPS 1997/98 rebate was due to a number of equally important and interrelated factors. The combination of regulatory amendments, perceived subsequent reinforcement of the regulation, publicity, and the rebate provided the incentive required to increase ROPS fitment (Day & Rechnitzer, 1999). "While the regulatory amendments and the perceived subsequent reinforcement, were significant factors, the effect would not have been as dramatic had these strategies been used in isolation" (Day & Rechnitzer, 1999, p. 11). Other factors contributed to the effective implementation of this program, including:

- development of the necessary partnerships between the VWA, the VFF, and the FMDA over previous years;
- community familiarity with previous rebate schemes, which served as pilots for this largest effort;
- the fact that the proportion of tractors fitted with ROPS was already more than 50%; and
- attitudinal change in the acceptance of compulsory ROPS fitment within the VFF, prior to the move made by the VWA towards regulatory change (Day & Rechnitzer, 1999).

Perhaps the only strategy that could have enhanced the implementation of the ROPS Rebate Scheme 1997/98 would have been to follow up with enforcement of the regulation. There was a reluctance to do so because of logistics and farmers' attitudes towards legislation in the past.

Two factors contribute to the effectiveness of ROPS as an intervention for tractor rollover deaths. "First, ROPS have varying degrees of effectiveness e.g., a cabin meeting the rollover standard will be more effective than a four post or two post ROPS in keeping the tractor operator within the safety zone during a rollover incident. Second, the effectiveness of ROPS, particularly four and two post ROPS, is greatly enhanced by the use of seat belts" (Springfeldt, 1993 as cited in Day & Rechnitzer, 1999, p. 11). Many tractors, especially older ones, are not equipped with seat belts, and when tractors do have seat belts, there is a general reluctance among owners to use them.

Actors in Decision Making and Planning

The Victorian WorkCover Authority, the Victorian Farmers Federation, and the Steering Committee (whose membership included the VWA, VFF, and FMDA) were involved in the decision making and the planning. Discussion and negotiation were used to resolve any conflicts that arose, and final decisions were reached through consensus.

Outcome

Evaluation

The Monash University Accident Research Centre was contracted by the VWA to carry out an evaluation of the 1997/98 tractor rollover protective structure rebate scheme. The evaluation used a combination of qualitative and quantitative methods to describe the effect of the program. Included in the evaluation were short- and long-term benefits of the scheme; potential lives saved; psychological trauma averted; general effects on farm safety; and a cost outcome analysis.

Short- and Long-Term Benefits

Potential lives saved
Based on data available from Sweden, it was predicted that "the actual effect of the rebate scheme may be to prevent slightly less than 2 deaths per year" (Day & Rechnitzer, 1999, p. 30). "This scheme would be expected to have an enduring benefit until the 12,129 tractors retrofitted under the scheme are retired from service" (Day & Rechnitzer, 1999, p. 30). "If the effect of the scheme were considered to be constant for

the first 10 years, then a total of 20 deaths would be expected to be prevented, all other things remaining the same" (Day & Rechnitzer, 1999, p. 30).

Psychological trauma averted
Families and communities among whom rollover deaths occur experience psychological and emotional trauma. "The family, while still grieving for the deceased, may also face other significant losses i.e., the loss of property, employment, financial support and lifestyle" (Day & Rechnitzer, 1999, p. 31). A traumatic injury death, such as a tractor rollover, can also have profound effects on rural communities and affect the productivity within these communities. The rebate scheme is likely to have prevented the trauma described above from occurring for 2 farm families and their communities each year for at least the next 10 years (Day & Rechnitzer, 1999, p. 32).

General Effects on Farm Safety

The 1997/98 ROPS rebate scheme may have had some impact on other areas of farm safety. Based on interviews with farmers, "4 of the 18 farmers reported taking any other safety related action since fitting the ROPS, including improvements to a wool shed, maintenance of creek crossings and irrigation ditches, locking away firearms, creating a fire break, and ensuring the storage of chemicals in a cupboard" (Day & Rechnitzer, 1999, p. 32). The VFF also observed a greater interest in farm safety among its members since the ROPS rebate scheme started operating. Staff in the department believed that the "publicity campaign increased the perception that enforcement of the ROPS regulations would follow the scheme, and that the enforcement may cover farm health and safety more broadly" (Day & Rechnitzer, 1999, p. 32). It is expected that "any influence the rebate scheme may have had on farm safety behaviour in general would decline upon completion of the scheme, unless other measures are implemented" (Day & Rechnitzer, 1999, p. 32).

Cost Outcome Analysis

A cost outcome analysis of the 1997/98 rebate scheme was included in the evaluation. Its purpose was to provide data for the comparison of the impact of the 1997/98 ROPS rebate scheme with alternative approaches to reducing tractor rollover deaths. Two perspectives were provided: the societal perspective (taking into account the costs and benefits to all members of society), and that of the VWA (taking into account the costs and benefits to the VWA; Day & Rechnitzer, 1999, p. 16).

Societal perspective
"The total cost of the rebate scheme was $7,877,344 AU in 1997/98. If the effect is assumed to be constant for the first 10 years, then 20 deaths could be expected to be prevented. In economic terms, $393,867 AU will have been spent per life saved. If the effect of the scheme was constant for 20 years (i.e., if the protected tractors remain in operation longer than assumed), then 40 deaths could be expected to be prevented. In this case $196,934 AU will have been spent per life saved" (Day & Rechnitzer, 1999, p. 34).

In addition, a number of positive outcomes would arise, including the following:

- Justice system costs associated with coronial inquests would be reduced.
- Property damage to tractors involved in rollovers would be averted.
- Psychological and emotional trauma for families and rural communities would be averted (Day & Rechnitzer, 1999, p. 34).

Other outcomes that could arise include in the following:

- increased health care costs, should there be an increase in non-fatal injuries due to rollover events, or incidents associated with the retrofitted frames;
- reduced WorkCover insurance premiums for the agricultural industry; and
- an improvement in other areas of farm health and safety, resulting from the scheme (Day & Rechnitzer, 1999, p. 34).

Victorian WorkCover Authority Perspective

"The economic cost of the rebate scheme to the VWA was $2,315,397 AU in 1997/98 (excluding VWA staff costs). If the effect is assumed to be constant for the first 10 years, then the prevention of 20 deaths can be expected. In economic terms, this amounts to $115,770 AU spent by the VWA per life saved. If the effect of the scheme was constant for 20 years, then 40 possible deaths could be prevented. In this case, $57,885 AU will have been spent per life saved" (Day & Rechnitzer, 1999, p. 34).

Other positive outcomes that could arise include:

- an improvement in other areas of farm health and safety resulting from the scheme; and
- strengthening of partnerships with other key players in farm safety (Day & Rechnitzer, 1999, p. 34).

Results

Demand for the ROPS rebates was substantially higher than in any previous rebate scheme, and penetration of the scheme extended well beyond the membership of the VFF, with 73% of applicants being non-members and 21% being self-nominated hobby farmers. All participant groups and organizations (farmers, farm machinery dealers, the VFF, and the FMDA) were satisfied with the scheme, and problems of obtaining ROPS for the older tractor models were not overwhelming (Day & Rechnitzer, 1999, p. 35).

Dissemination of Information

The Monash University Accident Research Center was contracted by the Victorian WorkCover Authority to document the history and results of the evaluation of the 1997/98 tractor rollover protective structure rebates scheme. The information was compiled in *Evaluation of the tractor rollover protective structure (ROPS) rebate scheme 1997/98* and disseminated through the network of Farmsafe Australia. A summary is available on Monash University Accident Research Center's website (http://www.general.monash.edu.au/muarc/rptsum/es155.htm). Information about the program has also been disseminated at national and international conferences.

PROMISING PRACTICES

Small Business Falls Prevention Project

Hume City Council, Hume, Australia

Main Key Informants:
Paul Wilson and Sue Bergin

Background

The Small Business Falls Prevention Project is an initiative undertaken by Hume City Council to provide a free occupational health and safety service to the local small business community. Working directly with the small business owner, project staff offer advice on how to identify, assess, and eliminate hazards that have the potential to cause slips, trips, and falls in the workplace. The effective management of these hazards has important benefits both to the small business owner and to the broader community at large, suggesting that this project would be directly applicable to other jurisdictions, such as Canada, where small businesses account for a significant proportion of total business activity.

In 1997, a total of 25,451 Australians were injured as a result of a fall in the workplace (Local Government Focus, 2000). Falls are a leading cause of serious head and spinal cord injury and, as such, are a major concern for neurotrauma prevention initiatives. Hume City Council, recognizing that local government is increasingly expected to provide leadership on issues of health and safety, voted in favour of developing a prevention program to reduce the incidence of workplace injury in local small businesses.

Rather than defining the problem as a narrow, isolated issue pertaining largely to private business and industry, the council approached occupational health and safety as part of a broader concern for community safety. Indeed, the council is coordinating the integration of various safety-related services, including the Small Business Falls Prevention Project, through the Hume Safe City Task Force. The Task Force provides an umbrella approach to a diverse range of issues, including road safety, emergency management, injury prevention, alcohol and drug abuse, suicide prevention, homelessness, and crime prevention (Local Government Focus, 2000).

Moreover, a Health and Safety Advisory Forum is strategically linked to the Task Force and its multi-agency work teams allow for both agency and community input. The integration of services on this scale is touted as a ground-breaking, innovative approach. The manager of community services for Hume City explained: "We tried to look at a constructive process, having various agencies working together rather than all contributing individual efforts in isolation from each other, duplicating services and sometimes working at cross purposes. It is like a case management system for safety issues. Councils are ideally placed to implement such a system because they are already involved in all areas of community life. This is not just Australian best practice, but world best practice" (Local Government Focus, 2000).

The WHO Safe Communities Program

The concept of the safe community originated in 1989 at the first World Conference on Accident and Injury Prevention held in Stockholm, Sweden. The manifesto for the Safe Communities Program, which was the resolution of the conference, declares that "all human beings have an equal right to health and safety." This conviction is a fundamental aspect of the Health for All strategy of the World Health Organization (WHO).

Essentially, the safe community concept refers to approaching injury control and safety in a comprehensive way for all ages, environments, and situations. A community can be defined as a delineated geographical area, groups with common interests, professional associations, or the individuals who provide services in a specific location. As such, the principles of a safe community will vary somewhat from place to place (WHO Collaborating Centre website).

The overriding tenet of the Safe Communities Program – what differentiates it from other injury prevention initiatives – is that the leading role is played by the community itself. Indeed, the ability to mobilize the community as a whole and have its members define for themselves the important safety issues is critical: "The community that has established a context for building relationships, organizing community intervention, and achieving results has taken the valuable first steps toward becoming a safe community" (WHO Collaborating Centre website).

In September 1989 the Department of Public Health Sciences at the Karolinska Institutet in Stockholm, Sweden, was appointed a WHO

Collaborating Centre on Community Safety Promotion. It is the role of the Collaborating Centre to review all applications for official WHO accreditation as a safe community. To this end, a comprehensive set of criteria has been developed for assessing the eligibility of the particular community applying for accreditation. While it is recognized that it is not always possible to apply each criterion in every case, the 12 criteria listed below have evolved based on the experiences of existing safe communities.

1   A cross-sectoral group responsible for injury prevention should be formed.
2   The program should involve the local community network.
3   The program should address all ages, surroundings, and situations.
4   The program should address the concerns of high-risk groups (such as children and older adults) and high-risk environments, and aim to ensure equity for vulnerable groups.
5   The program should have a mechanism to document the frequency and causes of injuries.
6   The program must involve a long-term approach, not one of brief duration.
7   The program evaluation should include indicators that show effects and provide information on the process as it advances.
8   Each community should analyse its organizations and their potential for participation in the program.
9   Participation of the health care community in both the registration of injuries and the injury prevention program is essential.
10 All levels of the community should ideally be involved in solving the injury problem.
11 Information on the experience should be disseminated both nationally and internationally.
12 The committee should be willing to contribute to the overall network of Safe Communities.

As of 1999, 48 communities around the world had been designated safe communities. Six communities are projected to receive accreditation in 2000 and dozens more applications are currently under preparation (WHO Collaborating Centre website).

In recognition of its commitment to community safety, the Municipality of Hume, Australia, was one of the first 10 cities to receive official WHO accreditation. Hume was formally designated a WHO safe community in 1996. (The former Shire of Bulla, now the City of Hume, was originally designated in 1994.) Hume City Council considers its involvement with the WHO Safe Communities Program one of its greatest successes.

History and Development of the Small Business Falls Prevention Project

Development of the Small Business Falls Prevention Project marked a significant addition to the Hume Safe Community Program. The project was specifically designed to help fulfil 2 of City Council's highest priorities. First, it was developed to advance the council's commitment to a safe community (as described above). Second, as a free service to assist local small business owners in reducing workplace injuries (thereby also reducing costs), the project provides further incentive for businesses to establish in Hume.

The planning and design of the project began in July 1999. A conscious decision was made at the outset to target small business and industry. (A small business was defined as any business operation with fewer than 20 employees.) According to the project officer, small businesses were targeted for several reasons. First, big business has been the focus of most occupational injury prevention programs to date, so there is a pressing need for such work within the small business sector. Second, small business owners lack the extensive resources of big business to implement formal health and safety policies and procedures. As a result, there is often little attention paid to increasing risk awareness and reducing safety hazards in the small workplace (P. Wilson, personal communication, April 2, 2000).

The Small Business Falls Prevention Project was officially launched during Community Safety Week in September 1999. The launch involved the start of a 6-week pilot phase in which the project officer began visiting local small businesses to promote and generate interest in the project. Business owners were provided with an information kit containing WorkCover posters and the project pamphlet.

A total of 100 businesses were visited during the pilot phase and 12 requested a formal risk assessment, thereby exceeding the expected strike rate of 10%. It was determined that cold-call visits often caught people at a bad time and resulted in the project officer being unable to get past the secretary. Follow-up telephone calls proved effective in enhancing the participation rate. It was decided that for future phases each business would receive a letter describing the project prior to the on-site visit.

Goals and Objectives

In 1998 180 WorkCover claims were filed in Hume Municipality as a result of an injury suffered in a fall at work (Small Business Falls Prevention Project, 2000). Hume City Council implemented the Small Business Falls Prevention Project to help tackle what it viewed as a community safety problem. The stated goal of the project is "to facilitate improved outcomes for the prevention of falls injury in local small business" (Australian Injury Prevention Database website).

In order to achieve this goal of reducing workplace injury, a series of specific objectives were developed:

- to target high-risk small industry through a community-based injury prevention program;
- to engage selected industries and employers to participate in a partnership with the community through the Safe Community Program, aimed at reducing risks and preventing falls injuries;
- to develop a strong culture of falls prevention within the small business community; and
- to evaluate the role of local government contributing to small business workplace safety (Australian Injury Prevention Database website).

Implicit in this statement of goals and objectives is the contribution the project makes to the broader Community Safety Program, designed to enhance the health and safety of all citizens of Hume Municipality.

Resources

This section of the report presents a discussion of the model underlying the Small Business Falls Prevention Project, as well as its sources of funding.

Model

The Small Business Falls Prevention Project is based upon the model of risk assessment, which is consistent with Haddon's (1980) matrix model in that it emphasizes injury prevention at both the primary and secondary levels (i.e., at the pre-event and event phases). The specific assessment procedure utilized in the Small Business Falls Prevention Project was developed by Workforce Information Network. According to this procedure, risk assessment is an evaluative process, involving 3 distinct stages:

Stage 1: identifying hazards (by using a standard checklist);
Stage 2: assessing hazards (considering the risk of the hazard); and
Stage 3: controlling hazards (implementing controls to reduce the risk of the hazard).

Each individual hazard identified by the project officer in the first stage is assessed in order that it can be assigned a priority rating. This second stage is critical as it allows for high-risk hazards to be attended to before those with lower priority ratings.

The priority rating is calculated on the basis of 3 specific characteristics of the identified hazard. The likelihood of an accident involving the hazard (e.g., remotely possible, quite possible) is assessed first. Next, the frequency of exposure to the particular hazard is determined (e.g., occasional, continuous). The third consideration is the potential consequence of an accident involving the particular hazard (e.g., disaster, noticeable outcome). Each hazard is ultimately assigned 1 to 5 priority ratings: very high, high, substantial, medium, and low.

Stage 3 involves the recommendation of changes to control the identified hazards on the basis of the control hierarchy shown below:

- elimination: involves removal of the hazard altogether;
- substitution: involves using another less hazardous chemical or machine;
- isolation: involves limiting exposure to the hazard;
- engineering: involves guarding the hazard with fixed/lockable guards or with red-eye cut-out switches;
- administration: involves reducing the time personnel are exposed to the hazard and/or providing training to personnel; and
- personal protective equipment: involves issuing ear muffs, safety boots, goggles, respirators, etc.

While elimination of the hazard is the most effective control, it is not always practical or feasible. Issuing personal protective equipment is the least desired method of control.

A central assumption underlying the risk assessment model is that all workplaces will always have hazards. The aim is to reduce the risks associated with those hazards. For some hazards, several options may be recommended to help reduce the risk; in such cases, a combination approach may be appropriate. In other cases, owing to either cost or impracticality, none of the recommendations are adopted, although the risk assessment process will have served to educate employees about the hazard. Thus, by emphasizing proper training (i.e., pre-event phase) along with the use of protective equipment (i.e., event phase), the Small Business Falls Prevention Project aims to reduce both the incidence and the severity of unintentional injury outcomes. This approach to injury prevention is in agreement with Haddon's (1980) matrix model, which depicts the interaction of risk factors over pre-event and event time to cause neurotrauma injuries.

Funding

The Small Business Falls Prevention Project is funded entirely by the Victorian WorkCover Authority. In early 1999, WorkCover approached Hume City Council with an idea for a workplace injury prevention program. The council then returned to WorkCover with a detailed proposal and, following a period of revision and discussion, funding was granted for the period July 1999 to June 2000.

Additional funding was requested from WorkCover in August 1999 to cover the expense of contracting an experienced researcher to conduct an external evaluation of the project. Further to this, an application was recently submitted to WorkCover for renewal of funding for a second 1-year period. A decision on this application has not yet been announced.

Office space and business equipment and supplies are furnished by the Health Services Business Unit of Hume City Council.

Implementation

The Small Business Falls Prevention Project employs a community-based approach to risk awareness and injury prevention. There is no obligation on the part of small business owners to participate; however, there are numerous advantages to doing so. Implementing the changes recommended during the on-site visit will provide a safer environment for workers employed by the small business owner, and it goes without saying that a safer work environment significantly reduces the likelihood of an employee sustaining an injury. On-the-job injuries result in many costs to the employer, both direct and hidden. Loss of production, replacement hiring, and training are some of the hidden costs involved (Small Business Falls Prevention Project, 2000).

Furthermore, reducing common hazards that have the potential to cause a slip, trip, or fall in the workplace decreases the likelihood of having to submit a WorkCover claim for an injured employee. Participation in the project may result in reduced WorkCover premiums for the business owner (Small Business Falls Prevention Project, 2000).

Effective Practices

According to the project officer, the success of the project has been due largely to the flexibility built into the way businesses are approached. As with any other product or service, the business owner must be sold on its merits. The project officer discovered that approaching a specific type of owner called for a specific type of sell. For instance, owners in the urban/suburban areas of the municipality were much busier than those in the rural districts and therefore less likely to express immediate interest in the project (P. Wilson, personal communication, April 2, 2000).

Age differences among the business owners also influenced willingness to participate in the project. Older owners, most of whom had successfully operated their own small businesses for many years, were much more reluctant to spend time on safety issues. Often the older owners claimed that health and safety are simply not issues in their workplace, to which the project officer would reply, "Well, you must be doing something right then. Could I take a look around so that I can tell other small business owners about your success?" Not surprisingly, this technique often resulted in the owner consenting to a de facto risk assessment.

In other cases, older business owners were clinging to the myth that there are no immediate tangible benefits to improving occupational health and safety. This is an example of an issue that, although not anticipated during the planning of the project, was successfully managed because of the flexibility inherent in the program. Conversely, an initial concern regarding potential language barriers proved unwarranted as fully 98% of business owners contacted could speak fluent English.

There is a tremendous willingness to work directly with the small business owner to achieve the mutually desired outcome of a safer workplace. The on-site risk assessments are conducted only upon the request of the owner; that is, there is no obligation. Nor is there any sense that this is another government inspection program. The fact that the service is entirely free makes the project easier to sell: many small businesses have limited resources.

With regard to enhancing the project, more resources must be devoted to re-visiting the workplaces over time. Not all the relevant issues can be addressed in a single visit and repeat visits would allow for the appraisal of any safety improvements implemented on the basis of the initial risk assessment. The project officer noted, "it must become an on-going process if we want to implement a progressive safety culture" (P. Wilson, personal communication, April 2, 2000).

Decision Making and Planning

The Small Business Falls Prevention Project established a steering committee to facilitate ongoing decision making and planning processes. The committee, which meets regularly every 2 months, is chaired by the coordinator of the Health Services Business Unit for the City of Hume. Other committee members include: the Small Business Falls Prevention Project Officer, a Victorian WorkCover Authority official, a Hume City Council employee with prior experience with occupational health and safety projects, a representative from the local insurance industry (QBE Mercantile Mutual), and the external evaluator.

Representation on the Steering Committee from the Hume City Council Economic Development Department was sought but Economic Development officials had little interest in the project. This department works closely with the local small business community on a daily basis and it was hoped that their relationship would enhance the participation rate of small business owners. According to the project officer, the involvement of several other local organizations might also have proven useful in terms of project planning and decision making. Like the Economic Development Department, the Chamber of Commerce and the Rotary Club have contacts with the local small business community.

Ongoing Evaluation of Prevention Strategy

The project officer has conducted informal checks regarding the implementation process during the course of the project. To date, 5 small business owners have been interviewed, following their participation in the risk assessment procedure, in order to assess their level of satisfaction with the project. Four of the owners expressed tremendous satisfaction and were very happy to have participated. One owner believed that the nature and number of changes recommended by the prevention officer during the course of the risk assessment greatly exceeded the capacity of his resources.

This feedback resulted in an adjustment of the expectations placed upon the small business owner. Following a consultation with WorkCover officials, changes were made in terms of the amount of flexibility within the risk assessment process. The project officer expressed an increased understanding of the pressures and demands facing small business owners (P. Wilson, personal communication, April 2, 2000).

Outcome

In this section the external evaluation of the Small Business Falls Prevention Project is described and an overview of the methods of dissemination of information provided.

Evaluation

An external evaluator (Small Business Research Unit, Victoria University) has been contracted to conduct a formal evaluation of the Small Business Falls Prevention Project. The evaluation plan calls for both formative and summative evaluation efforts, as described in the *Guide to Program Design and Evaluation Planning* (Ontario Neurotrauma Foundation, 1999). An assessment of the structure and implementation process will be included; however, the main focus will be an evaluation of the impact of the project, that is, the extent to which specific objectives have been met (Small Business Research Unit, 2000).

The evaluation team are to:

- assess the extent of actual changes implemented by employers in attempting to reduce risks in their workplace as a result of their participation in the project;
- review the implementation characteristics of the project;
- propose further strategic directions for Hume City Council, which would enable it to build on its role as a safe community;

- ascertain whether there were any unintended outcomes; and
- assess the overall worth of the project.

A combination of both qualitative and quantitative methods will be employed. The evaluation will include post-intervention observations utilizing comparative data from participating and non-participating small businesses. There will be 3 phases:

1 The process evaluation will measure the activities of the project and its reach. Data on activities and business participation will be collected from a survey, project reports, the project officer's diaries and records, interviews with small business owners, and through consultation with key project administrators.
2 The impact evaluation will involve the use of a survey developed and mailed out by the evaluation team. The questionnaire will be designed to assess the impact of the project over the past year (or the period of involvement with the project). The survey will also provide quantified responses to the risk assessment. Two matched samples (one of the businesses who were approached and chose not to participate and one of the businesses who were not approached) will serve as comparisons to participating businesses in order to evaluate the impact of the project.
3 The outcome evaluation is the final phase of the evaluation; it relates to the stated objectives of the project. The outcome measures – injury rates and severity of injury – are long-term effects and may prove difficult to collect. As a result, data collection in this phase will be limited to self-report measures.

To assist in evaluating the Small Business Falls Prevention Project, an attempt will be made to identify any similar best practice programs. These other programs will be investigated through an intensive literature search and through discussions with selected contact individuals and key informants. This process will assist in the identification of relevant performance indicators for workplace injury prevention programs (Small Business Research Unit, 2000).

Dissemination of Information

Monthly reports are written by the project officer and distributed to all stakeholders. Each report provides a brief update on the progress being made and the obstacles encountered. Also, at the 6-month point, an executive summary was prepared in order to report the results of the project to date.

There has been widespread promotion of the project through the media. When the project was first being launched, articles were published in many local newspapers as well as in *Safe Living News*, a Hume City Council newsletter. More recently, the project was promoted in the March 2000 issue of *Hume Economic Update*, distributed to over 700 businesses in Hume. Extensive information regarding the Small Business Falls Prevention Project is available via the Internet. A detailed description of the project has been added to the Hume City Council website (http://www.hume.vic.gov.au) and to the Australian Injury Prevention Database, a comprehensive listing of prevention programs compiled by researchers at the University of Queensland, Australia (http://www.spmed.qu.edu.au/aipd/progs0.asp). There is also a link to the Hume Safe Community Program through the website for the WHO Collaborating Centre on Community Safety Promotion at the Karolinska Institutet in Stockholm, Sweden (http://www.ki.se/phs/wcc-csp).

North American Guidelines for Children's Agricultural Tasks (NAGCAT)

Main Key Informant:
Dr William Pickett

Background

From 1991 through 1995, 74 childhood (19 years and younger) farm fatalities were reported in Canada (Canadian Agricultural Injury Surveillance Program [CAISP], 1997). The Canadian Agricultural Injury Surveillance Program also reported that 391 children (aged 0–14) were hospitalized for farm machinery injuries from 1990 through 1996 (CAISP, 1999). "Farm machinery injuries sometimes cause brain and spinal cord injury" (L. Hartling, personal communication, February 15, 2000). It is not clear which of these fatal and nonfatal injuries were directly related to children's active participation in agricultural work. As there is a lack of general standards or guidelines indicating appropriate work for children in the field of agriculture, children who live, work, or visit farms are at risk of agricultural unintentional injuries. "Many unintentional injuries occur because parents and children mistake physical size and age for ability, may overestimate developmental capabilities, and may underestimate levels of hazard and risk" (North American Guidelines for Children's Agricultural Tasks, 1999, p. 14).

The North American Guidelines for Children's Agricultural Tasks (NAGCAT) came about at the request of farm parents and the 1996 National Action Plan for Childhood Agricultural Injury Prevention. In 1996 steps were taken to pilot test the feasibility of developing agricultural work guidelines. The pilot test proved successful and the decision was then made to further develop a series of guidelines for children's agricultural tasks.

Resources

Collaborators

A core group of individuals from the National Farm Medicine Centre and the National Children's Center for Rural and Agricultural Health and Safety in Marshfield, Wisconsin, initiated the planning, implementation, and evaluation of the guidelines. The National Institute for Occupational Safety and Health (NIOSH) in the United States and the Canadian Coalition for Agricultural Safety and Rural Health in Canada were also involved. Participants on the project team were from the United States, Canada, and Mexico. Members of the team had a series of in-person and teleconference meetings between March 1997 and June 1999.

Funding

Funding was provided in 1996 by the National Institute for Occupational Safety and Health (NIOSH) to the Midwest Center for Agricultural Research (Marshfield, WI) and the Centers for Disease Control-funded Injury Prevention Research Center at the University of Iowa to pilot test a process for developing guidelines. From 1997–1999, the NAGCAT project team was supported by the Canadian Coalition for Agricultural Safety and Rural Health, NIOSH-funded Midwest

Center for Agricultural Research (Marshfield, WI), the NIOSH-funded National Children's Center for Rural and Agricultural Health and Safety, the federal Maternal and Child Health Bureau, and the employing agency of project team members (NAGCAT, 1999).

Implementation

By June 1999, there were 62 guidelines covering a variety of agricultural tasks focusing on the most common jobs children do on the farm (NAGCAT, 1999). Guidelines were not developed for children younger than 7 years because children of that age are not developmentally ready to engage in productive agricultural work. The guidelines are divided into 7 categories: animal care, tractor fundamentals, implement operation, manual labour, haying operations, general activities, and specialty production. The goal of the guidelines is to help children to do agricultural jobs safely; thus, they were developed with the best interests of the child as the focus. "This will enable children ages 7–16 years to have safe, meaningful work experiences in agriculture" (NAGCAT, 1999, p. 14).

The guidelines address primary prevention of unintentional injury. They are intended to help parents match a specific child's physical, mental, and psychosocial abilities with the requirements of a specific agricultural job. "They should also enable children to understand the rationale for an adult's decision whether or not to assign a specific job to a child" (NAGCAT, 1999, p. 11).

Two manuals were developed, one for parents and one for professionals. "Each parent resource manual includes an illustration of the agricultural job, a list of adult responsibilities, a checklist to assess a child's mental, physical and psychosocial skills to conduct the job, important steps necessary to do the job safely, identification of key hazards of the task, and a description of the level of supervision recommended" (NAGCAT, 1999, p. 14). "Each professional resource manual includes a comprehensive description of all findings from the consensus-development project involving more than 150 individuals from the U.S. and Canada. Content includes: background, methodology, terminology, principles of child development, and references, plus the job hazard analysis framework and accompanying child development checklist for 62 different agricultural jobs" (NAGCAT, 1999, p. 14).

Outcome

Method of Evaluation

Formal evaluation of the validity of the guidelines has not been completed to date. The Center for Disease Control in the United States has issued a call for proposals to conduct evaluations of the NAGCAT guidelines. These are being reviewed now, and evaluations of the guidelines will take place over the next 3 years. It is expected that the guidelines will be evaluated in multiple populations, using multiple types of approaches (e.g., randomized trials through more qualitative methods) (W. Pickett, personal communication, May 11, 2000).

Dissemination of Information

The results of NAGCAT were disseminated in 4 forms: final report to the funding agencies; a *Professional Resource Manual* designed for agricultural safety specialists; illustrated posters for parents; and selected elements of project results posted on the Internet.

Every year children are killed or seriously injured in agricultural settings. The North American Guidelines for Children's Agricultural Tasks look very promising, as they serve as a valuable resource for parents, agricultural safety specialists, farm owners, educators, youth groups, health professionals, and the media. The guidelines, however, need to be evaluated to determine the extent of their effectiveness in preventing injuries and fatalities among children in the field of agriculture.

Farm Response Program

Main Key Informant:
Lori Lockinger

Background

Agriculture continues to be one of the most hazardous occupations in Canada, resulting in serious injuries and fatalities every year. It also poses a concern for neurotrauma prevention specifically, as "farm machinery injuries sometimes cause brain and spinal cord injury" (L. Hartling, personal communication, February 29, 2000). Moreover, when "a rural resident is the victim of an accident, the increased time that it takes for care to be provided can affect the severity and outcome of the injury" (Lockinger, Hillier, Hagel, Chen, McDuffie, & Dosman, 1997, p. 388).

Factors that contribute to increased response times include the absence of central dispatching (911) in rural areas, the possibility of lengthy extrication time, the remote location of farms, and the judgment of the rescuer. The rescuer is usually a family member or friend, whose emotional involvement with the victim and lack of professional rescue training may hamper judgment at a critical time. Despite admirable intentions, a rescuer who does not use good judgment may cause additional injury.

Farm Response

Farm Response started in 1996 in Saskatchewan and evolved out of an existing program in Ithaca, New York. It is "an accident preparedness course, that provides rescuers with the knowledge to make appropriate decisions upon reaching a farm accident situation and also forewarns them of potential dangers of the scene" (Lockinger et al., 1997, p. 387). This program focuses on the event phase of unintentional injury. The objective is to train farmers and their family members in what to do or not to do in the case of an emergency.

This 4-hour course provides those first on the scene of a farm emergency with the skills to make appropriate decisions. The program warns rescuers of the potential dangers at an accident scene and covers situations specific to the farm, including: machinery entanglement, suffocation in grain bins or silos, pesticide spills or inhalation, electrocution, and animal handling. For each possible situation, algorithms illustrate proper sequencing of decisions and actions. Participants are also taught how to report unintentional injuries to Emergency Medical Services, what to include in a first aid and pesticide safety kit, and how to shut off a diesel tractor. Farm Response includes limited first aid instruction. However, "participants are encouraged to obtain first aid and cardiopulmonary resuscitation (CPR) training" (p. 389).

Participation in the program is voluntary. The course is offered every winter in Saskatchewan and over 1,000 people to date have taken it.

Resources

Collaborators

Farm Response was initiated by M.D. Ambulance Care Ltd of Saskatoon in cooperation with Saskatoon District Health and the Centre for Agricultural Medicine. Trainers were recruited from emergency medical service personnel in the province to provide instruction for farmers and their families.

Funding

Expenses for the program are covered by the Agricultural Health and Safety Network. For Network members, the only cost for participants is $10 for the course manual.

Implementation

At the conclusion of the course each participant was asked to complete an evaluation form and to rate various aspects of the course on a 5-point scale, with 1 representing poor and 5 representing excellent (Lockinger et al., 1997). More than 80% rated the student materials, instructor's knowledge, logical presentation of the information, discussions, and overall presentation of the program at scores of 4 or 5. Participants also indicated that the course made them more conscious about farm safety, stating plans to post emergency numbers by the phone, purchase first aid kits, and learn more about machinery on their farms (Lockinger et al., 1997).

Outcome

Farm Response is a promising program that has the potential to reduce the risk of further injury in the event stage of neurotrauma by teaching those first on the scene of an emergency situation to be aware of potential dangers, to respond in a timely fashion, and to react calmly in a difficult situation. This program has yet to be evaluated to determine its impact upon rural injury rates and long-term benefits for the behaviour and knowledge of participants. The Farm Response program has been replicated in agricultural regions of British Columbia and Ontario, and it is hoped that it can be extended to other parts of rural Canada.

Prevention of Fall-Related Injuries

A fall is defined as "occurring when a person loses balance causing them to hit the ground or other object at lower level" (Healthy Ageing Research Unit, 1998, p. 12). Falls from heights are a major cause of accidental death and injury in urban children (Barlow, Niemirska, Gandhi, & Leblanc, 1983). One study of child mortality showed that 12% of all deaths of children under the age of 15 resulted from falls from heights. The enactment of legislation governing window guards, including education in their use, is profiled as a best practice for effective child falls prevention.

Over the course of the lifespan, the occurrence of head injury follows a U-shaped curve (Horan & Little, 1998). The very high rates of head injuries in childhood drop to considerably lower levels throughout much of adulthood, and rise again in old age. Given current Canadian demographics, there is an increasing necessity for programs to address the needs of older people. "In Canada accidental falls are the second leading cause of hospitalizations for senior women and the fifth leading cause of hospitalizations for senior men" (Robson, Edwards, Lightfoot, & Bursey, 1999). Falls account for a major proportion of cervical spinal fractures and brain injury in older people (Horan & Little, 1998; SMARTRISK, 1998; Hyde, 1996); prevention of these types of injuries is thus of utmost importance. In Ontario alone, falls account for nearly 60% of the $870 million spent in direct health care costs, of which 45% are for care of older adults (SMARTRISK, 1999). The prevention of fall-related injuries in older adults can reduce the incidence of neurotrauma in the older adult population and can also result in substantial savings in health care costs. It has been estimated that falls prevention in older adults could result in a decrease of approximately 3,000 hospitalizations and 700 permanently disabled people over the age of 65 in Ontario (SMARTRISK, 1999).

Two of the following 4 cases addressing falls in the older population describe intervention strategies from a set of studies collectively called the FICSIT (Frailty and Injuries: Cooperative Studies on Intervention Techniques) trials. The objective of these trials was to determine the most effective prevention strategies. The other 2 cases utilize existing community resources in their intervention strategies. As well, they take into consideration both behavioural and environmental risk factors in the design of their programs. All strategies profiled attempt to reduce the incidence of falls and their resultant injuries through the implementation of interventions that target the major risk factors of falls.

Best Practices

- Children Can't Fly: A Window Falls Prevention Program
- Tai Chi and Computerized Balance Training for Falls Prevention in Older Adults
- Multiple-Risk-Factor Reduction Strategy for Falls Prevention in Older Adults
- No Falls! No Fear! Falls Prevention Project

BEST PRACTICES

Children Can't Fly: A New York Department of Health Initiative

Window Falls Prevention Program

Background

Falls from one level to another are a major cause of accidental death and injury in urban children (Barlow et al., 1983). In the early 1970s, the incidence of child mortality and morbidity due to falls from windows was recognized as high after a study of child mortality due to falls from heights was conducted between January 1965 and September 1969 in New York City (Spiegel & Lindaman, 1977). The study showed that 123 or 12% of all deaths of children under age 15 were the result of falls from heights. As a result, in 1972, the New York City Health Department (NYCHD) launched the educational and preventative program Children Can't Fly in the South Bronx. The success of this program led to the passing of legislation under the New York City Health Code in 1976 that requires owners of multiple dwellings to provide window guards in apartments where children under 11 years reside.

The Children Can't Fly program, now known as the Window Falls Prevention Program, remains in effect today and has had only one amendment since its inception and inclusion in the Health Code 9. The program targets any New York City adult responsible for the care of a child under 11 years of age, for any period of time. The pilot program targeted only high-risk regions of New York City, which tended to be areas of low socio-economic status (SES) and tenements. The program was subsequently expanded to include all of New York City, due to the extremely high incidence of mortality and morbidity in children due to falls from a window in the city. Table 1 illustrates the head and spine injury incidence rates for 61 children admitted to the Harlem Hospital Center over a period of ten years after the Window Falls Prevention Program began. These numbers represent only 4% of incidence rates before the program was implemented.

TABLE 1.   Major Injuries in 61 Children Who Fell from a Height

Type of injury	No. of patients	Specific injury	No. of patients
Head	56	Concussion	25
		Skull fracture	17
		Brain contusion	13
		Subdural	1
Fractures	70	Spine	2

Source: Barlow et al., 1983

History and Development

The Department of Health initiated the Children Can't Fly program in the Tremont Health District of the Bronx. This area was seen as having the greatest need for intervention, after 23 deaths of children under age 15 occurred in one year: 1971. Following the initial 2-year pilot project that began in the South Bronx in 1972, the program was expanded and covered all 5 boroughs by 1975. In 1976 the window guard requirement was made law through an amendment to the NYC Health Code.

Program Description

The 2-year pilot test of the Children Can't Fly program included 3 components that address the agent in the event, pre- and post-event phases of injury as described by Haddon (1980):

1 data collection through voluntary reporting of window fall incidents by area police and hospitals as well as through public health nurse follow-up visits to victims;
2 education and outreach through door-to-door safety audits and distribution of free window guard applications, as well as through the involvement of community organizations and a media campaign; and
3 the provision of easy to install, free window guards to families in high-risk areas.

Data Collection

During the first 4 years of the program, hospital emergency rooms and police precincts were asked to report window falls using postal card forms supplied by the program. Further data was collected by public health nurses in the form of a family profile that included demographic and sociological information. The nurse visits also served educational and preventative functions.

Education

Outreach workers made door-to-door visits during which they identified hazards, provided counselling to parents on prevention, and distributed applications for free window guards as needed. Both private and public community-based groups were enlisted for the distribution of prevention literature and instruction. A media campaign to raise awareness and provide prevention education was conducted through print, radio, and television in both Spanish and English.

Prevention Efforts

Free, easy to install window guards were distributed to families with pre-school age children living in tenements in high risk areas. Between 1972 and 1976 more than 16,000 window guards were distributed annually, particularly in areas of highest risk. While Environmental Health personnel installed 25% of the window guards, the majority were installed by the recipient. Audits of the installations were made and no falls were reported from windows where guards had been installed.

Stakeholders and Collaborators

The program was developed and implemented by the NYCHD but required the participation of law enforcement agencies and hospital emergency room staff as well as community interest. The joint efforts of these groups led to the passing of related legislation and the development of the NYCHD Bureau of Window Falls Prevention.

Resources

This initiative was supported at the outset by the NYCHD and continues to be supported by this department today. The ongoing success of the program relies on tenant and landlord cooperation in reporting methods, as well as continued enforcement of the window guard law.

Implementation

The Pilot Project

In accordance with recommendations made in Chapter 1 of the ONF *Guide to Program Design and Evaluation Planning*, the Children Can't Fly program was developed with the clear purpose to reduce child falls from windows and utilized a rationale grounded in technical reports and accident rates. The program did not induce increased risk or injuries from fires but ensured that at least 1 exit in first floor dwellings remained unbarred and that windows to fire escapes were not barred.

The program was first implemented in the area of greatest need and then expanded throughout the city over a period of 2 years, with higher-risk areas receiving the program first and low-risk areas receiving the program last. It was recognized that areas of low SES and tenement-type buildings posed the greatest risk of child falls. The provision of free window guards to families identified as most at risk was an effective and thoughtful intervention.

Data was continually collected during the pilot study through voluntary reports. This data was corroborated by city-maintained vital statistics that document deaths by cause and age. An evaluation design that incorporated archival data and pre- and post-data, as well as time series data (see the ONF *Guide to Program Design and Evaluation Planning*, p. 20, for a description of these designs) produced robust data for evaluation.

The Window Guard Law

In 1976, after the success of the Children Can't Fly pilot project had been demonstrated, the New York City Board of Health enacted legislation known as Health Code Section 131.15 (NYCHD, February 1999). The law faced and won a constitutional challenge from a property owner in October 1976. The challenge charged that the legislation shifted the obligation for care and protection of children from parents and placed it on the real estate industry (Spiegel & Lindaman, 1977). The law requires owners of multiple dwellings (buildings of 3 or more apartments) to provide and properly install approved window guards on all windows. This includes first-floor bathroom windows and windows leading onto a balcony or terrace in an apartment where a child (or children) 10 years of age or younger resides. Furthermore, guards must be installed in each hallway window, if any, in such buildings.

Any tenant may ask to have window guards installed (even if a child is not in residence) and no one may be refused, except for where the windows in question are required secondary exits or fire escapes. A one-time fee of $10 per guard may be charged to tenants, but payments may be amortized over as many as 3 years at the choice of the tenant. Tenants who receive public assistance do not have to pay these pass-along fees; instead, they are to submit the bill to the subsidizing agency. An annual reporting system is in place for both tenants and landlords to help ensure that the program is maintained and enforced (NYCHD, Lease Notice to Tenant).

Outcome

The Children Can't Fly pilot program succeeded in producing a reduction in window falls. One hundred and eight falls were reported in the Bronx in 1973; the following year the number declined to 64; in 1975 it had declined again to 54. Due to the voluntary nature of these reports, fatality statistics were also consulted. City wide, deaths from falls from heights over the same 3-year period declined from 57 to 45 and then to 37.

Medicaid costs for inpatient care in NYC in 1977 were $200/day. When compared to a cost of $3 for each window guard purchased by the Department of Health, the cost of saving lives and preventing injuries is clearly a bargain. The costs of after-care have not been included in any financial assessment of the program's success, but it is expected that these costs further support the cost effectiveness of the window guard program. Certainly, the passing of legislation is the hallmark of success for any injury prevention program. The Children Can't Fly program is exemplary in that it addresses education, engineering, and enactment within its program.

Dissemination

The NYCDH provides extensive information to landlords, tenants, and manufacturers through information phone lines, printed information, and a section in its website (http://www.ci.nyc.ny.us/html/doh/html/win/win.html). The available website information includes the following:

• Understanding the Basics – Window Guard Law
• General Information on Window Guards

- Window Guard Policy and Acceptance Board (Manufactures List 1998)
- Window Guard Regulations of the City of NY – Chapter 12
- Rent Information Telephone Numbers
- Education Material
- Window Guards – They Save Lives. They're The Law
- Required Forms

Through the website, all stakeholders are assumed to have access to information relevant to the project, including tenant rights and responsibilities, landlord responsibilities, approved window guards, the process for seeking approval, educational materials about window guards, and consequences for non-compliance.

Tai Chi and Computerized Balance Training for Falls Prevention in Older Adults

Main Key Informant:
Dr Steven L. Wolf

Background

Various falls prevention strategies for older adults have been targeted at diminishing the effects of physical deficits in older adults that contribute to falls, including changes in balance, strength, endurance, flexibility, and reaction time. Computerized balance training and the practice of Tai Chi are 2 interventions that target balance as a means to reduce falls in older adults.

Computerized Balance Training

Initially, the computerized balance training project evolved out of the principal investigator's longstanding interest in the phenomenon of biofeedback, and, specifically, in exploring the use of computerized balance training devices, which were relatively new at the time, as a tool for falls prevention. The device used in this project consisted of a force plate on top of a motorized platform, on which the individual would stand with both feet. Transducers, embedded in the force plate, are sensitive to shifts in weight and are used to gather data on an individual's postural sway. The resolution of changes in a person's centre of mass can then be displayed on a monitor as a cursor. The cursor moves proportionally in accordance to the individual's amount of sway. Training proceeds as the individual attempts to move the cursor to targets placed on the screen. This is achieved by shifting one's weight while standing on the platform. The platform can be moved in linear and angular planes, thus monitoring not only backward, forward, and sideways motions but also heel-to-toe pressures as the participant is moved in a toes up or down direction. Centre of mass displacements can be made more challenging as weight shifts are made with or without simultaneous movement from the supporting motorized platform. Because a streak showing the trajectory of the cursor can be displayed, the difficulty of these procedures can be further increased as they can also be performed with the eyes closed (Wolf, Barnhart, Ellison & Coogler, 1997; Coogler & Wolf, 1999; Wolf, Coogler, Green & Xu, 1993).

In 1990, when the United States National Institute on Aging and the National Institute for Nursing Research put out a request for proposals on novel interventions for ameliorating and understanding frailty and injuries in older adults, a potential opportunity to pursue the use of computerized balance training as a falls prevention strategy presented itself. To determine the details of the final proposal an interdisciplinary team, based primarily out of Emory University, was established. Representatives included experts in rehabilitation medicine, physical therapy, biostatistics, and public health. By chance, one of the team members was a Tai Chi grand master who also had an interest in investigating the use of Tai Chi as a falls prevention strategy.

Tai Chi

Tai Chi is a Chinese martial art that has a history of over 2,000 years. It has been practised as a form of exercise, particularly by older adults, for the past 300 years. Three basic principles are emphasized in Tai Chi (Wolf, Coogler, & Xu, 1997):

• the body should be relaxed and extended;
• the mind alert but calm; and
• the movements well coordinated and fluid.

Adhering to these principles, the practitioner can achieve proper posture and technique and can gain awareness of his or her body parts in space. The forms in Tai Chi are composed of movements that help to ameliorate restrictive changes in gait, posture, and movement patterns typically found in aging adults. These movements emphasize slow, continuous, and often circular movement, straight and extended posture of the head and torso, rotation of the head, trunk and limbs, and the shifting of body weight from one leg to the other. Through the repetition of these forms, flexed posture can be reduced, range of motion can be increased, strengthening of the lower limbs can occur, and balance and body awareness can be learned (Wolf et al., 1997).

Upon further consideration, the two strategies (Computerized Balance Training and Tai Chi) made for striking contrast: Western versus Eastern; modernity versus tradition; high technology versus low technology; expensive versus inexpensive; individual practice versus group practice. The interdisciplinary team seemed to have an opportune occasion to compare 2 diametrically opposing fall prevention techniques. The combination of these two strategies as a fall prevention intervention was named the Atlanta FICSIT trial.

FICSIT

Of the approximately 40 proposals submitted to the National Institute on Aging and the National Institute for Nursing Research, 8 were chosen and were collectively called the Frailty and Injuries: Cooperative Studies on Intervention Techniques (FICSIT) trials. The research teams of the intervention strategies selected worked together to establish a common data set of behavioural, functional, physiological, psychosocial, and environmental variables that affect older individuals. This information was gathered in addition to the data required for the specific variables studied in each particular intervention.

The hypotheses of the Atlanta FICSIT trial were as follows:

- primarily, both computerized balance training and Tai Chi would improve biomedical and psychosocial indicators of well-being;
- the magnitude of improvement in psychosocial indicators of well-being would be greater in the Tai Chi intervention group;
- these improvements would persist through a 4–month follow-up; and
- secondarily, the time to the occurrence of falls would increase (i.e., there would be a delay in the onset of falls).

Resources

Full funding for the Atlanta FICSIT trial was awarded jointly by the National Institute on Aging and the National Institute for Nursing Research. As with all sites included in the FICSIT trials, data for the common data set was collected. Before the start of intervention, all projects were approved and, if necessary, changes were made. However, no changes to the Atlanta FICSIT trial were needed. An external advisory board was in place to oversee the FICSIT trials, review all data and annual reports, and to intervene should problems arise.

Research Design

To be eligible for the Atlanta FICSIT trial, participants were required to be ambulatory, independently living adults over age 70, who were free of progressively debilitating conditions. In total, 200 individuals were recruited for this study. The majority of the participants (N = 128) were recruited through the placement of local advertisements. The remaining 72 participants were intentionally recruited from an independent living centre at Wesley Woods and were comparatively less active and more reclusive because of perceived limitations of their own mobility.

To insure that all candidates met the study criteria, a nurse practitioner screened each individual and confirmed his or her eligibility for the study, by verifying living arrangements, for example. Through a process of computer-generated fixed randomization, participants were then assigned to either the Tai Chi intervention group, the computerized balance training group, or the educational control group. Procedures were in place to promote adherence to the intervention and to determine necessary exclusion. All interventions were 15 weeks in length.

The study commenced in 1990 and concluded in 1994. Participants were assigned, in cohorts of 12, to each of the 2 intervention groups and the control group, and were monitored upon completion of the intervention. Participants from the earliest cohort were thus followed for 17 months in duration, while participants from the last cohort were followed for 4 months. The last cohorts were composed of the residents recruited from Wesley Woods (Wolf, Barnhart, Ellison, & Coogler, 1997).

Computerized Balance Training Intervention Group
Participants assigned to the computer balance training group met once a week for 1 hour. A harness was worn to safeguard against accident

falls, and breaks in training were taken as necessary. Training tasks become progressively more difficult over the 15-week period. While standing with both feet on the platform, participants attempted to move the cursor to the target on the screen while maintaining a stable centre of mass through weight shifts. The difficulty level in maintaining a stable centre of mass was increased through the following means:

- greater displacement of the platform;
- adding both linear and angular platform movements; and
- increasing speed and range of platform motion.

(A more detailed description can be found in Wolf et al., 1993)

Tai Chi Intervention Group
After examining the 108 movement forms of Tai Chi, 10 forms that were easy to learn were selected for the Tai Chi intervention group and modified when necessary to reduce stress for older adults. All forms intended for this older adult population were approved by Emory University School of Medicine's Human Investigations committee prior to the implementation of the intervention. These 10 forms increasingly challenged postural stability by shifting from bilateral to unilateral support, and worked to increased trunk and arm rotation while diminishing the individual's base of support. (Diagrams and instructions of forms, as well as a description of each form's therapeutic elements can be found in Wolf et al., 1997.)

Therapeutic Tai Chi programs for older people should be specifically tailored to their needs. It is of the utmost importance that the instructor be experienced in dealing with older adults. For successful implementation of such a program, special consideration must be given to accommodate issues such as medical problems, movement limitations, and the physical endurance of older individuals.

The participants in the Tai Chi group met twice a week with an experienced instructor, for an hour at a time. Two sessions were conducted instead of one, so that each participant could receive an adequate amount of individual attention to allow forms to be learned properly. However, the total time in contact with the instructor was no greater than in the other groups. In the first session, the forms were introduced. During the remaining weeks, proper technique was emphasized and the forms made progressively more complex. An instruction sheet of each form was given to each participant, and they were encouraged to practise their forms twice a day for 15 minutes.

Control Group
The control group attended weekly hour-long, exercise-free educational sessions. A gerontology nursing specialist led discussions on a variety of predetermined topics, including falls, bereavement, polypharmacy, memory loss, and sleep disturbances.

Implementation

As previously mentioned, a multidisciplinary team was formed and led by the principal investigator. Decisions were made through group discussion and consensus, with final decisions the responsibility of the principal investigator.

The investigators of this study recognized that the participants involved were healthy, and that it is the frail elderly who are most in need of intervention. Recognizing the need to evaluate the effectiveness of these interventions on a more frail and diverse population of elderly persons, the investigators have embarked on another study, with the express purpose of addressing these issues (S.L. Wolf, personal communication, 2000).

Measurements Taken

Baseline characteristics and sway data were collected prior to and immediately after completion of the interventions, and again 4 months after the intervention concluded (Wolf, Barnhart, Kutner, McNeely, Coogler, & Xu, 1996). Measurements were taken under the following 4 measurement conditions:

- standing quietly with eyes open;
- standing quietly with eyes closed;
- standing with toes up and eyes open; and
- standing with toes up and eyes closed.

The Chattecx Balance SystemTM was used to obtain sway data under these 4 different conditions. Although the same device was used in the computerized balance training group, participants in that intervention group did not receive any training on the tasks evaluated at post-intervention. Incidents of falls were continuously recorded for all participants as soon as they were assigned to a group. Various biomedical, functional, and psychosocial measures were also assessed prior to and following the study. Among the biomedical indicators measured were strength, flexibility, cardiovascular endurance, and body composition. Functionality was determined by use of the Lawton and Brody Instrumental Activities of Daily Living (IADL) scale, and psychosocial measures included completion of the Center for Epidemiologic Studies-Depression (CES-D) scale, Tinetti's fear of falling questionnaire, a mastery index, a perceived sleep quality rating, and an intrusiveness rating.

Outcome

Occurrence of Falls

While the computerized balance training intervention group did not exhibit improvements with regard to falls prevention, the Tai Chi intervention group experienced a delayed onset of falls and a 47.5% reduced risk of multiple falls, as compared to the educational control group (Wolf et al., 1996).

Biomedical Indicators

Loss of grip strength was significantly reduced in the Tai Chi intervention group as compared with the computerized balance training group and the educational control group (Wolf et al., 1996). Within the subset of the 72 relatively inactive older adults from the Wesley Woods independent living centre, ANCOVA analysis showed improved balance (as measured by a decrease in postural sway) for participants in the computerized balance training group (Wolf et al., 1996). Unexpectedly, however, those in the Tai Chi group showed an increased postural sway at the post-intervention evaluation. This led the authors to then speculate that postural sway may not be a useful indicator of balance, since the Tai Chi group did show a delayed onset in the occurrence of falls.

Psychosocial Indicators

The most marked changes between the groups, however, were observed in the self-report measures at the 4-month follow-up. Analysis using odds ratios indicated that those in the Tai Chi group were significantly more likely than those in the control group to report a beneficial effect as a result of their intervention strategy (Kutner, Barnhart, Wolf, McNeely, & Xu, 1997). They reported that the intervention had noticeably affected their life, had changed their feeling of confidence, and had positively affected daily and normal physical activities.

While participants in both the computerized balance training and Tai Chi intervention groups reported a significant change in their sense of confidence, this change was attributed to different causes (Kutner et al., 1997). For those in the computerized balance training group, the majority (75%) of individuals cited improved balance as the source of increased confidence; for those in the Tai Chi intervention group, the change was ascribed almost equally to improved balance (54%) and to an enhanced sense of well-being (46%).

Whereas statistical analysis of odd ratios showed individuals in the Tai Chi group to be less afraid of falling immediately following intervention, members of the computerized balance training and educational control groups displayed greater fear than the Tai Chi group after intervention (Wolf et al., 1997). However, all groups returned towards baseline measures at the 4-month follow-up, suggesting that a longer intervention period is necessary to retain enhanced perceptions of well-being. Given that the Tai Chi group showed increased sway but less fear of falling, and that Tai Chi appears to delay the onset of falls, the changes over time in fear-of-falling responses are interesting to note, as they may reflect attitudinal changes towards falls. While the majority (71%) of those in the computerized balance training group gave the same fear response over time, comparatively fewer (44%) individuals from the Tai Chi group did so, suggesting that Tai Chi may be able to change attitudes towards falls. The participants from Wesley Woods in the computerized balance training group also showed no significant changes in the psychosocial variables measured.

In addition to increased confidence and greater sense of well-being, Tai Chi also promotes socialization and is viewed as an enjoyable activity. This may facilitate the incorporation of regular exercise into the lifestyles of older persons. Unexpectedly, 40% of the Tai Chi group continued to meet informally on a weekly basis to practise their forms at the time of the 4-month follow-up, and 30% of the group continued to meet for weekly practice 2 years following the completion of the study (Wolf et al., 1997).

Future Directions

Both of these falls prevention techniques show promise. It appears that computerized balance training can be successfully adapted to falls prevention in older adults, but is restricted to people who have access to these fairly expensive machines. As well, while computerized balance training is conducted while standing on both feet, approximately 90% of falls occur while on one leg. Thus, there is a discrepancy between this training and the development of strategies for falls avoidance. However, computerized balance training can still be a valuable tool if the tasks can be diversified and incorporated into other strategies to improve balance. For example, tasks could test limits of stability to the point of near falls, movements could be made to be more dynamic, and the base of support could be progressively narrowed.

Unlike computerized balance training, Tai Chi is a highly social, low-cost, low-technology approach that can be readily implemented in the community. Through its slow, repetitive movements, Tai Chi has the potential to teach people how to control the relationship between their base of support and their centre of mass. Tai Chi also enables older adults to develop strategies for regaining a stable physical relationship as that relationship is compromised, that is, when their centre of mass approaches or exceeds their base of support.

When the FICSIT trials implementing different balance-, strength-, endurance-, and flexibility-based interventions were completed, and all the data from more than 2,000 participants involved were compiled, balance training strategies proved to be the most effective. And among the various FICSIT interventions targeting balance, Tai Chi was found to have the greatest impact in reducing the incidence of falls (Province et al., 1995).

As suggested, a more intense intervention may yield greater and more long-lasting effects. The participants in this study were of good general health, while those who are frail or in transition towards frailty, and thus most in need of intervention, may not have volunteered for such studies. Addressing the previously mentioned need to investigate the effects of a more intense Tai Chi intervention on a more frail and diverse population, the research group is now in the third year of a 4-year study involving 20 nursing homes and 300 participants. All participants in this study possess a defined diagnosis with immobilizing consequences. To reach this population, which might normally not agree to participate in a study, all participating individuals within particular congregate living facilities were assigned to either the intervention or control group by the process of randomization. Interventions are 48 weeks, with twice weekly sessions of 60 minutes increasing to 90 minutes.

To date, over 60 publications have resulted from the Atlanta FICSIT trials alone, including the primary 1997 outcome paper, "The effect of Tai Chi Quan and computerized balance training on postural stability in older subjects," as found in the journal *Physical Therapy*, and the project has generated coverage on national radio, television, newspapers, and magazines.

Multiple-Risk-Factor Reduction Strategy for Falls Prevention in Older Adults

Main Key Informant:
Dr Dorothy I. Baker

Background

Both intrinsic factors, such as irregular balance and gait, loss of muscle strength, and visual and cognitive impairments, and extrinsic factors, such as environmental hazards, contribute to falls. An incremental increase in fall rates has been reported in subjects with more risk factors (Tinetti, Baker, Garrett, Gottschalk, Koch, & Horwitz, 1993). Given that increased risk for fall-related injuries, as well as fear of falling and poor mobility, is strongly associated with an increased risk of falling (Tinetti et al., 1993), the need for a falls prevention strategy targeted at ameliorating the specific risk factors of each individual older adult is apparent.

Recognizing the prevalence and severity of falls in the older adult population, the National Institute on Aging and the National Institute for Nursing Research put out a request for proposals addressing this problem. The study of the selected intervention strategies was collectively called the Frailty and Injuries: Cooperative Studies on Intervention Techniques (FICSIT) trials. In addition to data collected for the specific variables studied in each particular intervention, the selected intervention teams also worked together to establish a common data set of behavioural, functional, physiological, psychosocial, and environmental variables on which data was also to be gathered.

The principal investigator of this study had been examining the occurrence of falls for a number of years. To address the problem of the global etiology of falls, a multifactorial risk abatement strategy was proposed as a possible FICSIT trial intervention. In this intervention strategy, the risk factors for falling of each of the participating older adults were identified on an individual basis, and the factors then treated. The effect of this multiple-risk-factor intervention in preventing falls was evaluated, and the relationship between changes in the risk factors studied and the occurrence of falls was also determined. To assess the feasibility of implementing this strategy in practice, cost analyses were to be included as well. Upon approval of the project, an interdisciplinary consensus group, including nurses, geriatric physicians, and physical therapists, was formed under the direction of the principal investigator to work out the final details of its implementation.

Resources

Funding for the majority of the project was provided by the National Institute on Aging and the National Institute for Nursing Research. The study commenced in 1990 and was completed in 1993.

Sample Population

Participants of the study were members of the three largest Health Maintenance Organizations (HMO) in the New Haven area. Eligibility for the study required that the participants be 70 years of age or older, be cognitively intact, live in the community, be ambulatory within their own home, expect to be in the New Haven area for the duration of the study, not be especially physically active, not be participating in any other ageing study, not possess any terminal illness, score at least 20 on the Folstein Mini-Mental State Examination, and be at risk for at least 1 of the identified fall risk factors. Risk factors were selected based on interrater reliability and on their feasibility of implementation in a home-based setting. They included the following:

- postural hypotension;
- use of any sedatives;
- use of 4 or more targeted medications;

- unsafe transfer skills (inability to transfer safely to bathtub or toilet);
- foot problems;
- problems of balance or gait; and
- low upper or lower extremity strength, and range of motion impairment.

Since robust individuals do not possess the targeted risk disabilities, and very frail individuals would not have tolerated or safely performed the intervention, individuals of intermediate risk were targeted for this study.

Pilot Trials

Prior to implementation of this strategy pilot trials were conducted to determine an appropriate length for the intervention, and the appropriate number and length of visits, based on clinical practice. A tracking system was used to note any differences in the assessment and implementation protocols used by the clinicians in the pilot study, as well as any recorded changes in the protocols made to allow for individual differences in the pilot study participants. These protocols were then standardized. A procedural manual of the final standardized assessment and intervention protocols was subsequently produced to ensure that the intervention strategy prescribed to participants with the same risk factors was identical.

Experimental Design

A match block design (Tinetti et al., 1993) was employed to prevent potential contamination of results that might have occurred because the physicians were caring for patients in both the control and intervention groups. Sixteen HMO physicians who cared for more than 100 patients aged 70 and over were frequency-matched and divided into low and high subgroups based on 2 characteristics: the average number of new medications prescribed per visit to an older patient, the actual percentage of patients over 70 within the physician's total patient domain. The number of prescription medications was a targeted risk factor, and thus an important criteria on which to insure uniform distribution of participants. The second criteria was felt to be important because physicians primarily treating older patients may approach them differently than physicians who have a wider age range of patients. Frequency-matched quartets (4 physicians each) were created; 2 physicians from each quartet were assigned randomly to the control group and 2 to the intervention group. Thus, group assignment of participants was determined by the group to which their physician had been assigned. In total, 300 participants were involved in this study, 150 in the intervention groups and 150 in the control groups.

Participant Assessment

All eligible participants were assessed by both a nurse practitioner and a physical therapist in their own home (Tinetti et al., 1993; Tinetti, Baker, McAvay, Claus, Garrett, Gottschalk, Koch, Trainor, & Horwitz, 1994). For the initial risk factor assessment by the nurse practitioner, postural blood pressure was obtained, tub and toilet transfers assessed, names and dosages of all prescription and nonprescription medications recorded, and environmental hazards for falling within the home evaluated. Gait, balance, transfer skills, muscle strength, and range of motion of the participant were then assessed by the physical therapist, within the week. Upon ascertaining the number of targeted risk factors for each individual, the required interventions were determined by use of decision rules and priority lists. To avoid overburdening subjects with an excessive number of simultaneous exercise programs, risk factors were prioritized by the consensus group according to likely contribution to falls and immobility. Home-based interventions targeting identified risk factors were carried out by the nurse practitioner and physical therapist and included adjustment of medication, education and training, behavioural instructions, and the assignment of balance and strength exercises which became progressively more difficult. For summary descriptions of the interventions and the required thresholds for their implementation see Tinetti et al. (1993). Illustrated, large-print instructions were provided for recommended exercises, which were to be performed twice daily for 15 to 20 minutes. Recommendations for changes in medication were reviewed with the participant's primary physician, who then made the final decision. Following initial assessment and the determination of the number of visits for potential intervention, the actual group assignment of participants was revealed. Targeted risk factors were then reassessed at a median of 4.5 months.

Intervention Phase

The intervention phase lasted a period of 3 months following baseline assessment, and was followed by a 3-month maintenance phase during which participants were expected to continue with their individualized risk abatement programs. Protocol was in place to deal with illness in participants and to outline methods for promoting compliance to the recommended interventions. Monthly contact was made with participants during the maintenance phase and adherence to the exercise program was reported weekly by each individual to the physical therapist. Cost effectiveness of this targeted risk abatement intervention strategy was also subsequently analysed.

To control for the amount of time and attention received by those in the intervention group, participants in the control group received home visits by social work students, during which a life-review interview was conducted using a standardized series of questions. Individuals in this group were assigned topics to contemplate for each session, and adherence to these assignments was monitored by the social work students. The number of visits was matched to the intervention that participants with comparable risk factors received.

Evaluation

The occurrence of falls was monitored by the use of a 2-year falls calendar, given to the participant at the beginning of the study. Magnets allowed the calendars to be easily attached to the refrigerator, and individuals were asked to record daily whether a fall had occurred or not, and to mail in each month's page at the end of the month. During the monthly follow-up phone calls, participants were asked about fall incidences occurring that month, the resulting injuries, and the circumstances of the falls. Change in mobility was assessed using the Performance Oriented Mobility Assessment, which involves observing position changes, balance manoeuvres, and gait manoeuvres required during daily activities. Change in self-efficacy – an individual's degree of confidence in the ability to perform activities in daily living – was also evaluated, as outlined in the article, "Development of the Common Data Base for the FICSIT Trials" (Buchner et al., 1993). Changes between baseline and reassessment values in targeted risk factors were also tracked. For this purpose, continuous measures of the risk factors for postural blood pressure, balance, and gait were created. Measures were also constructed for risk factors that were either inherently dichotomous (such as sedative-hypnotic use, safe tub and toilet transfers, and the use of 4 or more medications), or had a highly skewed data distribution (such as upper and lower extremity strength and range of motion).

Implementation

An interdisciplinary group, brought together by the principal investigator, collaborated to develop and test the protocol involved in implementing the strategy in a home-based community setting. Meetings were held on a weekly basis to work out details of the project and to discuss problems and provide feedback on concerns and issues that arose in the field (D.I. Baker, personal communication, March, 2000). Protocol was modified to ensure uniform implementation and uniform coding of data; it was also adjusted to the real-life needs, difficulties, and wishes of the older participants. A good monitoring system is required to record all the details involved and to identify problems at an early stage. The clinicians' skills and knowledge of working with older adults facilitated this process. Communication is key to the successful implementation of a project such as this, which involves an interdisciplinary team approach. Communication was especially important in this instance because, as a home-based study, team members were not in the office on a regular basis. Hence, regular meetings were essential. Individual team members must be given opportunity to voice their concerns and problems and to have the support of the team behind them.

The ability of the strategy employed in this study to be individualized to the needs of each particular person meant that it was well received by the older adult population. It allowed an ageing individual to retain a sense of control over his or her life.

Multifactorial interventions are more complicated to study and to implement clinically than single-stranded interventions. Nonetheless, a multifactorial approach to falls prevention most appropriately fits the multifaceted etiology of falls in older adults. While some investigators feel that it is not possible to identify which components of a multifactorial strategy played a contributing role in the observed treatment effect, this study has shown that such identification is not impossible.

In an environment of increasing budget constraints, where clinicians are being asked to make fewer visits and do more in less time, it is important that any intervention be shown to be cost effective. With this particular strategy, instead of having nurses and physical therapists travelling to individual homes, participants can be brought to a centralized site, thus effectively reducing the component incurring the greatest cost, that is, staff time. Fall prevention clinics for the various staff have already been run at a number of senior centres and adult day care centres, and the multi-risk-factor reduction strategy has been successfully implemented in these facilities. As well, less skilled, and consequently less costly, personnel such as physical therapy assistants could be employed to perform intervention protocol.

Outcome

Results indicate that the risk for falls was significantly reduced for those in the intervention group (Tinetti et al., 1994). As shown statistically by log-rank tests, the time until the onset of the first fall was significantly improved for those assigned to the targeted risk abatement strategy during the 1-year follow-up period. The proportion of participants who fell also decreased significantly in the intervention group (35%), compared to the control group (47%). There was also a trend towards less injurious falls and fewer falls requiring medical care. Scores from the Falls Efficacy Scale showed significant increases in self-confidence for individuals in the intervention group. Those in the intervention group also exhibited a reduction in the total number of risk factors possessed at time of reassessment.

Changes that occurred in targeted risk factors between the baseline and reassessment interview were examined using analysis of covariance on continuous measures and the Mantel-Haenszel chi-square test on categorical data. On the measures of postural blood pressure, unsafe transfers, stride length, and the use of 4 or more medications, the intervention group showed statistically significant improvements. Analyses of the effect of a reduction in each of the individual risk factors on the incidence of falling indicate that improved balance, stride length, transfer skills, range of motion, and lower extremity strength were at least marginally associated with fall rate. When participants were divided into tertiles, based on a composite risk factor change score, significantly more of those in the intervention group (42%) than those the control group (22%) where found to be in the tertile with the greatest risk factor reduction. Individuals in the intervention group showed progressively lower fall rates from the least, intermediate, and greatest risk reduction tertiles respectively. Although the same trend was seen in the control group, it was shown to be weaker. These results indicate that the specified intervention strategies directly contributed to a decrease in fall rate (Tinetti, McAvay, & Claus, 1996).

Cost Effectiveness

Efforts were taken to describe the cost effectiveness of implementing a targeted risk factor abatement program. Cost of intervention, including development, equipment, personnel, travel, and overhead costs, was determined for each participant for 1 year following enrolment to the study. For each participant, charge costs for hospitalization and emergency departments, outpatient services, home health care, and skilled nursing facilities were determined. Information from emergency departments, hospital and outpatient databases, and self-report data from follow-up questionnaires were used to uncover fall-related use of hospitalization and emergency departments, outpatient services, and home health care.

The use of a home-based multifactorial falls prevention strategy was indeed shown to be associated with lowered health care costs and both fewer total falls and fewer falls requiring medical care (Rizzo, Baker, McAvay, & Tinetti, 1996). Mean intervention costs per participant amounted to $925, and yielded a savings of $2,000 in mean health care costs. However, if median costs were compared, overall health care costs were approximately $1,100 higher in the intervention group. Participants were also divided into either a high-risk category (possessing 4 or more risk factors), or a low-risk category (possessing fewer than 4 risk factors). Total mean intervention costs in the high-risk category were shown to be substantially lower in the group receiving intervention ($10,537 as compared to $14,232 in the control group). Lowered health costs were attributed primarily to reduced hospitalization costs and, to a lesser extent, to reduced nursing home and home health care costs. This estimation of cost effectiveness is more conservative since the small number of very costly hospitalizations do not influence the figures. For those in the high-risk category, intervention either lowered health care costs and fall incidence, or only modestly raised costs, while substantially reducing fall rate. In the low-risk category, total costs were lower only when means were compared. Overall, each prevented fall cost $2,150 in intervention costs, while the overall cost per fall requiring medical care was $10,709. Given the cost analysis, multiple-risk-factor reduction fall prevention strategies seem to merit consideration, especially for those in the high-risk category.

To promote the use of a multifactorial falls prevention intervention in a clinical setting, demonstration projects have been funded in which the protocol developed in the study is appropriately modified for a particular setting, written in a manual, and then taught to the organization's clinicians. As well, at the time the first FICSIT paper was published, the National Institute on Aging notified the press and the FICSIT trials became publicized on *Good Morning America*. Consequently, the investigators of this project have received numerous telephone calls, interview requests, requests to speak and write articles on falls prevention, and the opportunity to share their protocol and procedure manual.

No Falls! No Fear! Falls Prevention Project
Queensland, Australia

Main Key Informant:
Nancye Peel

Background

Due to current Canadian demographics, there is an increasing necessity for programs to address the needs of older people. One area of particular concern among older people is falls. In Ontario, falls are a serious and common problem for seniors, resulting in high costs both to the individual and to society at large. Many falls, and their subsequent injuries, hospitalizations, and institutionalizations, are preventable.

A fall is defined as "occurring when the person loses their balance causing them to hit the ground or other object at lower level" (Healthy Ageing Research Unit, 1998, p. 12). A fall is not to be confused with either a slip or a trip. A slip is defined as "occurring when the foot slides from underneath the person" (p. 12). A trip "involves a stumble when an object obstructs the pathway" (p. 12). In both cases, balance is regained and the person does not hit the ground.

"Falls among older people are a target for preventive efforts because they are relatively common, carry a significant burden of morbidity and mortality, affect lifestyle choices, are a high cost to the community, and are potentially preventable" (p. 3). However, one type of falls prevention intervention does not necessarily fit all seniors. "Diminishing health status, which often is accompanied by limited mobility and increased medication use, becomes a major contributor to falls of frail seniors"

(Robson et al., 1999, p. 1). "These are not the major risk factors for falls of the healthy or even transitional seniors (between healthy and frailty), many of whose falls occur away from home in the presence of environmental hazards" (p. 1).

No Falls! No Fear! Falls Prevention Program

The No Falls! No Fear! Falls Prevention Program was a 2-year health promotion project in Queensland, Australia, in 1996/97. It focused on healthy, community-dwelling seniors. The program evolved from concerns expressed about older people and falls by both the Queensland Health Promotion Council and the Healthy Ageing Research Unit from an earlier pilot program called 60 and Better. Both organizations realized there were few programs that focused specifically on falls prevention among well, older, community dwellers, and that few programs utilized multicomponent falls prevention interventions. The strategy underlying the No Falls! No Fear! Falls Prevention Program addresses risk factors in the pre-event stage of injury. Risk factors associated with falls among older people include the following:

• decline in physical functioning;
• medication use;
• impairments to the sensory nervous system;
• disorders of the musculo-skeletal system;
• specific chronic diseases;
• environmental hazards;
• social and behavioural factors; and
• a history of falling (p. 5).

"The project goal was to reduce the number of falls, and their resultant injuries, experienced by older community members, by 10 percent after two years, using multi-interventions which targeted major risk factors for falls" (Healthy Ageing Research Unit, 1999, p. 24).

Participants

The target group comprised members of the National Seniors Association, a community group of active Australians aged 50 and over. Ten branches of the National Seniors Association committed to participation in the project. Participation was voluntary, with members indicating their willingness to take part by adding their name and address to a participant list.

There were 252 participants in the study. Information obtained from the baseline questionnaire indicated that the participants ranged in age from 51 to 87 years; 80% were female. Nearly half of the participants lived alone. Approximately 70% were pensioners. Self-rated health was reported as good to excellent in 76% of cases. In the majority of cases, participants owned their own homes.

Resources

Collaborators

The No Falls! No Fear! Falls Prevention Program was the result of a joint effort by the Healthy Ageing Unit, Department of Social and Preventive Medicine at the University of Queensland; the Queensland Health Promotion Council; and the National Seniors Association. The Department of Public Works and Housing and the Department of Occupational Therapy and Physiotherapy also provided services throughout the duration of the program.

The Healthy Ageing Unit played the leading role in the implementation of the program. Two committees were set up for the duration of the program: the Representatives' Committee and the Professional Advisory Committee. The Representatives' Committee consisted of participants nominated from each branch of the National Seniors Association. They met twice a year over the duration of the project to discuss planning, implementation, progress, and results. They also reported project details to their branch meetings and brought to the attention of the research team any issues raised by members concerning the project (Healthy Ageing Unit, 1998). Members of the Professional Advisory Committee were government, university, and health practitioner representatives who had interests and expertise in the health of the older community. This committee met 3 times over the duration of the project to discuss and advise on the conduct of the project (Healthy Ageing Unit, 1998).

The No Falls! No Fear! Falls Prevention Program utilized existing resources within the community (information services, exercise classes, home modifications, and medical assessments). Service providers recognized a need for a falls prevention program, and thus were cooperative and eager to become involved with this program.

TABLE 1.   No Falls! No Fear! Falls Prevention Program Budget, 1996/1997

Item	Year 1 (1996)	Year 2 (1997)
Staffing	$104,613 AU	$95,548 AU
Specific Costs	$7,328 AU	$3,328 AU
Administration Costs	$3,900 AU	$3,900 AU
Total	$115,841 AU	$102,776 AU

Funding

The Healthy Ageing Unit received funding from the Queensland Health Promotion Council to cover the costs of the program for 2 years. Staffing costs included salary for medical assessors, tradespeople, a home assessor, an exercise trainer, a research assistant, a project coordinator, and a project manager. Specific costs included travel expenses, video purchase, and staff development through seminar and workshops. Administration costs included telephone calls, postage, printing, and stationery. Table 1 provides cost details.

There were enough funds to cover the scope of the program. If more funds had been made available, however, the program could have been extended to include more people and to provide more exercise classes.

Implementation

Interview Strategies

"Four groups with approximately equal numbers of participants were formed by combining two or three National Seniors branches, and the groups were randomly allocated to receive the four interventions" (Steinberg, Cartwright, Peel, & Williams, 2000, p. 228). The intervention strategies consisted of the following:

- An information presentation, diary monitoring, and telephone follow-up of events designed to educate and inform the targeted community concerning falls prevention.
- An exercise program and access to a gentle exercise video, to encourage participation in exercise to improve strength, balance, and gait.

- A home assessment with recommendations for, and assistance with, any modifications of home hazards that may contribute to a fall.
- A medical examination to assess and advise on clinical factors that may predispose an individual to falling (Healthy Ageing Research Unit, 1998, p. 11).

An add-on approach was employed such that Group 1 (the control) used the first intervention strategy (A) only, Group 2 (A+B), Group 3 (A+B+C), and Group 4 (A+B+C+D). A member from each group drew a code to determine the intervention program for the group.

Each group used intervention strategy A. "Staff from the research team attended meetings of all participant branches as guest speakers, to present information concerning falls in the older community and discuss prevention strategies" (p. 12). During these presentations each participant was supplied with a calendar with tear-off months. Starting in April 1996, subjects were asked to record daily any slip, trip, or fall that occurred. For each day of the month, the calendar was marked with a tick if no incident occurred, or an S (for slip), T (for trip), or F (for fall). Details of the incident, including date, time, place, and circumstances, were recorded by the subject on the back of the monthly sheet. At the end of the month, the record was posted back to the Research Unit. If any incident was recorded, the subject was telephoned to confirm details, using a standard interview format. Details of the slips, trips, and falls were collected monthly for participants from April 1996 to August 1997 (p. 12).

Group 2 was offered, in addition, a 1-hour exercise class once a month, with the use of exercise handouts and a gentle exercise video encouraged between classes. In addition to the presentation and the exercise classes, Group 3 was offered a home safety assessment with financial and practical assistance to make home modifications. For Group 4, participants were offered a clinical assessment and advice on medical risk factors for falls, as well as the other 3 components (Steinberg et al., 2000, p. 228).

Effective Practices

The successful implementation of the No Falls! No Fear! Falls Prevention Program hinged upon the availability of community resources. The program did not use any new interventions but instead brought together existing resources (information, exercise classes, home modifications, medical assessments) and offered them as a package.

The multistrand interventions were the most effective in reducing the risk of slips, trips, and falls from occurring. It was the combination of all 4 interventions that made the program effective.

One thing that could have markedly enhanced the implementation and outcome of the program was funding. Additional finances could have been used to expand both the availability and the depth of the intervention. For example, if there had been more funding, the exercise program could have been more rigorous (N. Peel, personal communication, April 9, 2000).

Actors in Decision Making and Planning

The Representatives' Committee and the Advisory Committee were involved in the decision making and planning for the duration of the program. The 2 committees met to discuss the progress of the program. Any problems that participants encountered were reported to their representatives who, in turn, reported them to the Advisory Committee. As a result, there was constant feedback from the Representatives' Committee to the Advisory Committee. In addition, the researchers had ongoing interaction with participants throughout the program, contacting them by telephone regarding their monthly calendar recordings.

Outcome

"The program aimed to raise awareness of causative mechanisms and modify intrinsic and extrinsic factors that contribute to risk of falling" (p. 20). The evaluation design used retrospective data, pre- and posttest data, comparison and control group data (see the ONF *Guide to Program Design and Evaluation Planning*, p. 20, for a description of these designs). All participants in the program completed a baseline questionnaire. "Changes to behaviour and modification of risk factors were assessed from reports at monthly telephone interviews and by a follow up questionnaire at 12 months after commencement of the program" (Healthy Ageing Research Unit, 1998, p. 20). The results of the evaluation are as follows:

1 Awareness raising

Participants reported that having to fill in the calendar each day and record how incidents occurred made them more aware of factors contributing to the slip, trip, or fall. Fifty-one participants reported an increased awareness and knowledge of falls risk factors and prevention measures (p. 20).

2 Modification of behaviour

Participants reported altering activities of daily living over the 12-month duration of the program. "Fifty-six percent reported being more aware of falls prevention measures, 61 percent reported taking more care in particular circumstances, 16 percent reported avoiding specific activities, and 23 percent reported doing particular activities differently" (p. 21).

3 Modification of intrinsic risk factors

Fear of falling. The program improved confidence in participants. At the start of the program 58% of the participants expressed concern about the possibility of having a fall. At 12 months' follow-up, 41% expressed such concern. Similarly, at the beginning of the program, 25% reported that they restricted their activities either inside or outside the home due to their concern about falling. At 12 months, 17% reported restricted activity as a result of fear of falling (p. 21).

Physical activity. The percentage of participants undertaking daily exercise increased from 31% to 33%. The percentage of participants reporting no physical activity decreased from 18% to 12% (p. 22).

Medical conditions and medication. Participants reported taking action to decrease the risk of falls. Action included medication alterations, visiting the doctor, maintaining fitness and a good diet to control diabetes, using a walking stick for balance, and going to a podiatrist regarding foot problems (p. 22).

4 Modification of extrinsic risk factors

At 12 months' follow-up, participants reported making the following changes to the home environment during the program as a measure to prevent falls:

- 20% of participants installed grabrails in the bathroom/toilet;

- 7% installed handrails on stairs;
- 4% painted the edges of steps;
- 25% removed hazards such as loose mats, cords;
- 12% improved the lighting; and
- 6% made other modifications.

Both quantitative data (information gathered from the daily calendars) and qualitative data (information gathered from interviews with participants) were used in the evaluation. The multistrand interventions were effective in reducing the risks of slips, trips, and falls, far surpassing the program goal of a 10% reduction: "The results show statistically significant reductions in the risk of slips and trips in groups 2, 3 and 4 compared to group 1 (the control), with evidence also for reduction in the risk of falling" (p. 30). "The hazard ratios comparing the combined intervention groups with the control indicated a 58 percent reduction in the risk of slips, a 64 percent reduction in the risk of trips, and a 30 percent reduction in the risk of falls" (p. 30).

"Except for trips, there was no evidence to support the hypothesis that reductions in risk declined with increase in the number of intervention strategies employed" (p. 30), indicating that reductions were not in proportion to the number of strategies employed. "However, intervention group 4 (with all four components) showed the highest protective effect against slips, trips, and falls ..." (p. 30).

Both the quantitative and qualitative data also suggested that the program was effective in reducing incidence rates in the control group (p. 30).

All parties were satisfied with the program. Participants expressed high levels of satisfaction and enjoyment of the program, together with improved health and well-being. Over 80% of the group indicated that they wished to continue in the program beyond the 2-year funding period (p. 31). As well, coordinators of the program were pleased with the results.

Dissemination of Information

Information regarding the No Falls! No Fear! Falls Prevention Program was disseminated to participants of the program, members of the community, and to health care providers and health professionals. Participants in the program were kept up to date with progress reports at quarterly meetings. At the end of the program, each participant received an individual report. As well, a copy of an article published in the *Health Promotion Journal of Australia* was sent to each of the 10 participating branches of the National Seniors Association.

Members of the research team have addressed falls prevention meetings of older people's groups throughout the community. In addition, they have given presentations and participated in falls prevention workshops and seminars in which health care providers and health professionals form the target audience. The results of their program are also available on database programs so that people can contact them for information about their program.

The multistrand intervention approach, involving the combination of behavioural and environmental strategies, as well as the utilization and integration of existing community resources made the No Falls! No Fear! Falls Prevention Program a success. Members of the research team are currently looking for ways to integrate the No Falls! No Fear! Falls Prevention Program into the 60 and Better program or into other, similar programs which already exist for seniors.

Comprehensive Community-Based Prevention Strategies

The involvement of entire communities in injury prevention programs has been rare, as personal injuries have only recently come to be seen as a public health problem. The community itself is increasingly conceptualized as an actor in theoretical models of injury prevention. The health care community also now occupies a greater role in injury prevention, and a sophisticated interdisciplinary science of injury control and safety promotion has developed. Indeed, the World Health Organization initiated and supports the Organization of Networks for Community Programs.

In most industrialized countries, unintentional injury is the chief cause of death and a leading cause of disability among young people. In Canada, it is the 5–24 age group that is most at risk for brain and spinal cord injury (SMARTRISK, 1998). Although there have been dramatic reductions in injury-associated mortality rates over the past 100 years, much remains to be done. The profiles in this section represent the breadth and depth of the commitment to community-based injury prevention in North America and around the world.

Inner city communities present unique challenges to the control of unintentional injury. The success of the Harlem Hospital Injury Prevention Program in reducing the incidence of serious injury among children living in Harlem speaks to the value of employing a comprehensive community-based approach. The Think First Foundation serves an international network of local community chapters dedicated to the prevention of brain and spinal cord injury in young people. Beyond its school curriculum format, the program aims to increase community awareness and to encourage the development of healthy public policy. The Latrobe Valley Better Health Project targets home, playground, and sports injuries and alcohol misuse among youth. Based upon a successful Swedish model implemented during the 1980s, its primary aim is to utilize a community intervention approach to prevent injuries, reduce hazards, and increase public awareness of injury prevention

The final profile in this section is Risk Watch, a promising injury prevention program that brings together teachers and members of the broader community to educate children about risks to their well-being. The model was designed to allow for community input and local control over the curriculum. Participating communities have reported a high sense of ownership of and responsibility for the project.

Best Practices

- Harlem Hospital Injury Prevention Program: Safe Kids / Healthy Neigbourhoods
- Think First Foundation
- Latrobe Safe Communities: Latrobe Valley Better Health Project

Promising Practices

- Risk Watch

BEST PRACTICES

Harlem Hospital Injury Prevention Program: Safe Kids/Healthy Neighbourhoods

Main Key Informant:
Erik Cliette

Background

Preventing unintentional injuries to children is an important concern for communities, and one which presents unique challenges in inner city neighbourhoods. The Harlem Hospital Injury Prevention Program (HHIPP) is an example of an effective community-based effort, and one which is distinguished from similar efforts by its examination of injury rates as the chief evaluative measure. The HHIPP was launched in 1988 in response to several concerns:

- Injury is the leading cause of hospital admissions, morbidity, and mortality among children in the United States.
- These rates were found to be considerably higher among Harlem children than the national average or the rates for the rest of New York City.
- Response to the problem of child injury from communities and trauma centres was identified as inadequate.

While neurotrauma is not the exclusive concern of the HHIPP, this intervention warrants consideration by parties specifically targeting brain and spinal cord injuries. Data analysis used to measure the success of the program has found a substantial and statistically significant decrease in the rate of motor vehicle–related trauma since its inception, and this injury scenario is the leading cause of neurotrauma in many jurisdictions, including Canada (SMARTRISK, 1998a).

The program was initiated in 1988 by Dr Barbara Barlow, Director of Pediatric Surgical Services at Harlem Hospital. For more than 2 decades Dr Barlow had been acutely concerned with the need for trauma centres and hospitals to become leaders in the area of preventing, rather than simply treating, injury to children. Originally designed as a

4-year program, the intervention had the following goals:

- The reduction of childhood injuries through the provision of safety education, safe playing areas, and extracurricular activities.
- Reductions of health care and related costs.
- The development of new skills and self-esteem in children and adolescents.
- Fostering a sense of well-being in the community.
- The provision of safety equipment (bicycle helmets) at substantially reduced cost to residents of an economically disadvantaged community.

These objectives reflect a fundamental operating philosophy: if children are provided with enjoyable, safe, supervised activities, appropriate places to engage in them, and basic safety education, the emotional and societal tolls exacted by child injury can be substantially reduced. Moreover, it is believed that broadening these children's horizons through meaningful associations in organized activities such as art, dance, and sport will enable them to make a more positive investment in themselves and their world in general.

Since 1994, this initial project, based out of the Harlem Hospital and Columbia University in New York City, has been replicated in numerous U.S. urban centres. In addition to overseeing ongoing local initiatives the Harlem site now functions as the national office, developing and coordinating the replicate programs by serving as a model and by furnishing financial and technical assistance. Both of these functions are relevant to the overall impact of the project. Consideration of the success of the program should therefore take notice of its value as a template to which neurotrauma prevention interests can refer in other communities, as well as its outcomes in Harlem.

Consumers

The initiative has targeted children aged 6 to 16 residing in central Harlem, the upper Manhattan neighbourhood serviced by the Harlem Hospital. This community is predominantly Black and substantially less well off financially than the national or municipal average (Davidson et al., 1994a). Davidson et al. also report that the leading causes of unintentional injury among this population are falls and motor vehicle crashes. Injuries resulting from falls and car collisions are of particular concern to neurotrauma prevention interests. Recent data from the Harlem Hospital, for example, indicates that head trauma may occur in more than 42% of childhood injuries involving a motor vehicle (Durkin, Laraque, Lubman and Barlow, 1999). Replicate programs have been instituted in urban areas in which there exists an opportunity to address the needs of a similar population: a concentration of socio-economically disadvantaged children and adolescents, disproportionately at risk for injury.

History and Development

An important inspiration for the HHIPP was the success of New York City's 1976 window guard legislation, which resulted in a 96% decrease in window falls in Harlem. That initiative demonstrated the value of hospital and community members working in concert to bring about positive change. A grant obtained from the Robert Wood Johnson Foundation in 1988 followed 5 years of applications for funding for a hospital-based injury prevention program in Harlem. Initial funding from the RWJF consisted of two 2-year ad hoc grants, totalling $533,657 (US). These grants supported program development and were used to initiate activities to secure further funding from other sources. Central activities consisted of:

- Launching educational programs in violence prevention, and in motor vehicle, bicycle, street, and firearm safety.
- Providing extracurricular programs in art, dance, cycling, and Little League baseball and soccer.
- Initiating community-based coalitions with the goal of transforming numerous public spaces (e.g., parks and playgrounds) into safe play areas for children in Harlem.

Strategy

Notably, this program incorporates primary, or pre-event, injury reduction by emphasizing the prevention of injury scenarios. Also, it combines behavioural modifications such as safety education with an environmental strategy, through the transformation of the places and activities in which the target group would be at risk for injury.

Over its course, the program's success was evaluated using injury surveillance data from the Harlem Hospital. During the 5-year period

1988–1992 child injury admissions to the Harlem Hospital decreased by 41%, as compared to the baseline years 1983 through 1988 (RWJF, 1999, p. 7). These results have led to grant extensions from the RWJF for 2 additional endeavours:

1 Replication, beginning in 1994, of the HHIPP in the form of hospital-based injury prevention programs in 5 other cities with dispropor-tionately high rates of child injury: Pittsburgh, Chicago, Kansas City, Atlanta, and Torrance (California). Following these first 5 instances, programs supported through funding and/or technical assistance have been started in St Louis, Philadelphia, and Dallas. Additionally, technical assistance is being provided for the estab-lishment of replicate programs at Johns Hopkins Medical Center, the University of Miami, and the Babies' Hospital at the Columbia Presbyterian Medical Center.
2 The establishment and development of a nationally trade-marked network, mentioned briefly above, for the provision of technical assistance in paediatric injury prevention. Originally called Dis-semination of a Model Injury Prevention Program for Children and Adolescents, the network has since been renamed the Injury Free Coalition for Kids, and works with expansion sites to secure and develop their programs. Information about the coalition is available online at http://www.injuryfree.org. The National Program Office is housed at Columbia University, Harlem Hospital Center, New York, New York.

Stakeholders/Collaborators

In addition to the Harlem Hospital, the RWJF, and Columbia Univer-sity, numerous individuals and organizations have an interest in the HHIPP. The program associate director indicates that, as the Harlem Hospital is the caretaker for central Harlem, the HHIPP identifies the community at large as its most important stakeholders (personal com-munication, May 3, 2000). This group includes children and their par-ents as consumers of health care and injury prevention (health insurance concerns were also an issue, as in 1989 more than 60% of families in the targeted area received Medicaid), schools and educators, state and city health departments, and the New York City Department of Transporta-tion (Davidson et al., 1994b; Laraque, Barlow, Davidson, & Heagarty,

1994). Manhattan Borough Presidents and the New York City Parks Department and Board of Education are further examples of involvement of government offices. Finally, organizations dedicated to improving the quality of life of Harlem children have been important participants. The HHIPP has collaborated with 26 of these, notable among which are:

- Little League
- Soccer League
- One Hundred Black Men
- Black United Fund
- Boy Scouts of America
- Mothers Against Violence
- Project Oasis at the Central Board of Education
- Doing Art Together – Metropolitan Museum of Modern Art

Resources

The Robert Wood Johnson Foundation has provided major continuing funding for HHIPP. Significant additional funding for the Harlem effort has come from New York State and City government departments, Columbia University, and philanthropic corporate and individual donations (RWJF, 1999). These have accounted for more than $1 million in additional financial resources. Some of this funding is used for the establishment and support of replicate programs throughout the United States. For these more recent sites the availability of technical support and guidelines are also important resources, as the sites benefit from the experience of the 1988–1992 pilot program.

Injury Surveillance

Aside from funding, perhaps the single most important asset of the initiative, and a prerequisite for approval of additional sites, is the existence of a hospital-based injury surveillance system. This measure allows for the collection of data pertaining to changes in injury rates among the targeted population, and thus makes outcome evaluation possible. Statistical evaluation is relatively rare among community interventions and is an outstanding aspect of the HHIPP.

The Harlem initiative has relied upon the Northern Manhattan Injury Surveillance System (NMISS), which has monitored patterns in serious paediatric injury since 1983 (Davidson et al., 1994b). Moreover, this system was also implemented at the hospital that serves Washington Heights, a neighbouring community. Therefore, it was possible to examine pre-intervention and post-intervention data for both a control and a target community. The New York State Uniform Hospital Discharge Data (UHDD) and medical examiner data are used to develop population-based rates which increase the statistical validity of conclusions drawn from this evaluation.

Implementation

The commitment and skills of the individuals working to design and deliver the program are an important means of additional support. While the clear emphasis is upon injury prevention, the program associate director indicates that some of the staff at the Harlem site have university or graduate degrees in such areas as medicine, epidemiology, business administration, education, fine arts, early childhood education, and nursing (personal communication, May 3, 2000). Experience in mentoring, community development, and urban ecology is also evident in the literature reviewed. These various fields of expertise were beneficial resources for the original program and are also important for expansion sites. In both the original and the newer sites implementation can be understood as having 4 principal components:

1 Securing population-based injury data to raise awareness of the problem of child injury and to assess the effectiveness of programs.
2 Establishing coalitions of hospital, community, and government to pool resources. This is accomplished through:

- the identification of interested groups;
- participant agreement as to the process;
- acknowledgement of local perspectives;
- seeking community guidance with regard to practices;
- flexibility to variable circumstances; and
- acknowledgement of all contributions.

3 Creating safe activities and places to play and providing safety education for children and families.
4 Obtaining funding from local sources to augment and eventually replace the financial support of RWJF (RWJF, 1999).

HHIPP injury prevention activities can be understood as either environmental or educational. Environmental strategies include:

- the Playground Injury Prevention Program;
- the Unity through Murals Project;
- the Greening of Harlem Program;
- the Harlem Horizon Art Studio;
- the Harlem Hospital Dance Clinic;
- Harlem Little League Baseball;
- the Winter Clinic;
- the Harlem Soccer League; and
- Children Can't Fly.

Educational programs, which attempt to reduce injury through behavioural change, include:

- the Harlem Safety Program/Urban Youth Bike Corps;
- Harlem Safety City;
- the Harlem Alternative to Violence Program-Gunshot Wounds;
- Critical Incident Stress Management Teams;
- the Kids, Injuries and Street Smarts Program (KISS);
- First Ride, Safe Ride;
- the Youth Action Team; and
- Children Can't Fly (this program has both environmental and educational aspects).

Effective Practices

The major, and certainly understandable, concern of many parents in the early stages of implementation was that they be able to feel at ease leaving their children with program representatives (E. Cliette, personal communication, May 3, 2000). One significant measure taken to build this critical trust early on involved drawing many such representatives from the community; they are thus known, or known of, to parents. The program associate director, for example, was born and raised in Central Harlem; he comments that people are reassured by the fact that they know him and his family. The practice of involving local people clarifies the program's commitment to the community and therefore makes greater and repeated participation probable.

It might also be argued that the incorporation of evaluation represents a highly effective practice, because of the confidence in the program evaluation allows. Access to systematic injury data greatly benefits an intervention. It should also be noted here that the flexible but structured blueprint the HHIPP supplies has facilitated programs in numerous sites.

A final nod should be given to the Playground Injury Prevention Program, a project that directs energy to building safe urban play areas. This initiative offers a positive impact for all Harlem children. It also clearly illustrates an environmental strategy, and these have been shown to be generally more effective than education alone. Caution is warranted, however, as the implementation of new outdoor activities may in some cases have increased risk of exposure to hazards (Davidson et al., 1994a). This issue has not been directly investigated, and such investigation would be to the benefit of the intervention.

Outcome

HHIPP defines success in terms of its primary goal of reducing the incidence of serious injury in Central Harlem children. Measurement is accomplished through comparison of injury data in a target and a control community.

• a 14% drop overall, the first decrease since 1975, in child injury admissions after 1 year of intervention;
• a 23% decrease in motor vehicle trauma after 2 years;
• a 41% decrease in injuries among the targeted age group (6–16) after 5 years; and
• steady results, as, after 9 years, injuries to the targeted ages had fallen 55%, compared to 20% for all of New York City.

Proving a direct link between an intervention of this sort and outcomes is exceedingly difficult; however, there is cause for encouragement in this case. While the targeted age group showed a 41% decline in hospital admissions after 5 years, there was no decrease in nontargeted age groups and/or injury types. Additionally, Washington Heights, the control community, showed no decline in relevant injury rates between 1988 and 1995 (RWJF, 1999). The strong suggestion here is that where efforts were directed they had a positive impact (Davidson et al., 1994a).

One disappointing exception is seen in the case of falls. There was no significant change in the incidence of admissions resulting from injuries incurred in this way. While no specific effort was made to focus upon injuries incurred by falls, this is a major concern for neurotrauma and other injury prevention interests. Nonetheless, there is reason for confidence in the positive results reported and, so, cause for optimism. Also, a cost-benefit study reported that "for every dollar ($U.S.) invested in the Harlem Hospital Injury Prevention Program, $4 were saved in acute hospital costs and $85 in lifetime health care costs" (cited in RWJF, 1999). Financial savings pale, however, in comparison to the emotional trauma that stands to be averted through these expenditures.

Replication

The original HHIPP has been reproduced or is planned in 13 additional sites. Full discussion of results in these locations is available online at http://www.rwjf.org/health/013396.htm

Dissemination

Dissemination has occurred through peer-reviewed publications; national and local print, radio, and television media; and lectures by program staff. Additionally, the Injury Free Coalition for Kids website (http://www.injuryfree.org) distributes further information and contains web pages on each program.

Think First Foundation: A National Brain and Spinal Cord Injury Prevention Program

Main Key Informants:
Deborah Johnson and Eleanor Sam

Background

Traumatic brain injuries are the leading cause of death and disability among Canadian youth (Think First Foundation of Canada, 1999). Annual data from Statistics Canada indicates that young people between the ages of 5 and 24 years are most at risk for brain and spinal cord injuries (Think First Foundation, n.d.-a), with young males aged 15 to 25 at highest risk for brain and spinal cord injuries (Black, 1998). According to the president of the Think First Foundation of Canada, 37,000 new spinal and brain injuries are incurred each year across the nation (Black, 1998). The Rick Hansen Institute estimates the direct costs of these new injuries, along with the long-term costs of existing ones, at approximately 15 billion dollars a year (Black, 1998). The emotional costs of such injuries are immeasurable.

Think First Foundation

Many neurotrauma-producing events can be prevented through the education of individuals, community leaders, and policy makers (Sharman & Cusimano, 2000; Think First Foundation, n.d.-b) and by increasing community awareness and policy initiatives (Think First Foundation, n.d.-a). The Think First Foundation is a voluntary non-profit organization established to prevent brain and spinal cord injuries in youth. Think First employs 4 strategies to prevent neurotrauma injuries:

1 school-based education;
2 reinforcement activities;
3 general public education; and
4 healthy public policy.

Think First currently delivers 2 comprehensive injury prevention educational programs in school classroom or assembly formats: Think First for Kids, designed to influence behaviour early in a child's life, and Think First for Teens, a reinforcement program (Think First Foundation, n.d.-b).

The goal of the Think First programs is to prevent injury among young people by teaching them to use their minds to protect their bodies by thinking before acting (Think First Foundation, n.d.-a). The Think First programs are designed to address and prevent the leading causes of brain and spinal cord injuries in youth at the primary level of prevention.

Think First for Teens

Originally, the Think First program was only available for junior high and high school students as the Think First for Teens (TFFT) program. TFFT is a prevention presentation delivered in secondary schools. The program employs a health professional and an injury survivor to teach students about brain and spinal cord anatomy, mechanisms of injury, and prevention strategies. However, according to the program coordinator of the Think First Foundation in the United States, teenagers have deeply established habits that are difficult to change. Indeed, initial evaluations of this targeted program confirmed that changes in the measures of teenagers' attitudes towards safety or behavioural intentions were minimal. For this reason, the Think First For Kids program was introduced to enable younger students to develop good safety habits that would be reinforced by the TFFT program (D. Johnson, personal communication, April, 2000).

Think First for Kids

Originally designed by a curriculum specialist, the Think First for Kids (TFFK) program is based on the Oklahoma Elementary School Safety Education Program. TFFK is a comprehensive primary school program for children aged 6 to 8. This 6-week modular curriculum for grades 1–3 covers 6 important safety and injury prevention areas:

1 basic brain and spinal cord anatomy;
2 vehicular safety;
3 bicycle safety;
4 playground safety;
5 violence and conflict resolution; and
6 water safety.

Theoretical Foundations

Applied learning and behavioural research shows that exposure to similar messages repeated over time enhances learning and behavioural changes, which are more easily assimilated in childhood (D. Johnson, personal communication, April, 2000). In order to affect the greatest amount of change, this curriculum-based program utilizes modern concepts in cognition, development, and behaviour. The TFFK program's aim is to increase children's knowledge of injury mechanisms and their capacity for risk perception, through delivery of the program to children at their formative stage of development (Sharman & Cusimano, 2000).

History and Development of the Think First Foundation

The history of the foundation can be traced back to 1979, with the establishment of a spinal cord injury prevention program for high school students at West Florida, followed by a similar program in Columbia, Missouri, in the following year (Think First Foundation, 1999). Two neurosurgeons, one from each program, worked together to establish the national program in 1986. This program was originally called the National Head and Spinal Cord Injury Prevention Program; the name Think First was adopted as the program's new identity in May 1990 (Think First Foundation, 1999). The Think First for Kids curriculum was introduced across the United States in 1996 and in 1998 Think First underwent restructuring to promote implementation of programs and to facilitate the communication network among chapters, satellites, and advocates (D. Johnson, personal communication, April, 2000).

Presently headquartered in Rolling Meadows, Illinois, the Think First Foundation serves a national and international network of chapters and the public by developing and distributing educational materials, by providing training to program coordinators, and by offering ongoing technical support to chapter programs (D. Johnson, personal communication, April, 2000). The Think First program was brought to Canada by the Canadian Neurosurgical Society in 1992 (Think First Foundation, n.d.-b).

Resources

Think First for Teens: Program Components

Teens and young adults are at highest risk for brain and spinal cord injuries. The most frequent causes of these injuries are motor vehicle crashes, falls, sports, and recreation. The TFFT program consists of a multimedia presentation delivered, at no charge, to students in grades 7 through 12/13, in either a classroom or an assembly format. This presentation, which is designed to encourage careful risk taking, utilizes school-based education and reinforcement activities as the primary strategies to prevent neurotrauma (Think First Foundation, 1999).

School-Based Education

School-based education involves presentations that help define personal vulnerability and consequences of risk-taking behaviour. This educational portion consists of 4 segments (Think First Foundation, n.d.-b):

1 short films, which clarify the difference between exciting and dangerous behaviours and provide testimony from teens with brain and spinal cord injuries;
2 a discussion of anatomy of the brain and spinal cord, how injuries to these parts of the body occur, and how many of these injuries can be prevented;
3 a young person who has sustained a brain or spinal cord injury describes how life has changed; and
4 a discussion on proper bystander behaviour at the scene of an injury.

The final portion of the educational program is an optional wheelchair obstacle course. Volunteer students in wheelchairs negotiate a constructed obstacle course before the audience. The purpose of this is to raise awareness of the problems confronted by people in wheelchairs in everyday life (Think First Foundation, 1999).

Reinforcement Activities

Suggestions for follow-up activities that reinforce the basic educational program by providing options for continuous prevention education and practice within the school environment include: school and community billboards, health fairs, bike rodeos, alcohol-free graduation events, and essay and poster contests on skills in appropriate bystander behaviour.

In Canada, a new peer-to-peer approach strategy to reinforce the TFFT program has been proposed by the National Office: Making Connections: A Neurotrauma Prevention Appreciation Workshop. This pilot project will be implemented in 16 high schools in partnership with the Toronto Western Hospital and the Kingston General Hospital. Along with injury prevention, the primary objective of the program is to attract the brightest students to the field of neurotrauma research. Specific program components of Making Connections include:

• a Think First for Teens presentation;
• a neuroscience specific audiovisual presentation;
• a visit to a nearby specific intensive care unit;

- a visit to a neuroscience research laboratory;
- a visit to observe part of a surgical procedure on a brain or spinal cord injury (optional); and
- reporting on the experience to the class for peer-to-peer teaching.

Students participating in the pilot project will be selected by their teachers. Students who complete the program become ambassadors for it and present its content to their classmates.

Think First for Kids: Program Components

Included in this program are the following components (Think First Foundation, 1999):

- a curriculum manual with background material, lessons, and exercises;
- an animated safety video starring Street Smart, the safety hero;
- Street Smart comic strips that coincide with each of the curriculum units;
- classroom posters; and
- training and consultation with Think First staff.

Curriculum

The Think First for Kids curriculum is based on learning and behavioural theories that indicate that repeated, spaced messages enhance learning. The curriculum was written to meet learner competencies and some specific national student testing objectives for contact areas, such as language, math, and science (D. Johnson, personal communication, May, 2000). This original program was piloted in 1 or more classes in 22 schools, urban and rural, throughout the United States. Minor text revisions were made to enhance the curriculum, as a result of feedback. Through teacher evaluations and student tests, it was determined that the majority of students who complete the program will increase their knowledge of traumatic brain and spinal cord injury prevention and their use of good safety habits (D. Johnson, personal communication, April, 2000). Similarly, in Canada, pilot testing of the curriculum in 50 classrooms indicates that the TFFK program results in significant increases in knowledge pertaining to safe practices (A. Sharman, personal communication, May, 2000). Through curricular mapping studies, the Think First for Kids program was found to cover all of the mandatory elements that pertain to personal safety required by Ontario's new Health and Physical Education (HPE) Curriculum. Lessons also overlap other curriculum subject areas mandated in the new curriculum (Sharman & Cusimano, 2000).

Curriculum Manual

The curriculum manual includes 3 curricula (1 for each grade level). Each curriculum has 6 lessons: an introductory lesson introducing brain and spinal cord injury, and 5 lessons on key areas of injury prevention. Each lesson addresses the involved risks and the safety behaviours that help prevent injury, and each includes background information, lesson objectives, a lesson outline, a letter to parents, and suggested follow-up activities and resources. An outline of the key features of the introductory lesson and the safety and prevention lesson areas is provided below (Think First Foundation, 1999).

Lesson Areas

1 Introduction to the prevention of brain and spinal cord injury

- importance of brain and spinal cord
- use of safety habits to prevent brain and spinal cord injury

2 Vehicle safety

- safety belts
- vehicle safety habits

3 Bicycle safety

- bicycle helmets protect the brain
- bicycles are vehicles
- bicyclists ride safely and obey traffic rules

4 Safety around weapons and creative problem solving

- personal safety around weapons and creative problem solving are detailed

5 Playground, recreation, and sports safety

- appropriate use of playground equipment
- the use of protective gear and street safety

6 Water safety

- diving precautions and safe behaviours around pools, lakes, and other bodies of water

The aforementioned lesson areas are detailed on the Think First Website (http://www.thinkfirst.org). Inherent in both the TFFT and TFFK programs is the use of behavioural and environmental approaches to reduce the risk of unintentional injuries in childhood and adolescence. Behavioural approaches are evidenced in the Think First programs' approach to teaching and learning. Collaborative relations are developed by involving the extended community and families. Safety messages learned at school are, therefore, also reinforced by the environment that surrounds the students.

New Curriculum Developments

Think First for grades 4, 5, and 6 is a newly developed multifaceted curriculum that bridges the gap between TFFK and TFFT. This new curriculum is currently being piloted in Canada and the United States. The content areas of focus are: brain and spinal cord anatomy; injury prevention; violence and conflict resolution; risk taking; and alcohol use/abuse (E. Sam, personal communication, May, 2000).

According to the program consultant of the Think First Foundation of Canada, changes to the Canadian curriculum, developed by a Program Advisory Committee comprised of educators and neuroscience professionals, were implemented in order to address safety and injury prevention issues unique to Canada (E. Sam, personal communication, May, 2000). Focus groups were conducted with members of all levels of education (e.g., teachers, principals, superintendents) in order to improve the quality of the TFFK program. As a result of these discussions, changes to statistics, format, and methodology were made, and content is currently being revised to include 2 new modules: winter safety and strangulation (A. Sharman, personal communication, May, 2000). In addition, the Think First Foundation of Canada has produced a series of workbooks to involve families to help reinforce the school-based education component. This new aspect of the TFFK program is called TD Think First for Families (E. Sam, personal communication, May, 2000). Each family workbook complements the lessons taught in school. A more representative video of Canadian diversity entitled Dangerous

Games was produced to replace the videos used in the U.S. Think First for Teens presentation. To date, changes to the TFFK curriculum are still being implemented in Canada.

Funding

On the national level, the foundation was begun with seed money and other funding from neurosurgeons' organizations and corporations connected to neurosurgery. Additional resources were attained through donations and requests for funding to various groups (D. Johnson, personal communication, April, 2000). At the local level, program funding and development varies throughout the country. In 1998/99, with funding from Ronald McDonald Charities, the Think First Foundation of Canada implemented programs in 800 schools across the nation (C. Tator, personal communication, May 11, 2000). Recently, Think First Foundation has been successful in generating prominent sponsorship from TD Bank.

Resources Needed

The program consultant for Think First Foundation of Canada states that the national expansion of the program requires additional resources. For instance, increased financial resources would enhance the foundation's ability to monetarily reward brain and spinal cord–injured guest speakers. Creative strategies are employed to overcome financial barriers, however, such as the use of teleconferencing methods to communicate, and sharing travel costs for coordinator meetings and training sessions (E. Sam, personal communication, May, 2000).

Implementation

Effective Practices

Key informants from both the American and Canadian National Think First Offices cite many factors as vital to the successful implementation of the Think First programs (A. Burton, personal communication, April, 2000; E. Sam, personal communication, May, 2000). These include:

- skills of the individual implementing the program;
- support from and training provided by the National Office;

- open communication with the National Office;
- an alliance with educators;
- in-service (training) sessions with appropriate staff who deliver the programs; and
- the availability of learning opportunities for parents/guardians and other community members.

Specifically, elements of the foundations' programs that are notably effective in preventing brain and spinal cord injuries include (A. Burton, personal communication, April, 2000; E. Sam, personal communication, May, 2000):

- assessing community needs and resources prior to implementation;
- developing a business plan or implementation;
- having a consumer (brain or spinal cord injury survivor) speak with middle and high school students; and
- forming partnerships with like organizations (e.g., public health).

In addition, a process evaluation gave evidence that teachers held the program in high regard, with 85% of them rating it as very good to excellent. Many teachers found the peer-to-peer approach most effective, as students were more responsive to information coming from their peers rather than from adults (Sharman & Cusimano, 2000). Most importantly, this evaluation indicated that the most successful component to the effective implementation of the programs is the availability of personal contact in the delivery of the program.

Challenges

The challenges facing programs all across North America include (A. Burton, personal communication, April, 2000; E. Sam, personal communication, May, 2000):

- competing programs;
- limited paid personnel;
- finding an appropriate speaker with an injury; and
- lack of resources.

Governance

Two task force committees, one for Think First for Teens and one for

Think First for Kids, are in place to review the programs for updates, revision, and enhancement. Development of a Think First task force was coordinated through the National Office. Experts in selected fields were sought out by various means; for example, names were elicited by national contacts in the injury prevention field (A. Burton, personal communication, April, 2000). The committees are composed of chapter directors, board members, and National Office staff. Regular feedback to the committee occurs through chapter newsletters, email, correspondence by mail and phone, and national workshops.

While recommendations are often initiated by the National Office, final decisions are made by the Think First Foundation Board (D. Johnson, personal communication, April, 2000). Locally decisions are made by Provincial Chapter Directors (E. Sam, personal communication, May, 2000). The decision-making process also varies depending on the structure of the organization. At the local level, there are a variety of governing bodies, for example, advisory boards, board of directors, chapter director only, and so on (A. Burton, personal communication, April, 2000). Since the ultimate focus is to reach as many children and teens as possible with injury prevention education, collaboration in the decision-making process is emphasized. In the event that an issue cannot be resolved between two parties, the Think First Executive Committee will make a determination by voting on how the issues should be handled. Most conflicts are addressed locally and handled successfully at the local level (E. Sam, personal communication, May, 2000).

Dissemination

Information about Think First Programs is disseminated by various methods, including a Think First Foundation newsletter, *Prevention Pages*, and articles published in neurosurgical journals (D. Johnson, personal communication, April, 2000). Additionally, the foundation maintains a recently updated Website (http://www.thinkfirst.org), which is publicly accessible.

Outcome

Think First for Kids: San Diego, California

A study conducted by Gresham and Zirkle (1999) demonstrates the impact of the Think First for Kids (TFFK) curriculum-based injury prevention pilot program on student knowledge and self-reported be-haviours among 1st, 2nd, and 3rd grade children in San Diego, Califor-nia. This study is described below.

Research Design

A randomized pre-post comparative design was used to evaluate the impact of the TFFK intervention. Schools were chosen as the unit of randomization (so that the control classroom would not be exposed to the curriculum). Eight action (intervention) schools were assigned to receive the 6-week curriculum-based intervention from a trained edu-cator; 4 schools from each of the 2 school districts in San Diego. Eight control schools, which received no intervention, were then selected for comparison by matching on school district, socio-economic status, read-ing level, and race/ethnic composition. Eight action and 7 control schools participated in the pilot study (1 control school served as a control for 2 action schools).

Educational Intervention
The intervention curriculum was conducted during a 6-week period in the fall of the 1997 school year. One lesson, approximately 30 minutes in length, was delivered weekly.

Measurement of Program Effects
Action students completed a pre-test within 10 days prior to adminis-tration of the TFFK intervention and a post-test within 10 days after the completion of the curriculum. Control schools did not have the TFFK intervention; however, they followed the same pre- and post-test schedule. Univariate (t-tests) and multivariate techniques were used to assess changes in mean score of overall knowledge and self-reported behaviours. Both the pre- and post-tests were completed by 80% of the students.

Univariate Analysis
Students in the TFFK action schools exhibited significantly greater increases in knowledge than the comparison students for each grade level (p = .001) when comparing the pre- and post-test. This increase applied equally to both males and females. TFFK had the greatest impact on minority students' absolute change in score.

Multivariate Analysis

Adjusting for the covariates gender, socio-economic status (SES), and race/ethnicity, the TFFK educational intervention was a significant predictor of an increase in score from pre- to post-test for each grade level (p < .001). The TFFK intervention was associated with a significant decrease in self-reported risky behaviours for grades 1 and 3 and a significant increase in knowledge for all grades (p < .001). For grade 2, SES was also an independent predictor of change in the pre- to post-test scores. Similar results were depicted in a Canadian study evaluating the effects of the Think First 1–2–3 Canada program.

Think First 1–2–3 Canada

A questionnaire measuring students' knowledge gained and changes in self-reported behaviour was administered to both the action and control groups. The results of this pre/post-test design indicate that the intervention group showed significant changes in knowledge. Some self-reported behaviours were also changed significantly. Minimal changes in knowledge and self-reported behaviours were observed in the control group (A. Sharman, personal communication, April, 2000). The TFFT programs have not been as extensively evaluated as the TFFK. Currently, the Think First Foundation of Canada is working on evaluating beyond knowledge gained and changes in self-reported behaviour. Through the development of a computerized measure of behavioural intentions, the Think First Foundation of Canada plans to conduct short- and long-term assessments of the TFFK programs in terms of actual injury outcome.

Think First for Teens

Brain and spinal cord injuries are the most frequent cause of traumatic injuries and the leading cause of death and disability among Canadian youth. A Canadian study assessed the impact of this prevention program in terms of knowledge gained by the students who participated in a TFFT program.

A self-administered questionnaire assessing students' knowledge and behaviour was completed in a pre-test, post-test group design. Participants generally lacked knowledge of the causes and factors which increase their risk (Damba, Sam, Edmonds, Tator, & Cusimano, in press).

The post-test results indicate that, after participating in the TFFT program, students' knowledge of risk factors for these types of injuries and knowledge of prevention increased (Damba et al., in press). Future studies are needed to assess whether knowledge gain leads to reduction of injury (Damba et al., in press).

Preliminary results suggest that the intervention school-based injury prevention education offered by the Think First curriculum may have a public health impact. The combination of environmental and behavioural approaches inherent in the Think First Foundations' programs enhance the ability of program participants to positively reduce risk-taking behaviour and any resulting neurotrauma injuries.

Latrobe Safe Communities: Latrobe Valley Better Health Project

Main Key Informant:
Henk Harberts

Background

Successful community-based approaches to all-age, all-injury prevention have been applied in various parts of the world following successful reports from Sweden during the 1980s. In 1990 the Health Department of Victoria (Australia) released the Latrobe Valley Health Study, which revealed that Latrobe Shire, the municipality comprising the many smaller communities in the Valley, displayed a higher death rate than the rest of Victoria for diseases and injury resulting from circulatory, endocrine, and nutritional problems. This study, which utilized a comparative analysis of death rates between 1969 and 1983, identified poor nutrition, tobacco smoking, and lack of exercise as factors contributing significantly to this condition. Following a period of extensive community and literature consultation, the Latrobe Valley Better Health Project (LVBHP) Injury Prevention Program was launched in 1992 to address these problems.

History and Development

The Latrobe Valley Better Health Project operated from 1992 to 1996 in the state of Victoria, Australia. In recognition of its commitment to community safety and injury prevention, the Shire of Latrobe was formally designated a WHO safe community in 1996. Latrobe was only the fifteenth community worldwide to receive the official WHO accreditation (see Small Business Falls Prevention Project for a more detailed history of the development of the safe communities initiatives).

An initial period, funded by the Victorian Health Promotion Foundation, was dedicated to planning a specific course of intervening action. A steering committee was formed, including representatives of local governments and community health organizations, the Latrobe Regional Hospital, the State Electricity Commission of Victoria, the Gippsland Trades and Labour Council, the Directorate of School Education, and the Health Department of Victoria. Additional but infrequent participants included the Gippsland Aboriginal Cooperative, Latrobe Valley Migrant Resource Centre, and the Community Road Safety Council. During this phase, the LVBHP made extensive use of injury surveillance data to precisely describe the injury profile for the region, which for clarity's sake will be referred to here as "Latrobe." Although it later became possible to supplement this data with similar information compiled directly by medical practitioners, in association with a project called the Extended Latrobe Valley Injury Study (ELVIS), 1994–1995, initially, the Victoria Injury Surveillance System (VISS) was the major source of data. Based in 2 acute-care campus hospitals, this system compiles extensive information on types and degrees of injuries sustained in various scenarios and demographic information describing victims.

Model

The planning phase resulted in 2 key decisions: that reducing the risk of illness and disability should be a high priority and that a multiple-intervention approach should be adopted for the Latrobe Valley Better Health Project. Rather than implementing projects in isolation, a range of activities for the community as a whole should be planned. Research evidence indicated that, during the 1980s, this model had successfully reduced the incidence and prevalence of injury in Sweden over a 10-year period. The steering committee also decided that in order to evaluate the type and range of interventions to include in the project, the following criteria would be adopted for inclusion:

• There should be a focus on preventative measures.

- The extent of the problem being addressed should be quantifiable and the results should allow evaluation.
- There should be a balance of long- and short-term outcomes.
- Proposed activities should take into account social justice principles so that more equitable health outcomes are experienced by those from lower socio-economic status groups.
- Interventions should involve a variety of approaches, including the implementation of strategies that lead to better health choices because of environmental modifications.
- Interventions should not duplicate any health promotion program already underway in the area; actions chosen should initiate, coordinate, or contribute to health promotion in the Latrobe Valley.

Specifically, the proposed projects included:

- the Safety Features Display Home;
- the Youth Alcohol Action Campaign;
- Reducing Noise-Induced Hearing Loss: Ears Alive at 85;
- Reduction of Sports Injuries; and
- Playground Safety.

It should be noted that the wide variety of interventions applied within the context of this initiative address both the pre-event (prevention of occurrence) and the event (reduction of severity) phases of Haddon's (1980) injury-reduction matrix and employ prevention strategies designed to reduce trauma by modifying behaviour, host (victim), and environment. The LVBHP steering committee submitted for funding and, on December 23, was allocated $225,000 for injury and nutrition activities over an 18-month period. The project staff were appointed and 4 of the 5 proposed programs were funded. Ears Alive at 85 was excluded.

Consumers

While a wide range of groups stand to see their risk of injury reduced by the programs outlined above, data consulted by the steering committee suggested that young people were most precariously positioned. In particular, Latrobe had a high proportion of young families, and because children under the age of 5 years were proving to be a high injury risk group, significant improvements for this population were an important goal. Prevalent types of injuries among the targeted groups included falls, and sports- and alcohol-related unintentional injuries. These are leading causes of neurotrauma in many other parts of the world, including Canada and Ontario specifically (SMARTRISK, 1998).

Objective

The primary aim of the LVBH Injury Prevention Program was to utilize a community intervention approach to prevent injuries, reduce hazards, and increase public awareness of measures to reduce the incidence and severity of injuries in the Latrobe Valley community.

Resources

Initial funding, for both planning and the first year and a half of the actual intervention, was provided by the Victorian Health Promotion Foundation. More recently, the LVBHP (under its current title, Latrobe Shire Safe Communities) has operated with support from VICHealth (the Health Department of Victoria) and has sought funding from other public and private sources.

In addition to funding, this effort has made effective use of a variety of other resources. The Monash University Accident Research Centre, for example, was appointed to evaluate the impact and outcome of the injury prevention program, to provide advice on injury interventions, and to assist with the development of program plans. Early on, collaboration with the communities to be addressed was emphasized, as their input and proposals were solicited and considered. Further collaboration with formal organizations, noted above, was essential to the planning phase, which clearly demanded:

- taking steps to raise community awareness;
- seeking input on factors that are perceived to contribute to ill health; and
- gathering ideas about possible solutions.

Strategy

A strong argument can be made that the model followed in this intervention constitutes a resource in itself, in terms of implementation and content as well as planning. Based on a number of successful health promotion programs from around the world, the Latrobe Valley Better Health Project reflected a model of community development that incorporated the following steps:

- community analysis;
- design and initiation;
- implementation;
- maintenance; and
- reassessment.

Two project officers were employed during 1991 to survey needs, meet with local groups and individuals, and interact with the public at various community functions. In excess of 250 detailed individual consultations were carried out. This resulted in the development of 4 objectives, which took into account priority areas of Australia's National Better Health Program, namely:

- to increase community awareness of the risk factors which lead to ill health;
- to reduce the number of deaths related to cardiovascular disease;
- to improve the standard of nutrition in the community; and
- to reduce the incidence and severity of injuries.

The LVBHP focused on 4 safer practice interventions. Each of these interventions (the Safety Features Display Home, the Youth Alcohol Action Campaign, Reduction of Sports Injury, and Playground Safety) set goals and objectives and collaborated with individuals and services according to their needs.

Programs

Safety Features Display Home
The Home Safety Display collaborated with local fire brigades, services clubs, local government, public housing advocates, and tenants and Public Housing authorities. The Safety Features Display Home was opened to the public on March 2, 1993. It contained more than 50 safety criteria and was displayed for a period of 8 weeks in 1992. An 8-page newspaper supplement directed homebuyers and renovators to the display and included safety information about local injury statistics and interventions. Extensive television and radio news items men-

tioned the use of safety devices such as smoke alarms, electrical earth leakage devices, hot water controls, and pool fences.

Goal
To familiarize the community with home safety measures in order to reduce the incidence of child injuries in the home

Objectives
- To collaborate with the Latrobe Regional Hospital to provide a display of safety promotion in a home setting;
- to provide a central location for information on child safety products;
- to coordinate the dissemination of information about safety in the home and injury prevention strategies and equipment;
- to provide a venue for demonstrating child safety education; and
- to provide a venue for health promotion and education needs of parents with young children.

Safety issues were also addressed with Child Health Services to promote the use of Early Child Injury Prevention Program materials as well as with local government Children's Services staff. A safety checklist was developed with field officers in Latrobe Shire, and Child Safety Materials developed by Royal Children's Hospital Safety Centre were distributed to local and district child caregivers. Other "School Safe" materials were distributed and discussed with 6 local school communities, as well as with many undergraduate and student teachers. As 9% of the community under study had been determined to be from different parts of the world, multilingual children's safety educational materials were distributed.

The Youth Alcohol Action Campaign

An initial group of youth workers, young people, and agency representatives met between 1992 and 1993 to identify opportunities to address alcohol/injury in their community. Youth drop-in centres were established, where alcohol-free entertainment, music, and social activities were held.

Goal
To reduce the harm associated with alcohol misuse by young people.

Objectives
- To promote awareness and understanding of youth alcohol issues;
- to establish community-based Youth Alcohol Working Parties (YAPs) with membership drawn from a range of groups, e.g., young people, youth workers, and community representatives from the local Council, parents, schools, etc.;
- to provide information regarding attitudinal, behavioural, social, and environmental variables affecting the use of alcohol;
- to assist locally based YAPs to identify factors that foster alcohol misuse by young people in their town; and
- to assist locally based YAP's to address these factors via the development and implementation of action plans.

The Latrobe Valley Better Health project participated in a number of community meetings to draw attention to the topic of alcohol misuse. An Alcohol-Free Cocktail promotion was established and quickly became a vital part of street festivals and community promotions where pamphlets and free tastings were used. The promotion specifically addressed the issue of providing non-alcohol alternatives in many different community and social settings.

The implementation of local laws made it an offence to consume alcohol in public areas, with offender fines deposited in the Traralgon City Youth Development fund. There has been a subsequent ban on alcohol consumption in public places in each of Latrobe's central business districts of the Latrobe City.

Reduction of Sports Injury

The Sports Injury Reduction working party resolved to direct their efforts towards junior age groups in Australian Rules Football, as this sport accounted for 36–38% of all sports injury presentations at Latrobe Hospital.

Goals
- To reduce the incidence and severity of sports injuries in the Latrobe; and
- issues chosen to be identified through the VISS data collection system.

Objectives
- To implement a comprehensive sports injury control program and to publicize risks associated with athletic activity and the necessity for conducting programs;
- to bring together relevant representatives and to provide advice and assistance in reducing the injuries targeted; and
- to run an educational and consultative process throughout the Latrobe Valley.

Sports injury reduction materials were incorporated into coach accreditation courses, and a high level of publicity regarding sports injury reduction was promoted. Intervention packages with information about modified rules, warm/up, cool/down, codes of conduct, safety equipment and audits, and personal protection devices was made available. The promotion of a junior football helmet resulted in increased wearing rates for underage teams. The promotion of mouthguards through alliances with dental services, the local hospital, the school dental service, Community Health Promotions, private dental care providers, and football leagues was encouraged. The aim was to promote a no-wear, no-play mentality with respect to the wearing of mouth guards in football; this aim was incorporated into the Play Safe Sport sponsorship that still exists in the Gippsland Region.

Playground Injury Prevention Program

A Playground Safety working party was assembled, and specific attention was focused upon equipment and undersurface fall material maintenance. The Victorian Playgrounds and Recreation Association audited its most popular facility and then applied a checklist audit to all of its public playgrounds.

Goal
- To reduce the number of injuries sustained by young children while using playground equipment.

Objectives
- To collaborate with local government to ensure all municipal playgrounds are assessed against safety standards;

- to encourage all municipalities to produce a playground strategy that includes mechanisms for regular safety audits;
- to inform the community of the nature of injuries associated with playgrounds and to provide them with strategies to avoid such injuries;
- to provide injury prevention information to community groups with existing playgrounds and to those designing future play facilities; and
- to raise community awareness of playground safety issues generally.

After equipment upgrades, the most effective intervention appeared to have been the maintenance of the undersurface fall material. Upon completing the study, all participating councils implemented maintenance systems that included safety audits and the removal of outdated and unsafe equipment, which has continued to date. Because of the original audit, the councils used a checklist approach to playground maintenance that covered community needs and location, seating to promote adult supervision, height limits, fall materials, and play direction and challenge. Play equipment and recreational space was to be located within 400 metres of every urban residential address and equipment was to be powder-coated metal instead of treated pine. With the amalgamation of local government (December, 1994), however, the initial playground safety strategy became difficult to maintain, and playground facilities became the responsibility of City Parks and Gardens staff.

Implementation

The community consultation process largely determined the operational structure of the Latrobe Valley Better Health Project. This process took a series of methodical steps to plan, implement, and evaluate health promotion and health education programs. Numerous community-based injury prevention programs have used similar sequences in program development.

Decision Making and Planning

From September 1990 to July 1991 the original steering committee of the Latrobe Valley Better Health Project met monthly. The community consultation process largely determined the operational structure of the Latrobe Valley Better Health Project. One of these groups eventually

formed the Injury Prevention Reference group. In early 1992 the original planning phase steering committee became the Management Committee of the Project, which met on a monthly basis and was chaired by
a local mayor. The Injury Prevention Reference Group met on a bimonthly basis to ensure that the activities and working parties for each
of the 4 prevention objectives were established.

Ongoing Implementation

The project developed strategic plans for 1992–1996 and worked closely
with existing local groups to incorporate state strategies. The current
Latrobe Shire Council Municipal Public Health Plan (called Better Health
for Latrobe, 1997–1999) reflects the intentions and processes of community safety promotion and injury prevention. These plans are reviewed
and submitted to the Department of Human Services on a biennial
basis.

In 1996 the Latrobe Shire Council assumed responsibility and funding for the Safe Communities Program and incorporated the Better
Health Management Committee (which had previously overseen Safe
Communities) as an advisory committee. This committee continues to
meet monthly to pursue the ideal of promoting community injury
prevention and safety.

According to the Safe Communities coordinator, any persons on the
committee who disagree are encouraged to "work it out," because the
committee as a whole is responsible for representing community needs
and has to come to harmonious decisions and consensus for the benefit
of all stakeholders.

Legislation

The development of legislation in the early 1990s requiring all Victorian
local government to implement Municipal Public Health Plans and to
provide resources to support initiatives of this sort has resulted in a
network of activity. In September 1993 the Department of Health and
Community Services (now VICHealth) hosted a forum which saw some
80 participants, from a variety of injury-related fields, commence a
process of developing an overall strategy for the control of injury in the
State of Victoria. The LVBHP Injury Prevention Program contributed to
this plan and has continued to participate in various reviews and development of the strategy called Taking Injury Prevention Forward. This

state strategy is a response to the Australian National Health Goals and Targets, which list injury, cardiovascular disease, cancer, and mental health as priority areas of concern for all Australians.

Municipal Public Health Plans

The requirement for local Victoria governments to develop Municipal Public Health Plans during the early 1990s gave the program an effective protocol to establish a local response to injury control. Submissions incorporating injury prevention were made to numerous Latrobe Shire townships.

The LVBHP developed its own local strategic plans during 1992 and 1996; these accommodated community safety and injury prevention issues and acknowledged that close liaison with existing local groups was a legitimate process for dealing with the overall state strategy.

Outcome

The Monash University Accident Research Centre was appointed to evaluate the impact and outcome of the injury prevention program between 1992 and 1996, to provide advice on injury interventions, and to assist with the development of program plans. The evaluation design included pre- and post-intervention observations in a population of approximately 72,000. There was no single comparison community; rather, comparative data was used where possible.

- Process measures included key informant interviews with local organization representatives.
- Impact evaluation relied primarily on self-reported changes in injury risk and protective factors, gathered by a random telephone survey.
- Outcome evaluation was based on 5 years of emergency department injury surveillance data for the Latrobe Valley.

The program built strategic partnerships, increasing the emphasis on safety at the local level. Promotional and educational activities were implemented in the targeted areas of home, sport, and playground injuries and alcohol misuse among the youth. Some 51,000 educational contacts were made with the community and 7,470 resource items distributed. A 7.3% increase in the proportion of households purchasing home safety items was observed. Unsafe equipment was replaced and poor surfacing upgraded in municipal playgrounds. The demand for and availability of protective equipment for sport increased. The age standardized rate per 100,000 persons for emergency department presentations for all targeted injuries fell from 6,594 in the first program year to 4,821 in 1995–1996. There were significant decreases in the presentation rates for playground injuries among ages 5–14, sports injuries among 15–24 year olds, and home injuries among all age groups except for 65 years and above. The direct program cost per injury prevented was $272.

There were no decreases in alcohol purchases by liquor outlets and the rate of arrest for being drunk and disorderly increased among 10–24-year olds. These results, however, may reflect closer monitoring, stricter alcohol consumption laws, and more concerted enforcement of those laws. Moreover, significant reductions were observed in assaults among 10–24 year olds, compared to the number of assaults found in the over-25 age group.

Most program objectives were met to some extent. The lack of control community injury data limits the conclusions that can be drawn about the association between the program and the injury reductions observed. However, the reductions were associated with changes in injury risk and protective factors, and were greatest for the injury issues subjected to the most intense activity. Continued monitoring of the impact of the ongoing injury prevention program and improvement of the evaluation design by including a comparison community are merited. Presently, a senior research fellow from Monash University is collecting and evaluating more recent data from the Latrobe Valley Better Health Project. This evaluation has not yet been released to the general public.

Dissemination

To maximize coverage for the 4 main injury prevention objectives, the LVBHP utilized the mass media (television, radio, and newspapers) at every opportunity. Materials were distributed to appropriate parties in local communities and subsequently discussed. A number of approaches to local industry were made to promote the use of protective devices for injury prevention, and retail promotions on safety equipment and related information were made available to Latrobe Valley hardware stores. Word-of-mouth advertising ensures that the safe living message will continue to be reviewed and updated. An informative report on the Injury Prevention Program called *Community Cooperation Toward a Safer Future* was written by the coordinator of the Community Safety Program. This report is available to the general public and has proven to be a useful resource for replicating such a model. Evaluation of the Latrobe Valley Better Health Program indicates that the incidence of injury and trauma can be addressed successfully by comprehensive community action, and this approach should be encouraged by local and state governments.

PROMISING PRACTICES

Risk Watch
Quincy, Massachusetts

Main Key Informant:
Meri-K Appy

Background

Risk Watch (RW) is a primary injury prevention curriculum designed to create safer communities by joining teachers and the community to teach children the knowledge and skills required to avoid risks leading to unintentional injuries. The curriculum is appropriate for Canada because it is designed to address the 8 leading causes of unintentional injuries for North American children. RW is geared to schoolchildren for several reasons:

- Each year unintentional injuries kill more than 6,040 children and permanently disable more than 120,000 children (NFPA & Lowe's Home Safety Council, n.d.).
- Children are perceived to be receptive and open, and thus more likely to adopt the prevention message than older age groups (M.K. Appy, personal communication, March 23, 2000).
- Schools organize children into developmental levels, which facilitates teaching developmentally appropriate prevention messages. In the past safety information was not adjusted to reflect the developmental level of the audience (M.K. Appy, personal communication, March 23, 2000).

Generous co-funding from the Lowe's Home Safety Council, along with a supplemental evaluation grant provided by the Duke Endowment, enabled NFPA to create the Risk Watch curriculum with input from many of America's leading safety organizations. NFPA is a non-profit international membership association that facilitates the process through which fire codes and standards are developed (M.K. Appy, personal communication, March 23, 2000). Lowe's Home Safety Council is a non-profit organizational branch of Lowe's Inc., and a co-founder of RW (Wolf, 1997). NFPA has representation on the Lowe's Home Safety Council, which is how their partnership began.

History and Development

The idea behind RW stemmed from NFPA's well-received fire prevention curriculum, Learn Not to Burn. The effectiveness of the fire safety curriculum led members of the community to expect NFPA to combat the rise of other childhood injuries (M.K. Appy, personal communication, March 23, 2000). Although incidents of fire-related injury were declining, other types of child injury, like bicycle and car collisions, remained a problem that communities lacked the tools to manage (M.K. Appy, personal communication, March 23, 2000).

Despite initial resistance and fear of stretching NFPA's resources and expertise, it became clear that, to convey the fire safety message effectively, the message must be embedded within a broad educational package tackling the other risk areas leading to unintentional injuries in children (M.K. Appy, personal communication, March 23, 2000). Teachers recognized that, logistically, there is not enough time to allow the police, firefighters, and others to speak to the children individually (M.K. Appy, personal communication, March 23, 2000).

A comprehensive curriculum was needed yet, at the time, only topic-specific models or models that addressed a few risk areas were available (M.K. Appy, personal communication, March 23, 2000). Recognizing that media announcements and one-shot auditorium events were not enough to convey the safety message, the RW curriculum was developed to reinforce safety information throughout the school year (M.K. Appy, personal communication, March 23, 2000).

Neurotrauma Focus

The prevention of neurotrauma injuries was an important consideration in the development of RW, particularly as it pertains to motor vehicle collisions. Recognition that motor vehicle crashes are the chief cause of unintentional injury–related child deaths, and a leading cause of neurotrauma injury in children, led to the deliberate placing of the motor vehicle lesson as the first of the 8 risk areas to be taught (M.K.

Appy, personal communication, March 23, 2000). Included in the motor vehicle lesson is information about how to wear safety belts, use child car seats, and use booster seats correctly. RW tackles other risk areas to prevent neurotrauma injury through lessons in the prevention of falls, bike and pedestrian safety, and water safety.

Resources

RW employs the Haddon (1980) matrix by using environmental and behavioural strategies to reduce children's risk for unintentional injuries.

The environment is addressed by developing partnerships between the school, home, and community, with the expectation that children will learn safety messages at school and share the messages with peers and family through other RW activities.

Behavioural strategies are inherent to RW's experiential approach to learning, giving children the opportunity to rehearse making difficult safety decisions in a safe environment.

Program Model

RW is based on a program model that aims to develop knowledge, activity, and commitment in children.

- Knowledge is continually asking and finding out: What skills and information do I have and need to be safe?
- Activity provides opportunities to practise using skills, knowledge, and decision making, which lead to understanding and commitment to safe behaviours.
- Commitment refers to being able to say: I am willing to be responsible and take ownership for choosing and demonstrating safe behaviours.

The curriculum is divided into 5 teaching modules, indicative of the 5 age groups for which RW is intended: preschool to kindergarten; grade 1 to grade 2; grade 3 to grade 4; grade 5 to grade 6; and grade 7 to grade 8. Each module addresses the 8 risk areas. The most effective way to use RW is to implement the 5 modules with the same students, allowing each module to build on prior knowledge and strengthen safety attitudes and skills.

Program Components

The following components are present in each teaching module:

- Getting into Character: a set of warm-up exercises and tips to help students step into developmentally appropriate character roles that facilitate safety decision making (NFPA, 1998). For example, preschoolers and kindergarteners adopt the role of storytellers who share their ideas and experiences as they learn new injury prevention skills.
- Risk Area Lesson Cards: information cards that contain developmentally appropriate information about the 8 risk areas, and a lesson plan to teach the information.
- Risk Area Icon Cards: These contain illustrations and information that remind children of the essential prevention messages.
- RW in Action – Interactive Activities: a series of activities designed to help students practise decision making and actions that could save their lives in an emergency.
- Caregiver Letters: letters to parents and caregivers that provide information for making the home a safer place to live.
- Evaluation Instruments: evaluation techniques that measure student knowledge gain, and a form to provide recommendations to improve RW.
- Accessing Resources: a sample letter used to invite safety partners to take part in the RW curriculum, and a list of national organizations to contact for more information on matters of safety.

Sources of Funding

Lowe's Home Safety Council provided a $150,000 grant that NFPA matched and supplemented to develop the curriculum. In addition, NFPA is contributing more than $300,000 for an independent 3-year evaluation of RW by Interwest Applied Research, Portland, OR. Results of year 1 of the evaluation shows that "there is indisputable evidence that RW is effective in teaching important safety knowledge." Independent of the NFPA evaluation, the Duke Endowment, under the auspices of Duke University Medical Center, has contributed $300,000 to fund a 3-year evaluation in 2 North Carolina counties. In addition to the grants offered by external agencies, NFPA supports the process by publishing the codes and standards developed on fire safety (M.K. Appy, personal communication, March 23, 2000). Finally, RW costs $62.50 (U.S.) per teaching module and $265.50 (U.S.) for the complete 5-level Risk Watch set, including implementation support tools.

Sources of Information

The Technical Advisory Group is a distinguished coalition of private sector organizations, safety advocates, and national experts in the 8 risk areas who volunteered to inform the development of RW. Members of the advisory group provided research data, technical content, and appropriate prevention messages and reviewed curriculum lessons (NFPA & Lowe's Home Safety Council, n.d.). Constituents of the group were recruited by networking with the safety experts in the Lowe's Home Safety Council and National Safe KIDS Campaign. Members of the Technical Advisory Group were eager to participate in RW as many were not skilled in curriculum development but wanted to communicate to children the importance of safety (M.K. Appy, personal communication, March 23, 2000).

Teachers informed all stages of RW development to ensure that the final product was neither labour intensive nor time consuming. Field tests of the first iteration of RW were conducted to allow teachers to further shape the final document (M.K. Appy, personal communication, March 23, 2000). The pilot version differs from the current version of RW foremost in terms of its organization (M.K. Appy, personal communication, March 23, 2000). Teachers within the limited sample responded positively to the RW curriculum (Interwest, 1998; 1999).

Training

Through an application process, free training is provided to communities wishing to adopt the RW integrated model. NFPA trains Champion Management Teams (CMT) to create lasting collaborative ties to facilitate the implementation of RW. CMTs consist of state- or provincial-level representatives from the fields of fire, health, law enforcement, and the Board/Department of Education (M.K. Appy, personal communication, March 23, 2000). NFPA also assigns to each CMT a Risk Watch Field Advisor and a local champion to support the implementation process (Vice President of Public Education, NFPA, personal communication, March 23, 2000). CMTs agree to train 5 communities to use RW in the same collaborative mode (M.K. Appy, personal communication, March 23, 2000).

Other Resources

A number of other resources are available to support the implementation of RW:

- the RW *Leader's Guide*, a written document, walks the community through the process of forming a coalition to implement RW and explains how to work with a school;
- an RW video displays teachers who have implemented the RW model;
- *The Apple Corps*, a newsletter, highlights best practices of the RW model and is free to anyone who requests it;
- the RW website, showcases innovative lesson plan ideas submitted by teachers who have used RW, to prevent RW from losing its appeal and freshness;
- field advisors provide advice to communities; and
- NFPA staff offer seminars to introduce RW at the regional and state/provincial level.

Resources Needed

Despite the many resources available to support the implementation of RW, the following resources are needed:

- Funding to improve targeting of parents, because families "need more help than they're getting" when it comes to creating safer homes (M.K. Appy, personal communication, March 23, 2000).
- Robust audiovisual and internet components.
- Formal efforts to promote a learning exchange between RW communities and NFPA (M.K. Appy, personal communication, March 23, 2000).

Implementation

Partners

The partnership between the co-founders of RW, Lowe's Home Safety Council and NFPA continues to be a two-way street. (M.K. Appy, personal communication, March 23, 2000). Each organization tries to be a resource to the other through reciprocal committee representation and joint planning of events (M.K. Appy, personal communication, March 23, 2000).

Throughout the development of RW, there were minimal conflicts between the RW partners as a sense of urgency pervaded the group to address unintentional injuries in children (M.K. Appy, personal communication, March 23, 2000). Whenever differences of opinions arose, a consensus approach to decision making was used (M.K. Appy, personal communication, March 23, 2000). One advisory member described the RW project as "the most collaborative project I've ever worked on" (Wolf, 1998). At present, the Technical Advisory Group does not play a central role in RW but is likely to reassemble for future projects.

Effective Practices

The NFPA vice-president of public education notes several aspects of the RW model that have been effective in preventing injuries from occurring.

- Internally driven initiative: Community representatives must organize themselves into multi-agency coalitions. By doing so, communities develop a sense of ownership and responsibility for the RW project. Also, the multidisciplinary approach makes it easier for teachers to cover several injury risk areas (Wolf, 1997), and partners may draw from each others' strengths (e.g., grant writing) to further prevention initiatives.
- Community support: Include influential people in the coalition who have a similar vision (Wolf, 1998). To improve a community's receptiveness for RW include media coverage and "[plan] safety messages to coincide with holidays, changes in season, or a big news story that brings the issue of safety to the forefront" (Wolf, 1998, p. 90).
- Fit with the curriculum: RW was designed to be integrated into the standard school curriculum so that teachers may fulfil their state/ provincial mandates in language arts and health, while teaching safety.
- Flexibility: The teaching modules may be taught individually, sequentially, as part of a unit within a subject, or integrated into the standard curriculum of subjects like physical education, language, and health (NFPA, 1998).
- Developmentally appropriate and fun for kids.

Obstacles to Implementation

Obstacles to implementing RW include:

- Societal complacency: The public's lack of awareness of unintentional injuries and the notion that injuries are an inevitable part of childhood may be the biggest challenge to implementing RW (M.K. Appy, personal communication, March 23, 2000).
- Gatekeepers: Marketing the curriculum to school administrators and other gatekeepers has been a challenge (M.K. Appy, personal communication, March 23, 2000).

Ongoing Evaluation

Built into RW are tools that help to identify and address other obstacles to implementation: instruments that measure the knowledge gain of students before and after RW; Success Incident Reports that enable teachers and NFPA to track accounts of safety practices that result from RW. RW users are also invited to offer recommendations about how RW may be improved.

Outcome

Evaluation

The effectiveness of the RW approach is measured according to the level of children's knowledge gain. Evaluations were not able to measure behaviour change due to insufficient resources and because many of the behaviours addressed through RW are not regular occurrences that may be observed (Interwest Applied Research, 1998). NFPA contracted Interwest Applied Research to analyse the impact of RW on children's knowledge. This 3-year evaluation compares RW classrooms with classrooms that were not exposed to the curriculum in 6 communities in the United States and Canada.

Preliminary findings suggest the effectiveness of RW in improving children's knowledge of safety matters, although inadequacies in test materials taint the conclusion (Interwest Applied Research, 1998). Anecdotal accounts support the effectiveness of RW as new job positions devoted to the implementation of RW have been created in some U.S. states (M.K. Appy, personal communication, March 23, 2000).

The Duke University Medical Center is also conducting a 3-year evaluation of RW in a limited U.S. sample. Discussions are underway to implement and evaluate RW countrywide (M.K. Appy, personal communication, March 23, 2000). Another evaluation of RW is underway in Los Angeles, under the auspices of Harbor UCLA Medical Center and the Emergency Medical Services for Children. Findings have yet to be reported.

Lesson

An important lesson learned regarding the prevention of injury in children centres on conveying developmentally appropriate messages. Safety lessons should impart the importance of the matter and enable students to rehearse their newfound knowledge and skills.

Dissemination of Information

As previously described, the RW *Leader's Guide*, RW video, *The Apple Corps* newsletter, the RW website, field advisors, and NFPA staff are the means by which RW information is disseminated.

Discussion and Conclusion

Discussion and Conclusion

Previous sections of this *Compendium* emphasize 4 important points:

1 Unintentional injury is a major worldwide problem that is currently addressed through a variety of effective prevention strategies; the programs and strategies reviewed in this *Compendium* are highly pertinent to the Canadian injury context.
2 Systematic evaluation of injury prevention initiatives are establishing support for evidence-based practice; to improve this evidence base, the evaluation methods highlighted in the case studies presented in this *Compendium* are worthy of replication in Canada.
3 Because of the complexity of injury dynamics, best practices are not proven practices.
4 Best practices are strategies and programs that adhere to the best evidence of what is effective. Moreover, a "best practice" can change when a shift is made from individual clinical practice to the collective practice associated with implementing policy at the community level.

General Lessons Learned

Incidence versus Initiatives

Injuries occur across ages and in a variety of settings, and they reveal a range of causes. Consequently, prevention initiatives cover a wide range of forms. Further, interest and investment in these initiatives are not evenly spread. Available prevention resources and their evaluation (the size and scale of studies) vary with the type of injury and age of occurrence. No concentrated focus of attention correlates with the actual incidence of injuries; compare the amount of attention given to seat belts and helmets to that accorded to pedestrian injuries.

The Three Es

Prevention is most effective when the three Es (enactment, education, engineering) coexist in programs. That is, unintentional injuries appear to be preventable when education, engineering, and enactment components are combined. Not all forms of injury, however, are amenable to this combination. Health issues often conflict with individual life styles and political ideologies that limit legislative possibility.

Consider Context

Most initiatives are geared directly to the targeted high-risk group. However, the involvement of health, education, and social service professionals should be as great as that of parents and caregivers. Professionals need to be considered as part of the larger context because participative approaches have potential for greater success.

Going to Scale

The demonstrated effectiveness of many engineering advances has surprisingly not resulted in many manifestations of going to scale (attempting a massive implementation) in order to create preventative environments. Addressing this lack of going to scale may be the most important role for initiatives that cut across individual and collective solutions.

Buying In

No form of injury prevention is truly passive. Engineering solutions can be subverted and enactments can be ignored. For example, seat-belt legislation can be in place, but legislation alone cannot ensure that all drivers buckle up. Injury prevention initiatives must consider the importance of human intention in order to be successful. Public adherence to prevention initiatives requires widespread educational campaigns, as well as continuous attention to policy development.

Moving Towards Evidence-Based Prevention Practices

Prevention strategies require a multimethod approach to evaluating program effectiveness. This requirement is an important consideration when arguments are advanced for making randomized control trials (RCTs) the gold standard for determining success. In fact, both strong and weak interventions are amenable to the use of this design. While RCTs can yield robust support for some means of prevention, multiple strategies dealing with a diversity of forms of injury in a variety of settings are not amenable to this approach. More important are tailored replications of prevention strategies evaluated by multimethod designs.

Rather than adopting a narrow set of evaluation tools, the inclusion of multiple methods in program evaluation is becoming the norm. This technique is in keeping with the notion of an experimenting society advanced by the late Donald Campbell. Campbell suggested that continuous evaluation through a variety of appropriate methods offers the most promise of evolving effective forms of intervention and prevention; interestingly, the North American version of the Cochrane Collaboration for the provision of systematic research reviews is named after him (i.e., the Campbell Collaboration). The focus on continuous, multimethod evaluation has been supported as an extension of the Cochrane Collaboration because of the need to provide systematic reviews relevant to social and educational policies. The relevance of this development directly extends to unintentional injury prevention. Review of injury prevention strategies could not realistically be based on RCTs. The yield of research from the emerging science of research review and synthesis is needed to guide social policy makers and practitioners, as much as it is needed to guide the effects of medical interventions.

Injuries Are Preventable

Because prevention can be made to work, the real issues may lie in the areas of program implementation and utilization. Coleman et al. (1996) assert that the actual value of a program can only be confirmed if 3 staged conditions are met: efficacy, effectiveness, and implemention. For example, in laboratory trials the design of a bicycle helmet may be proven to adequately withstand impact; the second stage might be the determination of the effectiveness of helmets to protect real riders on the street; the third stage would involve creating conditions that increase helmet use. In each of these stages different forms of evidence may be obtained by utilizing a variety of evaluation methods. The legitimate truth value of the information produced through these stages, from different data sources, needs to be recognized (Volpe, 1998). Moreover, attention should be paid to encouraging coordinated interagency projects that involve widespread community participation. This sort of integration of services necessitates the inclusion of the various disciplines involved, and provides an assortment of ways of evaluating program effectiveness.

As was observed by SMARTRISK (1998), a national injury prevention strategy requires more than the identification of best practices, as supplied by this *Compendium*. Effective implementation of identified injury prevention best practices, nationally and locally, requires a thorough examination of, and a solid documented base describing, levels of investment in prevention and the necessary collaborative partnerships between government, non-government organizations, the public health infrastructure, and community-based organizations.

Although this *Compendium* has identified some co-requisites of successful prevention, it is more about what can be done than what should be done. The necessary political will, professional vision, comprehensiveness of stakeholder involvement, allocation of resources, collaboration of services, skill of providers, and wisdom of leadership must come together if we are to realize a true reduction in the incidence of neurotrauma.

Appendices

Appendix A: Interview Guide

All italicized points are probes and they are for your information only. These points highlight the types of information sought, and therefore do not need to be asked directly.

Introduction

Interview Details

- Name of person interviewed
- Job title
- Main professional responsibilities
- Name of initiative/institution/program
- Contact address/tel./fax/email
- Date

Notes for the interviewer:
As criteria for best practice, in this section we are trying to determine the following:

- Are prevention strategies committed to prevention at the primary and/or secondary level (i.e., at the pre-event and/or event phase)?
- Do these strategies take into account the interplay of the host, agent, and the environment (as described by Haddon (1980)) at the pre-event and event phases (see proposal for definitions)?
- Does previous research and/or local epidemiological data inform program objectives?

Background

According to the BRIO framework, exploring the Background of a program is intended to uncover its history and the environment and events that have shaped the program development and implementation (e.g., legal mandates in a community, special funding opportunities, community reactions to the program). Background inquiries aim to explain why the neurotrauma prevention program takes a particular form, and how for example, relevant policies, legislation, and community needs have influenced the objectives of the program.

Description of Consumers

1 Can you tell us about your target population?

- Demographic characteristics
- Socio-economic characteristics
- Most prevalent unintentional injuries

2 How was this population chosen?
3 What types of neurotrauma injuries (brain and spinal cord) are prevalent in this population?

- Rate of neurotrauma injuries (incidence and prevalence)

History and Development

1 When and how was the program/institution/centre founded?

- History and background to development

2 Please describe the types of prevention strategies (the term strategy will be used to include prevention-oriented programs, models, legislation, standards, product design etc. ...) currently available that have the potential to prevent (reduce/eliminate) neurotrauma injuries.

- History and development
- Description of the model(s) used
- Stakeholder participation
- Method(s) of implementation
- Primary or secondary prevention (pre-event or event phase)

3 Who initiated the development of these prevention strategies?
4 What events surrounded the development of this strategy?

   • For example, what was the impetus for the development of these
     strategies?

5 Why were the strategies designed the way they were?
6 What are stated goals and objectives of these strategies?
7 Are there any implicit goals connected to the objectives?

   • For example, community development

Stakeholders

1 Who are your stakeholders (the term stakeholders is used to include
   injury prevention consumers, legislators, professionals, etc., as
   defined by the interviewee)?
2 What types of issues were stakeholders facing at the time of development and implementation of these strategies?
3 How did the stakeholders react at the time of development?
4 How do associated stakeholders presently perceive the program?
5 What are implications of these perceptions for the future of the
   strategies employed in terms of the design and delivery?

Collaborators

1 Who were the key players/collaborators at the beginning of the
   initiative and are the same players involved at the present time?
   If not, why not, and how has the composition of collaborators
   changed?
2 What was (were) the process(es) by which these collaborators came
   together?

   • Legislation
   • Policies
   • Initiative by managers or professionals
   • Grass roots movement
   • Anything else?

3 Does any one discipline or partner take a leading role in the implementation and delivery of these strategies? (who, how, expand).

Resources

The Resources element of the BRIO model calls for an investigation of the program design and resource allocation, particularly, how the program intends to achieve the articulated objectives. Financial resources and the strategies adopted to prevent neurotrauma injuries are critical inputs to the program that should be clarified. Knowledge of alternative implementation and neurotrauma prevention strategies is useful to gauge the fit of the chosen strategies.

Notes to the interviewer
As criteria for best practice, we are trying to determine the following from this section:

- Does the prevention strategy employ a combination of environmental and behavioural strategies?
- Does altering the environment with the goal of reducing the risk of one type of injury increase the risk of another type of injury?
- Is the model grounded in credible and appropriate research (as obtained through literature and/or previous evaluation)?
- Are informed and appropriate approaches used to measure outcomes in order to establish sustainability, reliability, and replicability?

Resources to Implement Prevention Strategies

1 Who supported this initiative initially and who is supporting it now?

- Politicians
- Managers/administrators
- Professionals
- Community (including business)
- Consumers
- Anyone else?

2 What kind of support do they provide?
3 What kinds of resources were developed for and allocated to implement these strategies?

- Funding

- Training
- Personnel
- Buildings
- Office equipment
- Information systems
- Anything else?

4 How were these resources attained?
5 Are there any resources lacking?

Inputs to the Prevention Model(s)

1 How have the prevention strategies used changed from initial implementation?

- Outline changes to the model(s) to date
- Why and how have these changes occurred?

2 Were there, or are there, any pilot projects initiated to measure or assess the benefits of using these particular strategies?
3 Was the development of these strategies based on successful implementation anywhere else, or were they grounded in research or academic reviews?

Implementation

Implementation refers to the operationalization of a program, comparing the intended program design and actual practice. How and why does a neurotrauma prevention program adhere (or not) to the original plans for program governance, administration, management, implementation, and practice?

Notes for the interviewer
As criteria for best practice, we are trying determine the following from this section:

- Does the model use a multidisciplinary framework or approach?
- Is there a collaborative commitment to expanding the foundation of injury prevention from different disciplines?
- How is internal coherence managed; for example, what practices

and policies are in place to deal with the differences that arise within the multifaceted and multidisciplinary context in which injury prevention is practised?
- Does the program incorporate a developmental perspective that is both flexible and adaptable?
- Populations are diverse and have changing needs; are the strategies proposed sufficiently flexible to incorporate and address these changes?

Effective Practices

1 What practices do you feel have been most effective in:

- implementing the prevention strategies? (*process*)
- preventing injuries from occurring? (*outcome*)

2 What types of practices do you feel would enhance:

- implementing a prevention strategy? (*process*)
- preventing injuries from occurring? (*outcome*)

3 How do the strategies used account for cultural and/or other diversity issues?
4 What factors facilitate the implementation of these strategies?
5 What are some of the obstacles to implementing these strategies?
6 What mechanisms are in place to incorporate change, for example, changes in the environment or in the needs of the targeted population?

Actors in Decision Making and Planning

1 Who is currently involved in the decision making and planning?

- Politicians
- Managers/administrators
- Professionals
- Community/ business
- Consumers
- Anyone else?

2 What other individuals/groups/etc. do you feel should be involved in the decision making and planning?

3 What is the nature of your interaction with other professionals?

- Structural (decision making, power issues, procedures)
- Relationship (harmonious, friendly, power issues, respect, communication)

4 Describe what mechanisms (procedures) are currently in place to enable decisions to be made.

- How are final decisions reached?

5 What procedures are in place to resolve disputes when they arise?
6 How is responsibility shared or divided?

- accountability

Ongoing Evaluation of the Prevention Strategy

1 What sorts of checks are made on implementation?
2 How is feedback structured and given to management and front-line workers, to consumers and other stakeholders?
3 How and when are adjustments made to design and implementation of these strategies?
4 Provide some examples of adjustments made to date.

- Try to illuminate the processes involved in change.

5 What evidence exists as to the relation between what was intended in the design of the strategy and what exists today?

Outcome

To understand a program's Outcome is to determine the impact of the program. This component asks how practitioners, participants, and observers judge the attainments of the program. Long- and short-term outcome measures of the program, including intended and unintended positive (e.g., improved awareness of safety standards in the workplace) and negative outcomes are of interest.

Notes for the Interviewer
As criteria for best practice, we are trying to determine the following from this section:

- Does the program employ a cost-benefit analysis?
- Does the program employ a cost-effectiveness analysis?
- Determine whether and, if so, why the strategy is successful in preventing (reducing/eliminating) injury.
- How is success defined?

Evaluation

1 How do the practitioners, consumers, supporters, and observers evaluate the attainments of the prevention strategies?
2 Are any specific methods in place for measuring the success or effectiveness of this initiative?
3 What criteria are used in measuring effectiveness of the strategy?
4 What types of data are collected during the implementation of the strategy, if any, that contribute to its evaluation?
5 What are the short-term and long-term outcomes?
6 Describe any unanticipated positive or negative outcomes of the strategies used.
7 How have the results been used to make changes to the model(s)?
8 What procedures are in place to incorporate lessons learned from existing evaluations?
9 What are the lessons learned?

Dissemination of Information

1 How do you disseminate information to stakeholders?

Appendix B: Injury-Producing Events by Age Group

Age	Events Leading to Unintentional Brain and Spinal Cord Injury – Related Hospitalization	Events Leading to Unintentional Brain and Spinal Cord Injury – Related Death
Less than 1 year	• Falls • Choking suffocation	• Choking/suffocation • Motor vehicles and other road vehicles (occupants)
1–4 Years	• Falls (playground equipment, cycling) • Motor vehicles and other road vehicles (occupants/pedestrians, cyclists) • Choking and suffocation (anoxia to the brain) • Farm injury (tractors)	• Motor vehicles and other road vehicles (occupants/pedestrians) • Choking and suffocation (e.g., drowning)
5–9 Years	• Falls (playground) • Pedestrian injuries caused by moving road vehicles (cyclists, pedestrians, occupants)	• Motor vehicles and other road vehicles (occupants, pedestrians, cyclists)
10–14* Years	Falls (sports, recreational) Motor vehicles and other road vehicles (cyclists, occupants, pedestrians)	• Motor vehicles and other road vehicles (occupants, pedestrians, cyclists)
15–19 Years	• Motor vehicle and other road vehicles (occupants)	• Motor vehicle and other road vehicles (occupants)
Adults (20–60)	• Falls	• Motor vehicle crashes
55–79	• Falls • Motor vehicle crashes	• Motor vehicle crashes • Falls
80+	• Falls • Motor vehicle crashes	• Falls • Motor vehicle crashes

*40% of fall-related injuries for children under 11 years of age are the result of falls from playground equipment, stairs, sports, chairs/beds, or buildings.

Appendix C: Summary Tables of Case Studies

- Asphyxiation-Related Injury Prevention
- Motor and Other Road Vehicle–Related Injury Prevention
- Sports, Playground, and Recreation-Related Injury Prevention
- Farm-Related and Occupational Injury Prevention
- Fall-Related Injury Prevention
- Comprehensive Community-Based Injury Prevention

Asphyxiation-related injury prevention

Age group served	Prevention area	Program name	Contact information	Background	Resources	Implementation	Outcome	Evaluation	Engineering	Enactment
Toddlers	Drownings and near-drownings	Pool fencing: effectiveness of legislation and education	Dr W. Robert Pitt Director, Pediatric Emergency Mater Children's Hospital Annerley Road South Brisbane Queensland 4101 Australia Tel: 61-7-3840-3825 Email: rpitt@mater.org.au	• toddlers at risk of drowning and near-drowning; incidents in domestic pools • means of prevention include pool alarms, pool covers, and/or pool fencing • isolation pool fencing appears to be the most effective in preventing drowning and near-drowning incidents involving toddlers	• received funding from the Australian government	• combination of legislation, information and awareness campaigns, and education	• legislation combined with the awareness campaign resulted in a decrease in the number of drownings • high level of awareness • modification of behaviour (pool owners accepted the legislation) • main problem continued to be the failure of pool owners to maintain the pool gate (to prevent un-intended access)	✓	✓	✓

Motor vehicle and road-related injury prevention

Age group served	Prevention area	Program name	Contact information	Background	Resources	Implementation	Outcome	Evaluation	Engineering	Enactment
All drivers and pedestrians	Road safety	Red light cameras	John Veneziano Traffic Engineer Department of Public Works City of Fairfax 10455 Armstrong St Fairfax, VA 22030 Tel: (703) 385-7810 Email: Jveneziano@ci.fairfax.va.U.S.	• red light running the most common type of crash; accounts for 22% of all urban crashes and 27% of all injury crashes • developed and maintained by outside sources • ongoing program implemented in 1997 in City of Fairfax	• City of Fairfax invested approximately $100,000 • collected over $1 million in revenue as of the end of February 2000	• campaign employed mass media and direct contact • 30-day warning period in which cameras were used to photograph but not ticket violators vpreceded actual enforcement	• red light running violations decreased at all camera and non-camera sites one year after implementation • overall, violations decreased 9% after three months and 40% after one year • drivers more willing and ready to stop for all red lights, not just those equipped with cameras	✓	✓	✓
All drivers and pedestrians	Road safety	Roundabouts	Per Garder Associate Professor, Transportation Dept of Civil & Environmental Engineering University of Maine	• ongoing program implemented in 1991 for Vaxjo and in 1997 for Gorham • roundabouts developed, main-	• City of Vaxjo paid about 2 million Swedish Kroners ($140,000 U.S.)	• short-term and long-term studies conducted • intersections with high accident rates	• accident rates and speeds reduced • roundabouts increased intersection's capacity, resulting	✓	✓	✓

Motor vehicle and road-related injury prevention—(Continued)

Age group served	Prevention area	Program name	Contact information	Background	Resources	Implementation	Outcome	Evaluation	Engineering	Enactment
			Orono, ME 04469-5711 U.S.A. Tel: 207-581-2177 Fax: 207-581-3999	tained, and implemented by the cities of Vaxjo, Sweden, and Gorham, Maine	for the installation of 21 temporary roundabouts • City of Gorham paid $259,000 for 1 permanent roundabout	chosen for the implementation of roundabouts in each city	in significant cost savings			
Drivers	Road safety	Rumblestrips	John J. Hickey Research Manager Pennsylvania Turnpike Commission PO Box 67676 Harrisburg, PA 17106 U.S.A. Tel: 717-939-9551 ext. 3620	• drift-off-road accidents were increasing by over 50% on the Pennsylvania Turnpike • developed in the 1980s, rumble-strips maintained and implemented by the Pennsylvania Turnpike Commission	• development, research, and evaluation completely funded by the Pennsylvania Turnpike Commission • outside contractors were used for implementation	• full testing at test sites and actual turnpike sections • print and television media were used to publicize the innovation • positive test results led to implementation on the whole system	• 60% reduction in drift-off-road accidents • no degradation in the product after extended use • awarded the IBTTA Innovation Award • now used widely on many American interstates and 4-lane highways	✓	✓ ✓	✓

Motor vehicle and road-related injury prevention—*(Continued)*

Age group served	Prevention area	Program name	Contact information	Background	Resources	Implementation	Outcome	Evaluation	Engineering	Enactment
Children aged 5–9 years	Pedestrian safety	Child Pedestrian Injury Prevention Project	Mark Stevenson, PhD Chief Investigator, Child Pedestrian Injury Prevention Project, Department of Epidemiology and Biostatistics, School of Public Health Curtin University of Technology GPO Box U1987 Perth, WA 6845 Australia Tel: 08-9266-7121 Fax: 08-9266-2958 Email: mark@health. curtin.edu.au	• project based out of School of Public Health, Curtin University, Perth, Australia • developed and implemented during 3-year period 1995–1997 • target population: school-aged child pedestrians • long-term goal: to reduce pedestrian injury rates among children in western Australia	• funded by the Western Australia Health Promotion Foundation (Healthway), with additional funding from the Traffic Board of Western Australia and Main Roads Western Australia • project based on a modified version of the PRECEDE-PROCEED model	• a quasi-experimental community intervention trial in Perth metropolitan area • employed a multifaceted approach combining behavioural and environmental interventions (2 intervention groups and a comparison group) • "High Intervention Group" received both a school-based pedestrian safety education program and a community/environmental road safety intervention	• children in 2 intervention groups were significantly more likely both to cross the road with adult supervision and to play away from the road • significantly greater road safety activity was observed in the high intervention group • volume of traffic on local roads was significantly reduced in the high intervention group, but not in the other 2 groups • pedestrian safety curriculum materials were incorporated into a Kindergarten–Year 10 education pro-	✓	✓	✓

Motor vehicle and road-related injury prevention—(Continued)

Age group served	Prevention area	Program name	Contact information	Background	Resources	Implementation	Outcome	Evaluation	Engineering	Enactment
					• "Moderate Intervention Group" received only the school-based pedestrian safety education program while "Comparison Group" received no intervention		gram and disseminated state-wide			
Children via caregivers	Child passenger safety	SafetyBeltSafe U.S.A.	Stephanie M. Tombrello, LCSW Executive Director SafetyBeltSafe U.S.A. 1124 W. Carson Street, REI, Bldg. B-4 Torrance, CA 90502 U.S.A. Tel: 310-222-6860 Fax: 310-222-6862 www.carseat.org	• organization developed in 1960 • many initiatives in the area of child passenger safety including certification, check-ups, voucher programs and education	• independently funded through initiatives, contracts and grants	• campaigns involve law enforcement, health services and community • programs have evaluations but are not controlled studies	• organization has had successes in many areas including legislation and regulation changes, design changes, improved assessment techniques, training programs and education	✓	✓	✓

Motor vehicle and road-related injury Prevention—(Concluded)

Age group served	Prevention area	Program name	Contact information	Background	Resources	Implementation	Outcome	Evaluation	Engineering	Enactment
All ages	Road safety	RoadWise	Dennis Bell Manitoba Public Insurance Road Safety 9 THF Ir-234 Donald Winnipeg, MB R3C 4A4 Canada Tel: 204-985-7000 Email: dbell@mpi.mb.ca	• ongoing program implemented 1996 • developed, maintained, and implemented by MPI • target population: all Manitoban drivers and pedestrians • program is a group of incident/population-specific programs	• road safety formal MPI Department • program has corporate support and funding from MPI	• campaigns employ mass media and direct contact • programs are data-driven and revised and evaluated accordingly • program strives to find fresh approach to an old issue	• program has strong brand-awareness that obviates some of initial introductory work • program has forged partnership with Manitoba Department of Education • reduction in casualty crash reduction since 1996 may be attributable to program • program likely had strong role in self-reported changes in attitude towards safety	✓		

Sports, Playground, and Recreation-Related Injury Prevention

Age group served	Prevention area	Program name	Contact information	Background	Resources	Implementation	Outcome	Evaluation	Engineering	Enactment
All ages	Increasing use of bicycle helmets	Victoria Bicycle Helmet Initiative	Max H. Cameron Senior Research Fellow Monash University Accident Research Centre Melbourne, VIC Australia Tel: 61-3-9905-4373 Fax: 61-3-9905-4363 Email: Max.cameron@ general.monash.edu. au	• broad legislation requiring cyclists to wear approved safety helmet introduced in 1990, following a decade of promotional efforts • developed and implemented by Victorian Road Traffic Authority (VicRoads) • likely benefited from earlier and concurrent injury-prevention campaigns, research, and developments (e.g. motorcycle helmets; drink-driving; helmet engineering)	• major public funding supplemented by various types of private support, including funding • early creation of steering committee of experts, stakeholders, and other interests	• combines educational and legislative approaches • helmet rebate schemes highly effective • dissemination through mass media, private sector, and school system • uses ongoing injury-surveillance data to assess impact of initiative • data collected and analysed by university and public research interests	• dramatic increase in helmet-wearing rates • corresponding reduction in head injuries to cyclists • legislation appears to have reduced number of cyclists	✓	✓	✓

Sports, Playground, and Recreation-Related Injury Prevention—(*Concluded*)

Age group served	Prevention area	Program name	Contact information	Background	Resources	Implementation	Outcome	Evaluation	Engineering	Enactment
Ages 12 and up	Snowmobile safety	Snowmobile Trail Officer Patrol (STOP) Program	Sgt. Lynn Beach, Regional Co-ordinator, STOP OPP 3767 Hwy 69 South, Suite 1 McFarlin Lake Complex Sudbury, ON P3G 1E3 Canada Tel: 705-564-6900 Fax: 705-564-3115	• initiated 1992 • reduction of snowmobiling-related fatality and injury through new legislation and specialized education and enforcement programs • targets ages 12 and older; particular emphasis on males aged 18–35	• provincial and municipal funding • corporate and small business sponsorship • benefits from region-al police ex-pertise and partnership • supported by local in-terest orga-nizations	• collaboration of police, governmental, health care, community, and recrea-tional orga-nizations • new rider safety and licensing pro-gram created • community and mass media dissemination local and pro-vincial coordi-nation	• a 45% decrease in snowmobile-related hospital admissions • estimated an-nual savings of $72,960 in acute health care costs • out-of-province interest	✓		✓

Farm-Related and Occupational Injury Prevention

Age group served	Prevention area	Program name	Contact information	Background	Resources	Implementation	Outcome	Evaluation	Engineering	Enactment
Adult males	Farm	Tractor Rollover Protective Structure (ROPS) Rebate Scheme 1997/98	Dr Lesley M. Day ROPS Rebate Scheme Senior Research Fellow Accident Research Centre Monash University Wellington Rd Clayton, VIC 3168 Australia Tel: 61-3-9902-6000 Email: lesley.day@general.monash.edu.au	• 1-year program (1997/98) • created to facilitate the fitment of ROPS to all previously unprotected tractors in the state of Victoria	• funds were provided by the Victorian WorkCover Authority (VWA), participating farmers, and the Victorian Farmers Federation (VFF)	• combination of regulation, information and awareness programs, and education	• demand for ROPS rebates- was substantially higher than in any previous scheme • penetration of the scheme extended beyond the VFF to include non-members • potential to save lives and to avert psychological trauma for families of victims • general effect on farm safety • decrease in economic cost	✓	✓	✓

Fall-Related Injury Prevention

Age group served	Prevention area	Program name	Contact information	Background	Resources	Implementation	Outcome	Evaluation	Engineering	Enactment
Children via caregivers	Falls from heights	Children Can't Fly	Window Falls Prevention Program Center for Integrated Prevention Programs New York City Department of Health 2 Lafayette Street / 20th Floor New York, NY 10007 Tel: 212-676-2162 Fax: 212-676-2161	• pilot program to prevent falls to children in NYC established in 1972 • expanded from high-risk areas to all of city after first 2 years • developed by the NYC Department of Health in response to high morbidity and mortality rates of children due to falls from heights • included hospital staff and law enforcement agencies in data collection	• a NYCHD program	• media campaign to raise awareness • door-to-door outreach • distribution of vouchers for free window guards to high-risk families in need • ongoing evaluation via data collection through voluntary reports for health and law enforcement agencies	• a decrease in incidence of window falls by 50% in just 3 years • introduction of legislation that requires window guards in all multi-unit dwellings • successful defense of constitutionality of the legislation	✓	✓	✓

Fall-Related Injury Prevention—(*Continued*)

Age group served	Prevention area	Program name	Contact information	Background	Resources	Implementation	Outcome	Evaluation	Engineering	Enactment
Older adults	Falls	Tai Chi; Computerized balance	Dr Steven L. Wolf Professor of Rehab Medicine Centre for Rehab Medicine Emory University School of Medicine 1441 Clifton Rd NE Atlanta, GA 30322 U.S.A. Tel: 404-712-4801 Fax: 404-712-4809 Email: swolf@emory.edu	• part of FICSIT trials	• randomized control trial funded jointly by National Institute on Aging and the National Institute for Nursing Research	• comparison of the use of computerized balance training, Tai Chi, and an educational control group	• delayed onset of falls and reduced risk of multiple falls in Tai Chi intervention group • improved balance in computerized balance training group • increased sway in Tai Chi group • improved psychosocial indicators of well-being in Tai Chi group	✓		

Fall-Related Injury Prevention—(Continued)

Age group served	Prevention area	Program name	Contact information	Background	Resources	Implementation	Outcome	Evaluation	Engineering	Enactment
Older adults	Falls	Multiple-Risk-Factor Reduction Strategy	Dr Dorothy I. Baker Research Scientist, Chronic Disease Epidemiology, School of Public Health Yale University School of Medicine Program in Aging 1N – 129 York St New Haven, CT 06520 U.S.A. Tel: 203-769-9800 Fax: 203-764-9831 Email: dorothy.baker@yale.edu	• part of FICSIT trials • randomized control trial	• matched block design • funded jointly by National Institute on Aging and the National Institute for Nursing Research	• home-based individual assessment of falls risk factors • individually tailored program targeting identified risk factors	• significant reduction of falls as compared with control group • specified intervention strategies directly contributed to the the decrease in falls • associated with lowered health costs	✓	✓	

Fall-Related Injury Prevention—(*Concluded*)

Age group served	Prevention area	Program name	Contact information	Background	Resources	Implementation	Outcome	Evaluation	Engineering	Enactment
Older adults	Falls	No Falls! No Fear! Falls Prevention Program	Nancye Peel Senior Research Officer Healthy Ageing Unit Dept of Social and Preventative Medicine University of Queensland Herston, QLD 4006 Australia Tel: 61-7-3365-5383 Email: n.peel @spmed.uq.edu.au	• 2-year program in 1996/1997 • developed, maintained and implemented by Queensland Health Promotion Council and the Healthy Ageing Research Unit • target population: members of the National Seniors Association • program utilized a multistrand intervention approach to falls prevention • to reduce the number of falls, and their injuries	• Healthy Ageing Unit received funding from the Queensland Health Promotion Council to cover the costs of the program for 2 years	• participants were divided into 4 groups • group 1 was the control group • each group was randomly allocated to receive interventions • Interventions included: information, exercise classes, home modifications, and medical assessments • add-on approach was used	• results showed a significant reduction in the risk of slips and trips in groups 2, 3, and 4 compared to the control group, with evidence also for reduction in the risk of falling • modification of behaviour • modification of intrinsic risk factors • modification of extrinsic risk factors	✓		

Comprehensive Community-Based Injury Prevention

Age group served	Prevention area	Program name	Contact information	Background	Resources	Implementation	Outcome	Evaluation	Engineering	Enactment
Children aged 6–16	Child injury	Harlem Hospital Injury Prevention Program	Erik Cliette Program Associate Director, Harlem Hospital Center 506 Lennox Ave 17102 New York, NY 10037 Tel: 212-939-4005 Email: ec221@columbia.edu	• local initiative implemented 1988 • national program launched 1994 • goal is to reduce child injury through safety education, safe play areas and extracurricular activities • seeks long-term positive impact upon quality of life	• multilevel public, corporate, and private funding • multidisci-plinary per-spective • hospital and university support	• uses hospital-based, on-going injury monitoring data to eval-uate impact • target/control community evaluation • emphasizes community in-put and trust • combines edu-cational and environmental strategies • coverage in-cludes peer-reviewed journals • wide variety of collaborations and programs developed	• substantial and steady decrease in many types of injuries to children • successful repli-cation in numer-ous sites • creation of national network	✓	✓	*

Comprehensive Community-Based Injury Prevention—(Continued)

Age group served	Prevention area	Program name	Contact information	Background	Resources	Implementation	Outcome	Evaluation	Engineering	Enactment
Elementary and high school students	Comprehensive community safety	Think First Foundation	Deborah Johnson Think First Foundation 5550 Meadowbrook Drive, Suite 110 Rolling Meadows, IL 60008 U.S.A. Tel: 1-847-290-8600 Fax: 1-847-290-9005 http://www.thinkfirst.org/ Eleanor Sam, Exec. Dir. Think First Foundation of Canada 2-435 McLaughlin Pavilion 399 Bathurst Street, Toronto, ON M5T 2S8 Canada Tel: 416-603-5212 Fax: 416-603-7795 Email: think1st @netrover.com	• ongoing program initiated in 1986 • school-based injury prevention curriculum • raises general awareness of preventable injury • influences policy initiatives	• private and charitable funding • modular classroom program is geared to children's developmental progression	• local initiatives supported by national offices • collaboration with educators • employs mass media for awareness raising	• significant increases in knowledge and significant decreases in self-reported risky behaviours	✓		*

Comprehensive Community Based Injury Prevention—(Concluded)

Age group served	Prevention area	Program name	Contact information	Background	Resources	Implementation	Outcome	Evaluation	Engineering	Enactment
All ages; focus upon children and youth	Community health and safety	Latrobe Valley Better Health Project	Henk Harberts, Coordinator – Community Safety Promotion Latrobe Valley Better Health Project Latrobe Shire Council PO Box 345 Traralgon, VIC 3844 Australia Tel: 61-03-51-731-506 Fax: 61-03-51-731-558 Email: henka@ latrobe.vic.gov.au	• launched in 1992 following developmental phase begun in 1990 • targets home, playground, and sports injuries and alcohol misuse among youth • based upon successful Swedish model implemented during the 1980s • primary aim was to utilize a community intervention approach to prevent injuries, reduce hazards and increase public awareness of injury prevention	• initial funding received from the Victorian Health Promotion Foundation; later received financial support from both private and public sources • collaborative planning • planned impact evaluation • proven community development model • utilized 2 separate injury-surveillance data collection systems	• methodical planning, implementation, and evaluation of health promotion and education programs • development of initial and ongoing steering committees • multifactorial intervention • close collaboration with community and governmental groups • utilizes both educational and legislative approaches	• evaluation was based on 5 years of emergency department injury surveillance data for the Latrobe Valley • significant decreases observed in all targeted injuries • increase in purchase of home safety items • public playground equipment and surfaces upgraded for greater safety • lack of comparison/control community	✓	✓	✓

Appendix D: Contact Directory

General/Other

Adams, Dr Brian J.
Accident Compensation Corporation
Program Manager
Prism
PO Box 1595
Wellington
New Zealand
Tel: +64-4-918-7911
Fax: +64-4-918-3979
Email: adamsb@acc.org.nz

American Academy of Neurology
1080 Montreal Ave
St Paul, MN 55116-2311
U.S.A.
Tel: 651-695-1940
Fax: 651-695-2791
Email: web@aan.com

Basset-Spiers, Kent
Executive Director
Ontario Neurotrauma Foundation
201 – 520 Sutherland Dr
Toronto, ON M4G 3Y9
Canada
Tel: 416-422-2228
Fax: 416-422-1240
Website: http://www.onf.org.ca

Brown, Jennifer
Senior Consultant
Safety Centre
Royal Children's Hospital
Flemington Rd
Parkville, VIC 3052
Australia
Tel: +61-3-9345-6983
Fax: +61-3-9345-5086
Email: brownje@
    cryptic.rch.unimelb.edu.au

Browne, Doug
Division of Acute Care Rehabilita-
   tion Research and Disability
   Prevention (DACRRDP)
4770 Buford Hwy NE
MS K63
Atlanta, GA 30341
U.S.A.
Tel: 770-488-4031
Email: drb7@CDC.gov

Chipman, Mary
Preventative Medicine & Bio-
   statistics
University of Toronto
12 Queen's Park Cres W
Toronto, ON M5S 1A8
Canada
Tel: 416-978-6150
Fax: 416-978-8299
Email:
   chipman@pmb.med.utoronto.ca

Conn, Dr Robert
President / CEO
SMARTRISK Foundation
301 – 658 Danforth Ave
Toronto, ON M4J 5B9
Canada
Tel: 416-463-9878
Email: rconn@SMARTRISK.ca

Dayler, Linda
Community Program Developer
Trauma Prevention Council Central
   West
Toronto, ON M4J 5B9
Canada
Tel: 905-535-7149
Fax: 905-525-4994
Email: ldayler@skylinc.net

Diamond, Kim
Director of Programs
SMARTRISK
301 – 658 Danforth Ave
Toronto, ON M4J 5B9
Canada
Tel: 416-463-9878
Email: kdiamond@SMARTRISK.ca

Elkington, Dr Jane
Jane Elkington & Associates
9 Chaleyer St
Willoughby, NSW 2068
Australia
Tel: +61-2-9417-5102
Fax: +61-2-9417-8513
Email: elkingtn@ozEmail.com.au

Emery, Laura
Project Officer, Injury Control
   Program
Health Dept of WA
PO Box 8172, Perth Business Centre
Perth, WA 6845
Australia
Tel: +61-8-9222-2166
Fax: +61-8-9222-4471
Email: icc@iccwa.org.au

Grover, Kelly
Health Promotion Specialist
Hospital for Sick Children
555 University Ave
Toronto, ON M5G 1X8
Canada
Tel: 416-813-5165
Email: kelly.grover@sickkids.on.ca

Hendry, Chris
Public Affairs
Clarke Institute
33 Russell St
Toronto, ON M5S 2S1
Canada
Tel: 416-535-8501

Jackson, Mark RS
Center for Disease Control
National Center for Injury Preven-
    tion and Control
Division of Unintentional Injury
    Prevention
4770 Buford Highway, MS K-63
Atlanta, GA 30341
U.S.A.
Tel: 770-488-4754
Fax: 770-488-1317
Email: mcj4@cdc.gov

Kids In Danger
PO Box 146608
Chicago, IL 60614-6608
U.S.A.
Fax: 773-296-9658
Email:
    linda.ginzel@gsb.uchicago.edu

Langley, Dr John
Director
Injury Prevention Research Unit
Dept of Otago Medical School
PO Box 913
Dunedin
New Zealand
Tel: +64-3-479-8511
Fax: +64-3-479-8337
Email: john.langley@
    stonebow.otago.ac.nz

Lantz, Sue
SMARTRISK
301 – 658 Danforth Ave
Toronto, ON M4J 5B9
Canada
Tel: 416-463-9878 x22
Fax: 416-463-0137
Email: slantz@SMARTRISK.ca

Loos, Colleen
Co-ordinator
Australian Injury Prevention Data-
    base
Dept of Social and Preventive
    Medicine
University of Queensland
4th Floor, North Wing, Diamantina
    House
Princess Alexandra Hospital
Woolloongabba, QLD 4102
Australia
Tel: +61-7-3240-5813
Fax: +61-7-3391 4874
Website: http://spmed.uq.edu.au/
    aipd

Marsh, Nigel
Neuropsychology – Injury Preven-
    tion Authority
University of Waikato
New Zealand
Tel: 011-64-78-56-2889, ext. 8399
Fax: 011-64-78-56-2158
Email: samiam@waikato.ac.nz

McCarthy-Kent, Beth
Sudbury General Hospital
Regional Trauma Network
St Joseph's Centre
700 Paris St
Sudbury, ON P3E 3B5
Canada
Tel: 705-674-3181
Tel: 705-675-4765
Email: bmmcarthykent@
    hrsrh.on.ca

Mills, Janice
Health Educator Northern Rivers
    Area Health Service
NSW Health Dept
Casino Memorial Hospital
PO Box 268
Casino, NSW 2470
Australia
Tel: +61-2-6662-2111
Fax: +61-2-6662-3774
Email: janm@nrhs.health.nsw.gov.au

Minuzzo, Barbara
Secretariat
AIPN (Australia Injury Prevention
    Network)
Safety Centre
Royal Children's Hospital
Flemington Rd
Parkville, 3072
Australia
Tel: +61-3-9345 5786
Email:
    safety@cryptic.rch.unimelb.edu.au

Morrison, Dr Luke
Junior Research Fellow
Injury Prevention Research Unit
University of Otago
Dunedin
New Zealand
Tel: +64-3-479-8503
Fax: +64-3-479-8837
Email: luke.morrison@
    stonebow.otago.ac.nz

Munro, James
Medical Care Research Unit
University of Sheffield
Regent Court
30 Regent St
Sheffield, S1 4DA
United Kingdom
Tel: +44-114 222 0759
Fax: +44-114 222 0749
Email: j.f.munro@sheffield.ac.uk

Ontario Brain Association
PO Box 2338
St Catharines, ON L2R 7R9
Canada
Tel: 905-641-8877
Fax: 905-641-0323
Email: obia@obia.on.ca

Paramore, Vivienne
Project Officer
South West Brain Injury Rehabilita-
    tion Service
PO Box 326
Albury, NSW 2640
Australia
Tel: +61-2-6041-9902
Fax: +61-2-6041-9928
Email: vivienne.paramore@
    swsahs.nsw.gov.au

Parsons, Daria
Canadian Institute for Health
  Information
300 – 90 Eglinton Ave E
Toronto, ON M4P 2Y3
Canada
Tel: 416-481-1616
Fax: 416-481-2950

Reeder, Tony
Cancer Society Research Fellow
Social and Behavioural Research in
  Cancer Group
Dept of Preventive and Social
  Medicine
Dunedin School of Medicine
PO Box 913
Dunedin
New Zealand
Tel: +64-3-479 7257
Fax: +64-3-479 7298
Email: treeder@gandalf.otago.ac.nz

Ritchie, Jill
Peterborough County Health Unit
10 Hospital Dr
Peterborough, ON K9J 8M1
Canada
Tel: 705-743-1000
Fax: 705-743-2897

Rivara, Dr Frederick MD, MPH
Director of Harborview Injury
  Prevention and Research Center
Box 359960
325 Ninth Ave
Seattle, WA 98104-2499
U.S.A.
Tel: 206-521-1530
Fax: 206-521-1562

Rock, Allan
Federal Minister of Health
613-947-5000
Government Health Care Promotions and Programs
1-800-O CANADA

Rosenberg, Mark L.
Executive Director
The Task Force for Child Survival
  and Development
750 Commerce Drive, Suite 400
Decatur, GA 30030-2622
U.S.A.
Tel: 800-765-7173
Tel: 404-687-5635
Fax: 404-371-1087
Email: mrosenberg@taskforce.org

Selby, Leigh
Executive Officer
Spinesafe
PO Box 3023
Putney, NSW 2112
Australia
Tel: +61-2-9808-9202
Fax: +61-2-9809-6521
Email: spinesafe@one.net.au

Servadei, Dr F.
Division of Neurosurgery
Hospital M. Bufalini
Cesena, Italy
Fax: 39047 304664
Email: servadei@mbox.queen.it

Smith, Dr Gordon S MB, ChB, MPH
Associate Professor
The Center for Injury Research and
Policy
The Johns Hopkins University
School of Hygiene and Public
Health
Baltimore, MD 21205
U.S.A.
Email: gsmith@jhsph.edu

Speller, Dr Viv M
University of Southampton
Dept of Public Health
Highfield
Southampton, SO17 1BJ
United Kingdom
Tel: +44-023-8059-5601
Fax: +44-023-8059-5662
Email: v.m.speller@soton.ac.uk

Stewart, Tanya Charyk
London Health Sciences Centre
800 Commissioners Rd. E.
London, Ontario N6A 4G5
Tel: 1-519-685-8500 ext 77797
Email: tanya.charyk@lhsc.on.ca

Sturtuvant, Derryl
Director
Ministry of Health
Hepburn Block
10th Floor
80 Grosvenor St
Toronto, ON M4S 5B8
Tel: 416-327-7719

Threat, Cecil
Centers for Disease Control
4770 Buford Hwy. NE
MS K63
Atlanta, GA 30341
U.S.A.
Tel: 770-488-1307
Fax: 770-488-1317
Email: Ctt3@cdc.gov

Thurman, Dr David J
Medical Epidemiologist
Division of Acute Care, Rehabilita-
tion Research and Disability
Prevention
National Center for Injury Preven-
tion and Control
Centers for Disease Control and
Prevention
Mailstop K65
4770 Buford Highway NE
Atlanta, GA 30 341-3124
U.S.A.
Tel: 770-488-4715
Fax: 700-488-4338
Email: dxt9@cdc.gov

Tremblay, Bill
Prevention Coordinator
Brain Injury Association
Violence and Brain Injury Institute
105 N Alfred St
Alexandria, VA 22314
U.S.A.
Tel: 703-236-6000
Fax: 736-736-6001
Email: btremblay@biausA..org

Vulcan, Peter
Professor
Accident Research Centre
Monash University
Wellington Rd
Clayton, VIC 3168
Australia
Tel: +61-3-9905-1816
Fax: +61-3-9905-4363
Email: peter.vulcan@
    general.monash.edu.au

Asphyxiation-Related Injuries

The Danny Foundation
12901 Alcosta Blvd
Suite 2C
San Ramon, CA 94583
U.S.A.
Tel: 1-800-83-DANNY
Email: dannycrib@earthlink.net

Dzugan, Jerry
Director, AMSEA (American Marine
    Safety Education Association)
    Program
PO Box 2592
Sitka, AK 99835
U.S.A.
Tel: 907-747-3287
Fax: 907-747-3259
Website: http://www.uaf.edu/
    seagrant/amsea/

Dworkin, Gerry
Consultant, Aquatics Safety & Water
    Rescue Lifesaving Resources
10 Main St, PO BOX 905
Harrisville, NH 03450
U.S.A.
Tel: 603-827-4139
Email: admin@lifesaving.com
Website: http://
    www.lifesaving.com

Gilbert, Ronald R.
Director, Aquatic Injury Safety
    Group
1555 Penobscot Building
Detroit, MI 48226
U.S.A.
Chairman, Foundation for Aquatic
    Injury Prevention
1310 Ford Building
Detroit, MI 48226-3901
U.S.A.
Tel: 313-963-1600
Email: info@aquaticisf.org
Website: http://
    www.aquaticisf.org/index.html

Karmol, David
National Spa and Pool Institute
2111 Eisenhower Ave
Alexandria, VA 22314
U.S.A.
Tel: 703-838-9983
Email: dkarmal@nspi.org
Website: http://www.nspi.org

National Swimming Pool Foundation
300 – 10803 Gulfdale
San Antonio, TX 78213
U.S.A.
Tel: 210-525-1227
Email: lknspf@aol.com

Pitt, Dr W. Robert
Director, Paediatric Emergency
Mater Children's Hospital
Annerly Road, South Brisbane
QLD 4101
Australia
Tel: 617-3840-3825
Email: rpitt@mater.org.au

Stay On Top of It
Washington State Drowning Prevention Project
Children's Hospital and Regional Medical Center
PO Box 5371
Mail Stop CM-09
Seattle, WA 98105
U.S.A.
Email: mmurp2@chmc.org

Swift, Ed
Founder of Children's Safety Zone
Swift Office Solutions
6 – 2429 W 12th St
Tempe, AZ 85281
U.S.A.
Tel: 1-800-522-3308
Email: sos@sosnet.com

Waxweiler, Dr Richard
Acting Deputy Director
National Center for Injury Prevention and Control
4770 Buford Hwy K02
Atlanta, GA 30341-3724
U.S.A.
Tel: 770-488-4694
Fax: 770-488-4422
Email: rjw2@cdc.gov

Motor- and Other Road Vehicle–Related Injuries

Ayton, Mark
Ontario Ministry of Transportation
301 St Paul St
St Catharines, ON L2R 7R1
Tel: 1-800-268-4686
Email: mark.ayton@mto.gov.on.ca

Banfield, Joanne, RN
Manager, Trauma Injury Prevention
PARTY Program
Sunnybrook and Women's College Health Sciences Centre
Office for Injury Prevention, Room H259
2075 Bayview Ave
Toronto, ON M4N 3M5
Canada
Tel: 416-480-5912
Fax: 416-480-6865
Email:
    joanne.banfield@swchsc.on.ca

Bell, Dennis
Manitoba Public Insurance
Road Safety
9 THF lr-234 Donald
Winnipeg, MB R3C 4A4
Canada
Tel: 205-985-7000
Tel: 204-985-7199
Email: dbell@mpi.mb.ca

Bierness, Doug
Director, Information and Commu-
  nication
Traffic Injury Research Foundation
200 – 171 Nepean St
Ottawa, ON K2P 0B4
Canada
Tel: 613-238-5235
Fax: 613-238-5292

Bihrensdorsf, Ing
Danish Council for Road Safety
  Research
Lersø Parkallé III
2100 København Ø
Tel: 011-45-39-68-04-44
Fax: 011-45-39-16-39-40
Email: rft@rft.dk
Homepage:
  www.faerdselssikkerhed.dk

Carsten, Dr Oliver M.J.
Director of Research and Principal
  Research Fellow
Institute for Transport Studies
University of Leeds
36 University Rd
Leeds LS2 9JT
United Kingdom
Tel: +44-113-233-5348
Fax: +44-113-233-5334
Email: ocarsten@its.leeds.ac.uk

Cavallo, Antonietta
Senior Psychologist Road Safety
VicRoads, 4th Floor North Wing
60 Denmark St
Kew, VIC 3101
Australia
Tel: +61-3-9854-2627
Fax: +61-3-9854-2668
Email:
  cavalla@vrnotes.roads.vic.gov.au

Chin, Hoong Chor
Associate Professor
Dept of Civil Engineering & Centre
  for Transportation Research
National University of Singapore
10 Kent Ridge Cres
Singapore 119260
Tel: 65-874-2550
Fax: 65-779-1635
Email: cvechc@leonis.nus.edu.sg

Corbo, Maria
Monash University
Accident Research Centre
PO Box 70A
Monash University, VIC 3800
Australia
Tel: +61-3-9905-1805
Fax: +61-3-9905-1809
Email:
  maria.corbo@general.monash.edu.au

Cross, Dr Donna, EdD
Chief Investigator, Child Pedestrian
  Injury Prevention Project
Centre for Health Promotion Re-
  search
School of Public Health
Curtin University of Technology
Perth, WA 6845
Australia
Tel: +61-8-9266-7944
Email: dcross@health.curtin.edu.au

D'Angelo, Dan
Director, Design Quality
New York Dept of Transportation
Albany, New York 12205
Tel: 518-457-6467

Diamond, Kim
Director of Programs
HEROES
SMARTRISK
301 – 658 Danforth Ave.
Toronto, ON M4J 5B9
Canada
Tel: 416-463-9878
Email: kdiamond@SMARTRISK.ca

Donnelly, Dr Bruce R PhD
Principal Engineer, Veridian Engi-
  neering
Research Associate Professor
Emergency Medicine
State University of New York at
  Buffalo
Box 400, Buffalo, NY 14225
U.S.A.
Tel: 716-631-6798
Fax: 716-631-6348
Email:
  bdonnelly@buffalo.veridian.com

Garder, Per
Associate Professor, Transportation
Dept of Civil & Environmental
  Engineering
University of Maine
Orono, ME 04469-5711
U.S.A.
Tel: 207-581-2177
Fax: 207-581-3888
Email: garder@maine.edu

Hall, Margaret, PhD
Program Director, Child Pedestrian
  Injury Prevention Project
Centre for Health Promotion Re-
  search
School of Public Health
Curtin University of Technology
Perth, WA 6845
Australia
Tel: +61-08-9266-2115
Email: mhall@health.curtin.edu.au

Hargrave, Martin W.
U.S. Dept of Transportation
Federal Highway Administration
Mail Code: HRDS-04
6300 Georgetown Pike
McLean, VA 22101
U.S.A.
Tel: 202-493-3311
Email:
  martin.hargrave@fhwa.dot.gov

Herrstedt, Lene
Danish Road Directorate
Traffic Research Division
Stationsalleeen 42
2730 Herlev
Denmark
Tel: +45-33-93-33-38
Email: leh@vd.dk

Hickey, John
Pennsylvania Shoulder Rumble
    Strips
Research Manager
Pennsylvania Turnpike Commission
PO Box 67676
Harrisburg, PA 17106
U.S.A.
Tel: 717-939-9551 x3620
Email: jhickey@paturnpike.com

Hoo, Viola
Technical Service Representative
Scotchlite Reflective Fabrics &
    Thinsulate Insulation Product
3M Canada Company
1840 Oxford St E
London, ON N5V 3R6
Canada
Tel: 1-800-265-1840
Fax: 519-452-6142

Howard, Ian
Professor
Dept of Mechanical Engineering
University of Sheffield
United Kingdom
Tel: +44-114-222-7740
Email: i.howard@sheffield.ac.uk

Hydén, Christer
Professor, Dept for Technology and
    Society
Division for Traffic Engineering
Lund Institute of Technology
Box 118
221 00 Lund
Sweden
Tel: +46-46-222-91-30
Fax: +46-46-12-32-72
Email: christer.hyden@tft.lth.se

Isler, Dr Robert
Traffic and Road Safety Group
New Zealand
University of Waikato
Private Bag 3105
Hamilton, New Zealand
Tel: 011-64-78-56-2889

Jack, Ronald, Peng
Project Consultant, Canadian
    Guide to Neighbourhood Traffic
    Calming
Manager, Transportation Division
Delcan Corporation
1233 Michael
Gloucester, ON K1J 7T2
Canada
Tel: 613-738-4160
Email: ottawa@delcan.com

Jakobsson, Lotta
Volvo Car Corp
Dept 98241 PV21
SE-405 31 Gothenburg
Sweden
Tel: +46-31-591814
Fax: +46-31-595922
Email: vcc2.lottaja@memo.volvo.se

Johnson, Mavis
Manager, Road Improvement
    Strategies
Insurance Corporation of British
    Columbia
151 West Esplanade
North Vancouver, BC V7M 3H9
Canada
Tel: 604-661-6426
Email: majohns@icbc.com

Kodama, Steven
Toronto Works & Emergency
 Services
Transportation Services
703 Don Mills Ave
Toronto, ON M3C 3N3
Canada
Tel: 416-392-9633
Fax: 416-392-4940
Email:
 steven_kodama@city.toronto.on.ca

Koepsell, Dr Thomas
Professor of Epidemiology/Health
 Services
Adjunct Professor of Medicine
Dept of Epidemiology
University of Washington
Box 357236
Seattle, WA 98195-7236
U.S.A.
Tel: 206-543-8830
Fax: 206-543-8525
Email: koepsell@u.washington.edu

Lam, Yvonne
Executive Secretary
Road Engineering Association of
 Asia and Australia
46B, Jalan Bola Tampar 13/14
Section 13
40100 Shah Alam
Email: reaaa@po.jar.my

Mongeon, Sheila
Program Coordinator
PARTY Program Ottawa
Ottawa Hospital, Trauma Services
501 Smyth Rd, MB# 304
Ottawa, ON K1H 8L6
Canada
Tel: 613-737-8848
Fax: 613-737-8470
Email: smongeon@ogh.on.ca

Mortimer, Nigel
Defects Investigator
Transport Canada
Tel: 1-800-333-0510

Newstead, Stuart
Research Fellow
Monash University
Accident Research Centre
Monash University
PO Box 70A
Monash University, VIC 3800
Australia
Tel: + 61-3-9905-4364
Fax: +61-3-9905-4363
Email: stuart.newstead@
 general.monash.edu.au

Nilsson, Annika
Institutionen för Teknik och
 Samhälle
Avdelningen för Trafikteknik
Box 11
221 00 Lund
Sweden
Tel: 046-2223101
Fax: 046-123272
Email: annika.nilsson@tft.lth.se

O'Rourke, Dominique
The Co-operators
130 Macdonnell St
Guelph, ON N1H 6P8
Canada
Tel: 519-824-4400
Fax: 519-826-2925
Email: dominique-orouke@
    cooperators.ca

Patterson, Eve
Insurance Bureau of Canada
1800 – 151 Yonge St
Toronto, ON M5C 2W7
Canada
Tel: 416-362-2031
Fax: 416-362-2602
Email: epatterson@ibc.ca

Retting, Richard
Senior Transportation Engineer
Insurance Institute for Highway
    Safety
1005 N. Glebe Rd
Arlington, VA 22201–4751
U.S.A.
Tel: 703-247-1582
Email: rretting@iihs.org

Rush, John
LTPP Customer Support
U.S. Department of Transportation
Federal Highway Association
Turner-Fairbank Highway Research
    Center
6300 Georgetown Pike, HRDI-13
McLean, VA 22101-2296
Tel: 865-481-2967
Fax: 202-493-3161
Email: john.w.rush@saic.com

Sakuma, Seiji
Director, International Affairs
VERTIS
Nishi-Shimbashi Tachikawa
    Building
2-11-4 Nishi-Shimbashi, Minato-ku
Tokyo 105-0003
Japan
Tel: +81-3-3519-2181
Fax: +81-3-3592-0091

Sayed, Dr Tarek PEng
Assistant Professor
Dept of Civil Engineering
University of British Columbia
2324 Main Mall
Vancouver, BC V6T 1Z4
Canada
Tel: 604-822-4379
Fax: 604-822-6901
Email: tsayed@civil.ubc.ca

Small, Martin
Road Safety Programme Manager
Accident Compensation Corpora-
    tion
Prism
PO Box 242
Wellington
New Zealand
Tel: +64-4-918-7975
Fax: +64-4-918-3979
Email: smallm@acc.org.nz

Smith, Bruce W.
Director of Traffic Engineering and
 Highway Safety Division
NYS Dept of Transportation
1220 Washington Avenue, 5-312
Albany, New York 12232-0748
Tel: 518-457-0271
Fax: 518-457-1780
Email: bwsmith@gw.dot.state.ny.us

Stewart, Sheilagh
Ministry of the Attorney General
729 Bay St, 9th Floor
Toronto, ON M5G 2K1
Canada
Tel: 416-326-4660
Fax: 416-326-2423
Email:
 sheilagh.stewart@jus.gov.on.ca

Stewart, Tanya Charyk
London Health Sciences Centre
Tel: 519-685-8500 ext 77797
Email: tanya.charyk@lhsc.on.ca

Stevenson, Mark, PhD
Chief Investigator, Child Pedestrian
 Injury Prevention Project
Dept of Epidemiology and Bio-
 statistics
School of Public Health
Curtin University of Technology
Perth, WA 6845
Australia
Tel: +61-08-9266-7121
Email: mark@health.curtin.edu.au

Taft, Camilla
National SAFE KIDS Buckle Up
1301 Pennsylvania Avenue, N.W.
Suite 1000
Washington, DC 20004-1707
U.S.A.
Tel: 202-662-0600
Fax: 202-393-2072
Website: http://www.safekids.org

Tombrello, Stephanie M., LCSW
Executive Director
1124 W. Carson Street, REI, Bldg. B-4
Torrance, CA 90502
U.S.A.
Tel: 310-222-6860
Fax: 310-222-6862
Website: http://www.carseat.org

Williamson, John P.
Program Manager
OBD (Operation Buckle Down)
ODWI (Operation Driving While
 Impaired)
NMSHTD Traffic Safety Bureau
Tel: 505-827-0904
Email: john.williamson@
 nmshtd.state.nm.us

Whittaker, Iris
Manager, Business Information
 Centre
VicRds
Ground Floor North
60 Denmark St
Kew, VIC 3101
Australia
Tel: +61-3-9854-2447
Fax: +61-3-9853-0084
Email: iris_whittaker@
 vrnotes.Rds.vic.gov.au

Van der Zijpp, Dr Nanne
Variable Message Signs
Dept of Civil Engineering
Delft University of Technology
Postbus 5048
2600 GA Delft
Netherlands
Tel: +31-15-278-5485
Fax: +31-15-278-3179
Email: zijpp@ct.tudelft.nl

Várhelyi, Dr András
University Lecturer
Dept of Technology and Society
Lund University
Box 118
221 00 LUND
Sweden
Tel: +46-46-222-48-24
Fax: +46-46-12-32-72
Email: andras.varhelyi@tft.lth.se

Veneziano, John
Traffic Engineeer
Dept of Public Works
10455 Armstrong St
Fairfax, VA 22030
U.S.A.
Tel: 703-385-7810
Email: jveneziano@ci.fairfax.va.us

Sports, Playground, and Recreation-Related Injury

Beach, Sgt Lynne
Regional Coordinator
STOP (Snowmobile Trail Officer
    Patrol)
Ontario Provincial Police
3767 Hwy 69 South, Suite 1
McFarlin Lake Complex
Sudbury, ON P3G 1E3
Canada
Tel: 705-564-6900
Fax: 705-654-3115
Email: lynn.beach@jus.gov.on.ca

Beringer, Carol
Coordinator
KIDSAFE Connection
Alberta Children's Hospital
Calgary Regional Health Authority
1820 Richmond Road S.W.
Calgary, AB T2T 5C7
Tel: 403-229-7833
Fax: 403-541-7533
Email: carol.beringer@
    crha-health.ab.ca

Besner, Norman
Director/Supervisor
FCMQ (The Quebec Federation of
    Snowmobile Clubs)
4545 Ave Pierre de Coubertin
PO Box 1000 Station M
Montreal, PQ H1V 3R2
Canada
Tel: 514-252-3076
Fax: 514-254-2066
Email: info@fcmq.qc.ca

Bisschop, Sean, MA
Psychometrist/Research Coordina-
  tor
Neurorehabilitation Program –
  Neurology Service
Toronto Rehabilitation Institute
550 University Ave, 7th Floor
Toronto, ON M5G 2A2
Canada
Tel: 416-597-3422 ext. 3608
Fax: 416-597-3044
Email:
  bisschop.sean@torontorehab.on.ca

Blitvich, Jenny
Lecturer, School of Human Move-
  ment and Sports Sciences
University of Ballarat
PO Box 663
Ballarat, VIC 3352
Australia
Tel: +61-3-5327-9690
Fax: +61-3-5327-9478
Email: j.blitvich@ballarat.edu.au

Cameron, Max H.
Senior Research Fellow
Monash University Accident Re-
  search Centre
Melbourne, VIC
Australia
Tel: +61 3 9905 4373
Fax: +61 3 9905 4363
Email: max.cameron@
  general.monash.edu.au

Comper, Dr Paul
Clinical Psychologist, Neuropsy-
  chology
Neurorehabilitation Program –
  Neurology Service
Toronto Rehabilitation Institute
550 University Ave, 7th Floor
Toronto, ON M5G 2A2
Canada
Tel: 416-597-3422 x3035
Fax: 416-597-3044
Email:
  comper.paul@torontorehab.on.ca

Foot, Richard
STOP (Snowmobile Trail Officer
  Patrol)
3767 Hwy 69 South, Suite 1
McFarlin Lake Complex
Sudbury, ON P3G 1E3
Tel: 416-383-2300, ext. 2282

Frantzell, Magnus
Manager
Volunteer License for Driving
  Program
Snowmobile Safety
Box 5516
11485 Stockholm
Sweden
Tel: 011-46-86-67-5834
Fax: 011-46-86-67-3491
Email: magnus.frantzell@quicknet.se

Garneau, Michel
Canadian Council of Snowmobile
  Organisations
4545 Ave. Pierre de Coubertin
P.O. Box 1000, Station M
Montreal, Que.
Canada H1V 3R2
Tel: 514-252-3002
Fax: 514-252-0361

Gilchrist, Dr Julie
Division of Unintentional Injury
  Prevention
National Center for Injury Preven-
  tion and Control
4770 Buford Hwy NE, Mailstop K63
Atlanta, GA 30341
U.S.A.
Tel: 770-488-4652
Email: jrg7@cdc.gov

Giles, Ken
U.S. Consumer Product Safety
  Commission
Washington, DC 20207
U.S.A.
Tel: 301-504-0580
Website: www.cpsc.gov

Goulet, Dr Claude
Conseiller en recherche
Direction de la sécurité
Secrétariat au loisir et au sport
Ministère de la Santé et des Services
  sociaux
306 – 100, rue Laviolette
Trois-Rivières, PQ G9A 5S9
Canada
Tel: 819-371-6140
Fax: 819-371-6992
Email:
  claude.goulet@msss.gouv.qc.ca

Green, Dr Robin
Clinical Psychologist, Neuropsy-
  chology
Research Associate
Neurorehabilitation Program – ABI
  & Neurology Services
Toronto Rehabilitation Institute
550 University Ave
Toronto, ON M5G 2A2
Canada
Tel: 416-597-3422 x3593
Fax: 416-597-3044
Email:
  green.robin@torontorehab.on.ca

Klim, Ed
President
ISMA (International Snowmobile
  Manufacturers Association)
170 – 1640 Haslett Rd
Haslett, Michigan 48840
U.S.A.
Tel: 517-339-7788
Fax: 517-339-7798
Email: snow@snowmobile.org

Kristman, Vicki L.
PhD candidate, Epidemiology
Dept of Public Health Sciences
University of Toronto
12 Queen's Park Cres. W.
Toronto, ON M5S 1A8
Canada
Tel: 416-767-8525
Fax: 416-978-8299
Email: v.kristman@utoronto.ca

Kuhn, Kelcy
Chair
Canadian Parks and Recreation
    Association
National Playground Safety Initia-
    tive
Tel: 506-325-4650
Fax: 506-325-4541
Email: kelcy.kuhn@gov.nb.ca

Lesage, Dominique
Agent de planification/
    programmation
Régie régional de la Santé et des
    Services sociaux
Direction de la santé publique
Prévention des traumatismes
    (ÉCOHS)
1301, rue Sherbrooke E
Montréal, PQ H2L 1M3
Canada

Longman, Rob
Director
War Amps – Play Safe Program
Playsafe/Drivesafe Program
The War Amps Key Tag Service
1 Maybrook Drive
Scarborough, ON M1V 5K9
Canada
Tel: 416-297-2665

Mack, Dr Mick G.
University of Northern Iowa
School of Health, Physical Education
    & Leisure Services
WRC 133
Cedar Falls, IA 50614-0241
U.S.A.
Tel: 319-273-6129
Email: mickey.mack@uni.edu

Mackenzie, Kevin
Canadian Playground Safety
    Institute
CSA International
178 Rexdale Blvd
Toronto, ON M9W 1R3
Canada
Tel: 613-748-5651 (general)
Tel: 416-747-2496
Fax: 416-747-2473

Mainwaring, Lynda
Assistant professor
Faculty of Physical Education and
    Health
University of Toronto
55 Harbord St
Toronto, ON M5S 2W6
Canada
Tel: 416-946-5134
Fax: 416-978-4384
Email:
    lynda.mainwaring@utoronto.ca

McLean, Glen
Director
Canadian Parks and Recreation
    Association National Playground
    Safety Initiative
306–1600 James Naismith Drive
Gloucester, ON K1B 5N4
Canada
Tel: 613-748-5651
Fax: 613-748-5854
Email: cpra@activeliving.ca

National Playground Safety Inspec-
tor Certification Course and Exam
22377 Belmont Ridge Rd
Ashburn, VA 20148
U.S.A.
Tel: 703-858-2148
Fax: 703-858-0794
Email: cflocke@nrpu.org

O'Rourke, Kevin
Safety Manager
OFSC (Ontario Federation of
Snowmobile Clubs)
12–106 Saunders Road
Barrie, ON L4N 9A8
Canada
Tel: 705-739-5005 or 705-739-7669
Fax: 705-739-5005
Email: korourke@ofsc.on.ca

Payne, Scott
Researcher
NC State University's Recreation
Resources Service
4012 – A Biltmore Hall, Box 8004
Raleigh, NC 276955-7118
Email: scott_payne@ncsu.edu

Pitt, Dr W. Robert
Director, Pediatric Emergency
Mater Children's Hospital
Annerley Rd
South Brisbane, QLD 4101
Australia
Tel: +61-7-3840-3825
Email: rpitt@mater.org.au

Richards, Dr Doug
Medical Director and Assistant
Professor
Faculty of Physical Education &
Health
University of Toronto
55 Harbord St
Toronto, ON M5S 2W6
Canada
Tel: 416-978-7377 (academic)
Tel: 416-978-4678 (clinical)
Fax: 416-971-2846
Email: doug.richards@utoronto.ca

Roberts, William O., MD
MinnHealth Family Physicians
4786 Banning Ave
White Bear Lake, MN 55110
U.S.A.
Tel: 651-426-6402
Email: rober037@tc.umn.edu

Roseveare, Christine
Regional Public Health
Hutt Valley Health Corporation Ltd
Wellington
New Zealand
Tel: +64-4-570-9140
Fax: +64-4-570-9212
Email:
christine.roseveare@hvh.co.nz

Schipilow, Bill
Fair Play in Minor Hockey
17 Canterbury St
Dartmouth, NS B2Y 1S8
Canada
Tel: 902-469-6203
Fax: 902-469-0062
Email: bschipilow@auracom.com

Sbeghen, Bart
Campaigns
Bicycle Victoria Campaigns
19 O'Connell Street
North Melbourne
GPO Box 1961R, Melbourne 3001
Australia
Tel: 03-9328-3000
Fax: 03-9328-2288
Email: barts@bv.com.au

Stubbington, Kevin
S.T.O.P. ("Safety Towards Other
    Players")
1716 Benjamin Ave
Windsor, ON N8X 4N6
Canada
Tel: 519-256-2318
Fax: 519-256-8349
Email: s.t.o.p@sympactico.ca

Tator, Dr Charles H.
Professor and Past Chair of Neuro-
    surgery
University of Toronto, Division of
    Neurosurgery
Toronto Western Hospital
2-435 – 399 Bathurst St
McLaughlin Pavilion
Toronto, ON M5T 2S8
Canada
Tel: 416-603-5889
Fax: 416-603-5298
Email: ctator@torhosp.toronto.on.ca

Thompson, Dr Donna
Project Coordinator,
NPPS (National Program for Play-
    ground Safety)
National Action Plan for the Preven-
    tion of Playground Injuries
University of Northern Iowa
School for Health, Physical Educa-
    tion and Leisure Services
Cedar Falls, IA 50614-0618
U.S.A.
Tel: 1-800-554-PLAY
Tel: 319-273-7529
Fax: 319-273-7308
Email: donna.thompson@uni.edu
Website: http://uni.edu/playground

Tsuji, Ayumi
Assistant
War Amps – PlaySafe Program
1 Maybrook Dr
Scarborough, ON M1V 5K9
Canada
Tel: 416-297-6220 x253
Fax: 416-297-2660
Email: playsafe@waramps.ca

Willer, Dr Barry S.
Professor of Psychiatry
Associate Professor of Rehabilitation
    Medicine, Psychiatry
University of Buffalo
197 Farber Hall
South Campus
SUNY at Buffalo
3435 Main St
Buffalo, NY 14214
U.S.A.
Tel: 716-829-2300
Fax: 716-829-2300
Email: bswiller@buffalou.edu

Farm-Related and Occupational Injury

Bergin, Sue
Research Co-ordinator
Small Business Research Unit
Victoria University of Technology
PO Box 197
213 Nicholson St
Footscray, VIC 3011
Australia
Tel: +61-3-9284-7082
Fax: +61-3-9284-7085
Email: sue.bergin@vu.edu.au
Website: www.business.vut.edu.au/
   sbru

Brehm, Nancy
Agricultural Safety Program
   Associate
National Children's Centre for Rural
   and Agricultural Health and
   Safety
Marshfield Clinic
1000 North Oak Ave
Marshfield, WI 54449-5790
U.S.A.
Tel: 1-888-924-7233
Tel: 715-389-4999
Email: brehmn@mfldclin.edu

Bryson, Dr Rob
Research Director
Department of Community
   Medicine
Queen's University
Kingston, ON
Canada
Tel: 613-549-6666 x3479

Day, Dr Lesley M.
ROPS Rebate Scheme
Senior Research Fellow
Accident Research Center
Monash University
Wellington Rd
Clayton, VIC 3168
Australia
Tel: +61-3-9902-6000
Email:
   lesley.day@general.monash.edu.au

DeBlois, Holly
Rural Youth Safety Specialist
National Children's Centre for Rural
   and Agricultural Health & Safety
Marshfield Clinic
1000 North Oak Ave
Marshfield, WI 54449-5790
U.S.A.
Tel: 1-888-924-7233
Tel: 715-389-4999
Email: debloish@mfldclin.edu

Dosman, Dr Jim
Director
Centre for Agricultural Medicine
University of Saskatchewan
Regina, SK
Canada
Tel: 306-966-8288
Email: dosman@sask.usa.sk.ca

Dyer, Bill
Manager, Workplace Training
National Institute of Disability
   Management and Research
Suite 240, 151 West Esplanade
North Vancouver, BC V7M 3H9
Canada
Tel: 604-646-7570
Email: bill.dyer@icbc.com

Farm Safety 4 Just Kids
P.O. Box 458
Earlham, Iowa
U.S.A.
Tel: 515-758-2827
Email: info@fs4k.org

Farmsafe Western Australia
ThinkSafe Campaign
Safety on the Farm
GPO Box 1577
Canberra, Act 2601
Australia
Tel: +61-8-9388-0019
Email: farmsafe@nohsc.gov.au

Gallagher, Susan Scavo
CSN National Injury and Violence
    Prevention Resource Center
Children's Safety Network
55 Chapel St
Newtown, MA 02458-1060
U.S.A.
Tel: 617-969-7101 x2207
Email: sgallagher@edc.org

Gillis-Cipywnk, Maura
Manager, Canadian Coalition for
    Agricultural Safety and Rural
    Health
329 – 3085 Albert St
Regina, SK S4S 0B1
Canada
Tel: 306-966-8288

Hartling, Lisa
Canadian Agricultural Survey
    Program
Kingston General Hospital
76 Stuart St
Kingston, ON K2L 2V7
Canada
Tel: 613-549-6666 x3479

Hillier, Tim
Head, First Medic Program
M.D. Ambulance Care Ltd
116 Ave
Saskatoon, SK S7L 2B6
Canada
Tel: 306-975-8808

Higginson, Jennifer
Canadian Federation of Agriculture
1101 – 75 Albert St.
Ottawa, ON K1P 5E7
Canada
Tel: 613-236-3633
Fax: 613-236-5749
Email: cfafca@fox.nstn.ca

Houlahan, James
Deputy Director of Education and
    Training
Australian Center for Agricultural
    Health and Safety
PO Box 256
Moree NSW 2400
Australia
Tel: +61-2-67-52-8210

Husseini, Ahkmed
Administrator
International Safety Standards
Manager Program
Environmental Program Standards
Canadian Standards Association
178 Rexdale Blvd
Toronto, ON M9W 1R3
Canada
Tel: 416-747-2697

I DEAL with Farm Safety Program
Frontenac, Lenix and Addington
    Health Unit
221 Portsmouth Ave
Kingston, ON K7M 1V5
Canada
Tel: 613-549-1232 x123

Johnson, Les
St John Ambulance
439 Churchill Ave. North
Ottawa, ON K1Z 5E1
Canada
Tel: 613-236-1283 x261
Fax: 613-722-7024
Email: ljohnson@nhq.sja.ca

Lee, Dr Barbara
Center Director
National Children's Centre for Rural
    and Agricultural Health & Safety
Marshfield Clinic
1000 North Oak Ave
Marshfield, WI 54449-5790
U.S.A.
Tel: 1-888-924-7233
Tel: 715-389-4999
Email: nccrahs@mfldclin.edu

Leefhead, Marian
Project Coordinator
Pre-School Farm Safety Program
Gardener College, ECD Dept
4704 – 55 St
Camrose, AB
Canada
Tel: 780-672-0171
Tel: 780-373-2467

Lockinger, Lori
Head, Farm Response Program
Centre for Agricultural Medicine
University of Saskatchewan
103 Hospital Drive
Saskatoon, SK S7N 0W8
Canada
Tel: 306-966-6643

Marlenga, Dr Barbar
Assistant
National Children's Centre for Rural
    and Agricultural Health & Safety
Marshfield Clinic
1000 North Oak Ave
Marshfield, WI 54449-5790
U.S.A.
Tel: 1-888-924-7233
Tel: 715-389-4999
Email: marlengb@mfldclin.edu

Pickett, Dr William
NAGCAT (North American Guide-
  lines for Children's Agricultural
  Tasks) ·
National Children's Center for Rural
  and Agricultural Health and
  Safety – U.S.A.
Canadian Agricultural Survey
  Program
Dept of Emergency Medicine
Queen's University
Angada 3, Kingston General
  Hospital
76 Stuart St
Kingston, ON K7L 2V7
Canada
Tel: 613-549-6666 x3788
Email: PinkettW@post.queensu.ca
Website: http://www.nagcat.org

Rich, David
Farmsafe Alliance Manager
VIC Farmers Federation
Level 4
24–28 Collins St
Melbourne, VIC 3000
Australia
Tel: +61-3-9207-5509
Fax: +61-3-9207-5510
Email: drich@vff.org.au

Ronnick, Steve
Farm Safety Association
Public Relations
Guelph, ON
Canada
Tel: 519-823-5600

Ruby, Harold
Manager, Farm Safety Tube
Ontario Soil and Crop Improvement
  Association
1 Stone Road West
Guelph, ON N1G 4Y2
Canada
Tel: 519-826-4217
Email: oscia@ontariosoilcrop.org

Safety Standards for Agricultural
  Machinery
CSA, Technical Committee
178 Rexdale Blvd
Etobicoke, ON M9W 1R3
Canada
Tel: 416-747-4000

Tormoehlen, Roger
Extension Specialist
Tractor Training Module for Kids
  Program
Dept of 4-H Youth
Purdue University
1161 AGAD Bldg
West Lafayette, IN 47907-1161
U.S.A.
Tel: 765-494-8429

Whalen-Ruiter, Theresa
North American Guidelines for
  Children's Agriculture Tasks
CFA Farm Safety Coordinator
Canadian Federation of Agriculture
1101 – 75 Albert St.
Ottawa, ON K1P 5E7
Canada
Tel: 613-731-7321
Fax: 613-236-5749
Email: ruiter@intranet.ca

White, Chris
WORKSAFE, Western Australia
Director, Information
ThinkSafe Towns
Farm Safe
Australia
Tel: +61-8-9327-8648
Email: white@worksafe.wa.gov

Wilson, Paul
Project Officer, Small Business Falls
  Prevention Project
Hume City Council
PO Box 119
1079 Pacoe Valley Road
Broadmeadows, VIC 3047
Australia
Tel: 03-9205-2525
Fax: 03-9309-0109
Email: hchealth@eisa.net.au
Website: http://
  www.hume.vic.gov.au

Witworth, Ted
Field Services Officer
Agriculture Safety Audit Program
22–23, 340 Woodlawn Rd West
Guelph, ON N1H 7K6
Canada
Tel: 519-823-5600
Fax: 519-823-8880

Young, Eric
Project Coordinator
Victorian WorkCover Authority
PO Box 1143
Geelong, VIC 3220
Australia

Fall-Related Injury

Baker, Dr Dorothy I.
Research Scientist, Chronic Disease
  Epidemiology, School of Public
  Health
Yale University School of Medicine
Program in Aging
1N – 129 York
New Haven, CT 06520
U.S.A.
Tel: 203-769-9800
Fax: 203-764-9831
Email: dorothy.baker@yale.edu

Barker, Dorothy
Trauma Patient Care Coordinator
Hospital for Sick Children
555 University Ave
Toronto, ON M5G 1X8
Canada
Tel: 416-813-8574
Email:
  dorothy.barker@sickkids.on.ca

Bernick, Laurie
Clinical Nurse Specialist
Baycrest Centre for Geriatric Care
3560 Bathurst St
Toronto, ON M6A 2E1
Canada
Tel: 416-785-2500 x2525
Fax: 416-785-2501
Email: lbernick@baycrest.org

Campbell, Dr John A.
Professor, Geriatric Medicine
Dept of Medicine
Dunedin School of Medicine
Otago Medical School
PO Box 913
Dunedin
New Zealand
Tel: +64-3-474-0999 x5056
Fax: +64-3-479-5459
Email:
    john.campbell@stonebow.otago.ac.nz

Cass, Lorraine
Senior Nursing Consultant
Population Health Service
Ontario Ministry of Health and
    Long Term Care
5700 Yonge St, 8th Floor
Toronto, ON M2M 4K5
Canada
Tel: 416-327-7389
Fax: 416-327-7438
Email: lorraine.cass@moh.gov.on.ca

Day, Dr Lesley
Senior Research Fellow
Accident Research Centre
Monash University
Bld 70, Wellington Rd
Clayton, VIC 3168
Australia
Email: +61-3-9905-1811
Fax: +61-3-9905-1809
Email:
    lesley.day@general.monash.edu.au

Edwards, Dr Nancy
Associate Professor, School of
    Nursing
Director, Community Health
    Research Unit
University of Ottawa
451 Smyth Rd
Ottawa, ON K1H 8M5
Canada
Tel: 613-562-5800 x8395
Fax: 613-562-5443
Email:
    nedwards@zeus.med.uottawa.ca

Falls prevention project: South
    Eastern Sydney
South Eastern Sydney Area Health
    Promotion Unit
Sutherland Hospital, Locked Bag 21
Taren Point, NSW 2229
Australia
Tel: +61-2-9382-9898

Gallagher, Dr Elaine RN, MScN,
    PhD
School of Nursing
University of Victoria
Box 1700
Victoria, BC V8W 2Y2
Tel: 250-474-7472
Fax: 250-474-7472 / 250-721-6231
Email: egallagh@hsd.uvic.ca

Gardner, Melinda M.
Research Physical Therapist
New Zealand Falls Prevention
   Research Team
Dept of Medical & Surgical Sciences
University of Otago Medical School
PO Box 913
Dunedin
New Zealand
Tel: +64-3-474-0999 x8523
Fax: +64-3-474-7641
Email: melinda.gardner@
   stonebow.otago.ac.nz

Haertlein, Dr Carol
Associate Professor, Occupation
   Therapy Dept
School of Allied Health
   Professionals
University of Wisconsin –
   Milwaukee
PO Box 413
Milwaukee, WI 53201
U.S.A.
Tel: 414-229-6933
Fax: 414-906-3933
Email: chaert@uwm.edu

Holliday, Pam
Research Associate
Centre for Studies in Aging
U-Basement
2075 Bayview Ave
Toronto, ON M4N 3M5
Canada
Tel: 416-480-6100 x3510
Fax: 416-480-5856
Email: pam.holliday@swchsc.on.ca

Hurley, Mary Jane
Co-Chair, North York Coalition for
   Seniors Falls Prevention
Program Coordinator, Sunnybrook
   & Women's College Health Sci-
   ences Centre
H228 – 2075 Bayview Ave
Toronto, ON M4N 3M5
Canada
Tel: 416-480-5960
Fax: 416-480-6838

Jaffe, David L.
Research Biomedical Engineer
Dept of Veterans Affairs
Palo Alto Rehabilitation, Research
   and Development Center
3801 Miranda Ave
Palo Alto, CA 97304–1200
U.S.A.
Tel: 650-493-5000 x64980
Fax: 650-493-4919
Email: jaffe@roses.stanford.edu

Lehner, Sheila H.
Program Director, Benevolent Ballet
1401 Winged Foot Dr
Apopka, FL 32712
U.S.A.
Tel: 407-889-7770
Email: lehners1@aol.com

Maki, Dr Brian
Associate Professor, University of
    Toronto
Senior Scientist, Sunnybrook &
    Women's College Health Sciences
    Centre
Centre for Studies in Aging
2075 Bayview Ave
Toronto, ON M4N 3M5
Canada
Tel: 416-480-6100 x3513
Fax: 416-480-5856
Email: brian.maki@swchsc.on.ca

Miller, Dr J. Phillip
Director, Coordinating Center,
    FICSIT, WUSM
Division of Biostatistics
Washington University School of
    Medicine
660 S. Euclid, Box 8067
St Louis, MI 63110
U.S.A.
Tel: 314-362-3617
Fax: 314-362-2693
Email: phil@wubios.wustl.edu

Newton, Dr Roberta A.
Professor, Dept of Physical Therapy
Temple University
3307 North Broad St
Philadelphia, PA 19140
U.S.A.
Tel: 215-707-4897
Fax: 215-707-7500
Email: rnewton@thunder.temple.edu

Peel, Nancye
No Falls! No Fear! Falls Prevention
    Project
Senior Research Officer
Healthy Ageing Unit
Dept of Social and Preventive
    Medicine
University of Queensland Medical
    School
Herston, QLD 4006
Australia
Tel: +61-7-3365-5383
Fax: +61-7-3365-5442
Email: n.peel@spmed.uq.edu.au

Radetsky, Michael
CHIPPS (Community Home Injury
    Prevention Program for Seniors)
Program Coordinator
CHIPPS Program
SFDPH
118 – 101 Grove St
San Francisco, CA 94102
U.S.A.
Tel: 415-554-2924
Email:
    michael_l_radetsky@dph.sf.ca.us

Robson, Ellie
Health Strategy Researcher
Capital Health Authority
Public Health Dept
300 – 10216 124th St
Edmonton, AB T5N 4A3
Canada
Tel: 780-413-7955
Fax: 780-482-4194

Sableman, Dr Eric
Biomedical Engineer, Musculo-
    skeletal Systems Section
Dept of Veteran Affairs
Palo Alto Rehabilitation, Research
    and Development Center
3801 Miranda Ave, m/s 153
Palo Alto, CA 97304-1200
U.S.A.
Tel: 650-493-5000 x63345
Fax: 650-493-4919
Email: sabelman@roses.stanford.edu

Smith-Lloyd, Donna
Stay on Your Feet: North Coast Falls
    Prevention Program
North Coast Public Health Unit
31 Uralba St
Lismore, NSW 2480
Australia
Tel: +61-2-6621-7231
Email:
    donnas@doh.health.nsw.gov.au

Stevens, Dr Judy A.
Epidemiologist
Division of Unintentional Injury
    Prevention
National Center for Injury Preven-
    tion and Control
Centers for Disease Control and
    Prevention
1600 Clifton Rd
Atlanta, GA 30333
Tel: 770-488-4649
Fax: 770-488-1317
Email: jas2@cdc.gov

Tinetti, Dr Mary
Professor, Medicine & Epidemiology
    and Public Health
Yale University School of Medicine
333 Cedar St
PO Box 208025
New Haven, CT 06520-8025
U.S.A.
Tel: 203-688-5238
Fax: 203-688-4209

Van Beurden, Eric
Research and Evaluation Officer
Stay on Your Feet Program
Health Promotion Unit
Institute of Health and Research
31 Uralbra St
Lismore, NSW 2480
Australia
Tel: +61-2-6620-7507
Email:
    evanb@doh.health.nsw.gov.au

Window Falls Prevention Program
Center for Integrated Prevention
    Programs
New York City Department of
    Health
2 Lafayette Street, 20th Floor
New York, NY 10007
U.S.A.
Tel: 212-676-2162
Fax: 212-676-2161

Wolf, Dr Steven L.
Professor of Rehabilitation Medicine
Center for Rehabilitation Medicine
Emory University School of Medi-
   cine
1441 Clifton Rd NE
Atlanta, GA 30322
U.S.A.
Tel: 404-712-4801
Fax: 404-712-4809
Email: swolf@emory.edu

**Comprehensive Community-Based
Strategies**

Appy, Meri-K
RISK WATCH
Vice President of Public Education
National Fire Protection Association
   (NFPA)
1 Batterymarch Park
Quincy, MA 02269-9101
U.S.A.
Tel: 617-984-7285
Fax: 617-984-7222
Email: bdunn@nfpa.org

Butchart, Alex
Deputy Director
Centre for Peace Action
P.O. Box 293
1812 Eldorado Park
Johannesburg, South Africa
Tel: +27-11-342-3840
Fax: +27-11-945-3956
Email: psych@icon.co.za

Burton, Ann
Board Member, Think First Founda-
   tion
Director, New York State Chapter
Sunnyview Hospital
1270 Belmont Ave
Schenectady, NY 12308
U.S.A.
Tel: 518-382-4520
Fax: 518-386-3675
Email: burton@sunnyview.org

Cliette, Erik
Program Associate Director
Injury Free Coalition for Kids
   (National)
Harlem Hospital Injury Prevention
   Program (Local)
Harlem Hospital Center
506 Lennox Ave 17102
New York, NY 10037
Tel: 212-939-4005
Email: ec221@columbia.edu

Comoletti, Judy
Education Director
Project Manager
National Fire Protection Association
PO Box 9101
Quincy, MA 02269–9101
U.S.A.
Tel: 617-984-7287
Fax: 617-770-0200

Cusimano, Dr Michael
St Michael's Hospital
38 Shuter Street, Rm 2004
Toronto, ON M5B 1A6
Canada
Tel: 416-864-6048

Donohue, Deanne
Plan-it Safe
Children's Hospital of Eastern
  Ontario
401 Smyth Rd
Ottawa, ON K1H 8L1
Canada
Tel: 613-738-3588
Fax: 613-738-4800
Email: ddonohue@uottawa.ca

Harberts, Henk
Coordinator, Community Safety
  Promotion
La Trobe Valley Better Health Project
La Trobe Shire Council
PO Box 345
Traralgon, VIC 3844
Australia
Tel: +61-3-51-731-506
Fax: +61-3-51-731-558
Email: henka@latrobe.vic.gov.au

Johnson, Deborah
Program Coordinator
National Think First Foundation
5550 Meadowbrook Dr
Suite 110
Rolling Meadows, IL 60008
U.S.A.
Tel: 1-847-290-8600
Fax: 847-290-9005
Email: thinkfirst@aans.org

Kall, Denise
Coordinator
Safe Communities Coalition of
  Brockville
1 King St W.
PO Box 5000
Brockville, ON K6V 7A5
Canada
Tel: 613-342-2917
Fax: 613-342-1785
Email: 2bsafe@brockville.com

Mione, Angela
FOCUS Community Project
200 – 336 Pine St
Sudbury, ON P3C 1X8
Canada
Tel: 705-674-4330
Email: focusgroup@on.aibn.com

Sam, Eleanor
Executive Director
Think First Foundation of Canada
2-435 McLaughlin Pavilion
399 Bathurst Street
Toronto, ON M5T 2S8
Canada
Tel: 416-603-5212
Tel: 416-603-5331
Tel: 1-800-335-6076
Fax: 416-603-7795
Email: think1st@netrover.com

Scott, Ian
Research Director
Kidsafe Australia
Level 1
222 – 224 Church St
Richmond, VIC 3121
Australia
Tel: +61-3-9427-1008
Fax: +61-3-9421-3821
Email: iscott@kidsafe.org.au

Seedat, Dr Mohamed
Director
Centre for Peach Action
PO Box 293
1812 Eldorado Park
Johannesburg, South Africa
Tel: 27-11-342 3840
Fax: 27-11-945 3956
Email: psych@icon.co.za

Sharman, Asheer
St Michael's Hospital
38 Shuter Street, Rm 2006
Toronto, ON M5B 1A6
Canada
Tel: 416-864-5312

Simpson, Dr Jean
Research Fellow
Dept of Preventive and Social
    Medicine
Dunedin School of Medicine
Health Sciences Division
University of Otago
New Zealand
Tel: +64-3-479-1100
Email:
    jsimpson@gandolf.otago.ac.nz

Sundstrom, Moa
Karolinska Institutet, Institutionen
    for
Folkhalsovetenskapm, Norrbacka,
    plan 2,
171 76 Stockholm
Sweden
Tel: +46-8-517-700-00
Fax: +46-8-30-73-51
Email:
    moa.sundstrom@socmed.sll.se

Nixon, Dr James
Associate Professor
Dept of Paediatrics and Child
    Health
Royal Children's Hospital
Brisbane, QLD 4029
Australia
Tel: 61-7-3365-5322
Email: j.nixon@mailbox.uq.edu.au

Zirkle, Dorothy
Program Manager
Think First Injury Prevention
    Program
SHARP HEALTH CARE
5555 Grossmont Center Drive
La Mesa, CA 91942
U.S.A.
Tel: 619-644-4661
Fax: 619-644-4128
Email: Zirdo@ops.sharp.com

Appendix E: URLs for Injury Prevention and Control Research Centres

Canada

- Injury Prevention Centre, the provincial resource centre for injury prevention in Alberta, Canada. http://www.health-in-action.org/ipc/
- Ontario Neurotrauma Foundation (ONF), a non-profit, granting organization dedicated to reducing the incidence, prevalence and impact of neurotrauma injuries. http://www.onf.org/
- SMARTRISK, committed to encouraging Canadians to adopt smart risk behaviour. http://www.smartrisk.ca/

United States

- Consumer Product Safety Commission (CPSC). www.cpsc.gov/
- National Highway Traffic Safety Administration (NHTSA) www.nhtsa.dot.gov/
- National Centers for Disease Control and Prevention. www.cdc.gov/
- National Center for Injury Prevention and Control. www.cdc.gov/nciprc/ncipchm.htm
- Harborview Injury Prevention and Research Center (HIPRC) – University of Washington, Seattle, WA. http://depts.washington.edu/hiprc/
- Southern California Injury Prevention Research Center (SCIPRC) – UCLA, Los Angeles CA. www.ph.ucla.edu/sciprc/sciprc1.htm
- Harvard Injury Control Center, New England Injury Prevention Research Center (HICC)- Harvard University, Boston, MA. www.hsph.harvard.edu/hicrc/

- Johns Hopkins Center for Injury Research and Policy – Johns Hopkins University, Baltimore, MD. http://www.jhsph.edu/Research/Centers/CIRP/contents.htm
- University of North Carolina Injury Prevention Research Center – Chapel Hill, NC. www.sph.unc.edu/iprc
- Colorado Injury Control Research Center – Colorado State University, University of Colorado & Colorado DPHE.
- Kentucky Injury Prevention and Research Center (KIRPC) – University of Kentucky, Lexington, KY. www.kiprc.uky.edu/

Targeted Injury Prevention and Control Research Centers (U.S.)

- University of North Carolina Highway Safety Research Center http://www.hsrc.unc.edu
- Agricultural Health and Safety Centers (National Institute of Occupational Safety & Health affiliated). http://agcenter.ucdavis.edu
- Neuromuscular Research Center – Boston University, Boston, MA http://agcenter.ucdavis.edu/agcenter/
- National Institute for Occupational Safety and Health (NIOSH) www.cdc.gov.niosh/homepage.html
- National Highway Traffic Safety Administration (NHTSA) www.nhtsa.dot.gov

International

Australia

- Australian National Injury Prevention Surveillance Unit www.nisu.flinders.edu.au/
- Monash University Accident Research Centre is one of Australia's leading road safety and injury prevention research organisations. www.general.monash.edu.au/muarc/
- Australian Injury Prevention Database, University of Queensland A database of injury-related health promotion programs implemented throughout Australia since 1988. http://www.spmed.uq.edu.au/aipd/progs0.asp

New Zealand

- Injury Prevention Research Unit: Dunedin, Otago www.otago.ac.nz/IPRU/home.html

Sweden

- The Swedish Karolinska Institutet Department of Public Health Sciences Division of Social Medicine lists their efforts in Research in Safety Promotion and Injury Prevention. www.phs.ki.se/socmed/

Appendix F: Research Team Profile

Richard Volpe, PhD, the project leader, is a professor and projects director, Life Span Adaptation Projects, and co-director of the Institute of Child Study, Department of Human Development and Applied Psychology (OISE), University of Toronto. He was a Laidlaw Foundation Post Doctoral Fellow, University of Toronto, Hospital for Sick Children, and the Clark Institute and is full member of the Graduate Department of Community Health, Faculty of Medicine. Volpe was formerly director, Dr R.G.N. Laidlaw Research Centre, University of Toronto, director of the Laidlaw Foundation's Evaluation and Conceptual Elaboration Unit of their Child at Risk Program, and an Organization for Economic Cooperation and Development (OECD) Evaluation Expert.

Jeannette L. Amio is a PhD candidate at OISE/UT in the Department of Human Development and Applied Psychology. Her research interests lie in the field of community psychology, with particular emphasis on integrated prevention programming. Her professional experience has centred on prevention program implementation and evaluation and Amio has worked on numerous projects with Better Beginnings, Better Futures as a research assistant. She is also a neurotrauma consumer, having been involved in an automobile accident that left her with a fractured skull, among other injuries.

Angela Batra, the project coordinator for this project, graduated with a Master's in Social Work from the University of Toronto in 1998. She was the project coordinator of an international survey of integrated services, which analysed exemplary models of integrating various services with schools using the BRIO, formerly CIPP, evaluation framework. Her background includes professional education and work experience in mental health with diverse populations. She has also worked with school-aged children in various settings on a clinical and research level, with the goal of enhancing overall school community well-being by promoting preventative and systemic approaches to service delivery and integration. Angela is currently a consumer of rehabilitation services (physiotherapy and chiropractic) for spinal cord-related injuries following a motor vehicle crash in January 1999.

Claire Howard has academic and professional experience in both the health care and education fields. Currently she holds an undergraduate degree in Gerontology and several years of work experience with the elderly. Howard is working on a Master of Arts in Curriculum, Teaching, and Learning with a specialization in Comparative, International, and Development Education.

Janice Ketley is a secondary school teacher employed by the former City of York Board of Education, now the Toronto District School Board. She taught Business Skills and Co-operative Education at the Adult Day School in the City of York for 9 years, the last 2 years as assistant and then department head. In 1997 she transferred to Weston Collegiate as Co-operative Education Department Head and taught the program to adolescents. Prior to teaching, she was employed as a Registered Respiratory Therapist over a period of 17 years at Vancouver General Hospital (Vancouver, B.C.), St Mary's Hospital (New Westminister, B.C.), University Hospital (London, Ontario), Woodstock General Hospital (Woodstock, Ontario), and Mississauga General Hospital (Mississauga, Ontario). Ketley is presently on a leave of absence from the Toronto District School Board and resides in Sydney, Australia, with her husband and 2 children.

Carly Leung graduated from the University of Toronto with an Honours Bachelor of Science degree in Microbiology. She is currently working in a pharmaceutical company for vaccine research.

Donna Louie is a recent graduate of the University of Toronto. Currently, she holds an Honours Bachelor of Science degree with a double major in biology and psychology. Her personal interests include web page development and design.

Julie Michelangelo graduated in 1999 from the University of Toronto with an Honours Bachelor of Science Degree in Psychology and Sociology. Her professional experience includes research, writing, and teaching. Previous volunteer experience with acquired brain injured individuals enhanced her interest in research related to brain and spinal cord injury prevention programs.

Nathaniel Paul is a PhD candidate in the Department of Sociology and Equity Studies in Education at OISE/UT. His research interests lie in the field of cultural production, risk assessment, and social aspects of the human body, and in medical sociology in general. His work experience includes advocacy research on social policy and child poverty in Canada.

Vera Roberts is a PhD candidate at OISE/UT. Her research interests include the applications of technology for education and the cognitive aspects of injury prevention. She is the curriculum coordinator for the Adaptive Technology Resource Centre's Special Needs Opportunity Windows (SNOW) web site (http://snow.utoronto.ca) and is involved in the development of online workshops for educators of individuals with special needs. Currently, she is also coordinating a research project, funded by the Office of Learning Technologies (OLT), that examines the effectiveness of online workshops.

Dara Sikljovan is a PhD candidate at the Human Development and Education Department at OISE/UT. Her research interests are in the field of early childhood education. Her background includes supervised work in the head injury classroom at the Ontario Crippled Children's School (now the Bloorview MacMillan Centre School). Her more recent experience includes holding a position as research assistant at the Hincks Institute for the *Growing Together Project*, an early intervention community based program in St James Town, Toronto.

C. Shawn Tracy is a graduate student in the Department of Public Health Sciences at the University of Toronto. He holds a degree in psychology from Trent University (Peterborough, Canada), where he studied adult development and psychometric theory. Among his current interests are healthy public policy, the social psychology of ageing, and the health of older workers.

Man Sang Wong graduated with a Bachelor of Commerce degree from McMaster University; he also obtained a BA degree from the University of Toronto. His professional experience extends to writing case studies and articles professionally. Currently he is writing about health-related issues for a student web site.

Appendix G: Consortium Members Profile

Burton L. Borthwick, PhD, is president/director of Education/Consultation Evaluation & Research (E-CER) at the Bloorview MacMillan Centre. He is a co-chair of the Special Education Technology Consortium (SEC). He was a principal/director of the Hugh MacMillan Board of Education, program consultant and Superintendent for Ministry of Education. His significant contributions to education include: establishing the first Provincial Demonstration School (The Trillium School) offering an "on-site" teacher education program for teachers of students with learning disabilities, and coordinating the implementation of Ontario Special Education Legislation (Bill 82).

Geoffrey Roy Fernie, BSc, PhD, MIMech E, CEng, PEng, CCE, is director at the Centre for Studies in Aging, Sunnybrook and Women's College Health Sciences Centre; a professor in the Department of Surgery, University of Toronto; and a director of research in aging, Sunnybrook and Women's College Health Sciences Centre. He has also held concurrent appointments with the Institute of Biomaterials and Biomedical Engineering, Departments of Occupational and Physical Therapy at University of Toronto, for the past 15 years. A number of his remarkable innovations, especially considering the needs of elderly users (e.g., SturdyLift, SturdyGrip, SturdyWalker), have been patented and many of them awarded.

Gretchen Kerr, PhD, is an associate professor and associate dean of the Faculty of Physical Education and Health at the University of Toronto. She is also a member of the Graduate Department of Community Health, Faculty of Medicine. The health of children and youth in sports is the focus of her research.

Professionally, Gretchen contributes to coaching education in the areas of psychosocial development of children, harassment, and injury prevention.

Yves Lajoie, PhD, is an assistant professor at the School of Human Kinetics, Laurentian University. Postdoctoral specialization focused on physical and occupational therapy. Areas of expertise relate primarily to spinal cord injuries.

John Henry Lewko, PhD (Sport Psychology), is a full professor of the Human Development Department and a director of the Centre for Research in Human Development at Laurentian University. His significant contributions have been in the field of handicapped children and adolescent development research. Lewko was a recipient of the Research Excellence Award for 1993–1994.

Geraldine A. Macdonald, EdD, is a lecturer at the Faculty of Nursing and academic adviser for the Case Management Program at Woodsworth College, University of Toronto. She is also a freelance health writer, a full member of the RNAO Nursing Education Interest Group Committee and Voice of Women (NGO). One of her most recent projects involves planning a workshop: "Participatory Approaches to Community-Based Health Communication."

C. William L. Pickett, PhD, is an assistant professor in the Community Health and Epidemiology Department, and Emergency Medicine at Queen's University. He is the recipient of the Career Scientist Award (1994–2004) from the Ontario Ministry of Health. One of his current research activities is with the North American Guidelines for Children's Agricultural Tasks Project.

Peter G. Rumney, MD, FRCPC is physician director of the Neuro Rehabilitation Program (formerly: The Paediatric Acquired Brain Injury Program) and a staff paediatrician at the Bloorview MacMillan Centre. He also holds a concurrent appointment with the Hospital for Sick Children Staff in the Department of Paediatrics and Neurology. He is a member of the Acquired Brain Injury Program, Paediatric Sub-Committee to the Ministry of Health. His current research interests (e.g., risk-taking behaviour and later closed head injury, advocating for bicycle helmet use in the community, assessing outcome measures in paediatric ABI) are mostly related to brain injury prevention. In 1995 he was selected as the Professional of the Year and received the Lloyd Loynes Award presented by the OBIA board of directors.

David A. Wolfe, PhD, ABPP, is a professor in the Department of Psychology, and the Department of Psychiatry (cross-appointment) at the University of

Western Ontario. He is a chair of the Sub-Committee on the Abuse of Children and Adolescents for the International Working Group on Trauma, United Nations, and a member of the advisory board, Canadian Incidence Study of Child Maltreatment, Child Maltreatment Division, Health Canada. One of his current research studies, preventing violence in relationships, involves adolescents with histories of abuse and neglect and is particularly aimed at preventing future violence towards women and children.

Appendix H: Partner List

Adair, William
Executive Director
Canadian Paraplegic Association
 Ontario
520 Sutherland Drive
Toronto, ON M4G 3V9
Canada
Tel: 416-422-5644
Toll Free: 1-877-422-1112
Fax: 416-422-5943
Website: http://www.cpaont.org/

Hayday, Brian
Executive Director
Canadian Health Network
180 Dundas Street West, Suite 1900
Toronto, ON M5G 1Z8
Canada
Email: b.hayday@inovaction.com

Kumpf, John
Executive Director
Ontario Brain Injury Association
P.O. Box 2338
St Catharines, ON L2R 7R9
Canada
Tel: 905-641-8877
Fax: 905-641-0323
Email: obia@obia.on.ca
Website: http://www.obia.on.ca/

Norquay, Jennifer
Executive Assistant
Ontario Brain Injury Association
P.O. Box 2338
St Catharines, ON L24 7R9
Canada
Tel: 905-641-8877
Fax: 905-641-0323
Email: obia@obia.on.ca
Website: http://www.obia.on.ca/

Steen, David
President and CEO
Society for Manitobans with
    Disabilities
825 Sherbrooke Street
Winnipeg, MB R3A 1M5
Tel: 204-784-3734
Canada
Email: dsteen@smd.mb.ca

Appendix I: Index of CD Contents

Documents

1 A Compendium of Effective, Evidence-Based Practices in Prevention of Neurotrauma
2 The economic burden of unintentional injury in Ontario, SMARTRISK
3 The economic burden of unintentional injury in Canada, SMARTRISK

Video Clips

1 HEROES, SMARTRISK
2 *Risk Watch*, National Fire Protection Association, Quincy MA
3 Think First for Kids, Think First Foundation
4 PARTY Program, Sunnybrook & Women's College Health Sciences Centre (2 clips)

References

1. Introduction, Conclusion, and General

Ammerman, R.T., & Hersen, M. (Eds.). (1997). *Handbook of prevention and treatment with children and adolescents: Intervention in the real world context.* New York: Wiley & Sons.

Baker, T.E., Rogers, E.M., & Sopory, P. (1992). *Designing health communication campaigns: What works?* Newbury Park: Sage.

Barss, P., Smith, G.S., Baker, S.P., & Mohan, D. (1998). *Injury prevention, an international perspective: Epidemiology, surveillance, and policy.* New York: Oxford University Press.

Bellnir, K. (1997). Spinal cord injuries: Causes and statistics. In K. Bellnir (Ed.), *Back and neck: Disorders sourcebook* (pp. 311–322). Detroit: Omnigraphics.

Black, N., Brazier, J., Fitzpatrick, R., & Reeves, B. (Eds.). (1998). *Health services research methods: A guide to best practice.* London: BMJ Books.

Bonnie, R.J., Fulco, C.E., & Liverman, C.T. (Eds.). (1999). *Reducing the burden of injury: Advancing prevention and treatment.* Washington, D.C.: National Academy Press.

Boulton, M., Fitzpatrick, R., & Swinburn, C. (1996). Qualitative research in healthcare: II. A structured review and evaluation of studies. *Journal of Evaluation in Clinical Practice, 2,* 171–179.

Breckon, D.J., Harvey, J.R., & Lancaster, R.B. (1998). *Community health education: Settings, roles, and skills for the 21st century* (4th ed.). Gaithersburg, MD: Aspen.

Bronfenbrenner, U. (1979). *The ecology of human development: Experiments by nature and design.* Cambridge, MA: Harvard University Press.

Brownson, R.C., Baker, E.A., & Novick, L.F. (Eds.). (1999). *Community-based prevention: Programs that work.* Gaithersburg, MD: Aspen.

Byers, B. (1999). *The Ontario drowning report 1999 Edition*. PHERO, 85–88.

Campbell, D.T., & Russo, M.J. (1999). *Social experimentation*. Thousand Oaks, CA: Sage.

Canadian Institute of Child Health (1994). *The health of Canada's children: A CICH Profile* (2nd ed.). Ottawa, ON: Canadian Institute.

Canadian Institute of Child Health and Canadian Association of Paediatric Hospitals. (1994). *Directory of Canadian programs and researchers: Child/youth injury prevention*. Ottawa, ON: Canadian Institute of Child Health.

Christoffel, T. (1989). The role of law in reducing injury. *Law, Medicine and Health Care, 12(1)*, 7–15.

Christoffel, T., & Gallagher, S.S. (1999). *Injury prevention and public health: Practical knowledge, skills, and strategies*. Gaithersburg, MD: Aspen.

Coleman, P., Munro, J., Nicholl, J., Harper, R., Kent, G., & Wild, D. (1996, February). *The effectiveness of interventions to prevent accidental injury to young persons aged 15–24 years: A review of the evidence*. Sheffield: Medical Care Research Unit, University of Sheffield.

Connolly, T., Arkes, H.R., & Hammond, K.R. (Eds.). (2000). *Judgment and decision making* (2nd ed.). Cambridge: Cambridge University Press.

Cowen, E.L., Hightower, A.D., Pedro-Carroll, J.L., Work, W.C., & Wyman, P.A. (with Haffey, W.G.). (1996). *School-based prevention for children at risk: The primary mental health project*. Washington, DC: American Psychological Association.

Doern, G., & Phidd, R. (1983). *Canadian public policy: Ideas, structure, processes*. Agincourt, ON: Methuen Publications.

Durlak, J.A. (1997). *Successful prevention programs for children and adolescents*. New York: Plenum Press.

Durlak, J.A., & Ferrari, J.R. (1998). Some exemplars of implementation. *Journal of Prevention and Intervention in the Community, 17*, 81–89.

Elkington, J. (1998). *Evaluation of the Spinesafe Education Program* (Unpublished report). Ryde, New South Wales, Australia: Spinesafe.

Ferrari, J.R., & Durlak, J.A. (1998). Why worry about implementation procedures: Why not just do? *Journal of Prevention and Intervention in the Community, 17(2)*, 1–3.

Gager, P.J., & Elias, M.J. (1997). Implementing prevention programs in high risk environments: Application of the resiliency paradigm. *American Journal of Orthopsychiatry, 67*, 363–373.

Garbarino, J. (1988). Preventing childhood injury: Developmental and mental health issues. *American Journal of Orthopsychiatry, 58(1)*, 25–45.

Garling, T. (1985). Children's environments, accidents, and accident prevention. In T. Garling & J. Valsiner (Eds.), *Children within environments: Toward a psychology of accident prevention* (pp. 3–12). New York: Plenum Press.

Gielen, A.C. (1992). Health education and injury control: Integrating approaches. *Health Education Quarterly, 19(20),* 203–218.

Gordon, J.E. (1949). The epidemiology of accidents. *American Journal of Public Health, 3,* 504–515.

Guba, E.G., & Lincoln, Y.S. (1989). *Fourth generation evaluation.* London: Sage.

Haddix, A.C., Teutsch, S.M., Shaffer, P.A., & Duñet, D.O. (Eds.). (1996). *Prevention effectiveness: A guide to decision analysis and economic evaluation.* New York: Oxford University Press.

Haddon, W. (1972). A logical framework for categorizing highway safety phenomena and activity. *Journal of Trauma, 12(30),* 193–207.

Haddon, W. (1973). Energy damage and the ten countermeasure strategies. *Journal of Trauma, 13,* 321–331.

Haddon, W. (1980). Advances in the epidemiology of injuries as a basis for public policy. *Public Health Reports, 95(5),* 411–421.

Haddon, W., & Baker, S.P. (1981). Injury control. In D. Clarke & B. MacMahon (Eds.), *Preventative and community medicine.* Boston: Little Brown.

Haddon, W., & Goddard, J. (1962). An analysis of highway safety strategies. *Passenger car design and highway safety* (pp. 6–11). New York: Association for the Aid of Crippled Children and Consumers Union of New York.

Hawtin, M., Hughes, G., & Percy-Smith, J. (1999). *Community profiling: Auditing social needs.* Buckingham: Open University Press.

Health Canada. (1997). *For the safety of Canadian children and youth: From injury data to preventive measures.* Minister of Public Works and Government Canada.

Henderson, A., & Champlin, S. (Eds.). (with Evashwick, W.). (1998). *Promoting teen health: Linking schools, health organizations, and community.* Thousand Oaks, CA: Sage.

Horan, M., and Little, R. (1998). *Injury in aging.* Cambridge: Cambridge University Press.

Jennett, B. (1996). Epidemiology of head injury. *Journal of Neurology, Neurosurgery, and Psychiatry, 60,* 362–369.

Kneger, N. (1999). Questioning epidemiology: Objectivity, advocacy and socially responsible science. *American Journal of Public Health, 89(8),* 1151–1152.

Laflamme, L., Svanstrom, L., & Schelp, L. (Eds.). (2000). *Safety promotion research.* Stockholm: Karolinska Institutet, Department of Public Health Sciences, Division of Social Medicine.

Lynch, K.B., Geller, S.R., Hunt, U.R., Galano, J., & Semon Dubas, J. (1998). Successful program development using implementation evaluation. *Journal of Prevention and Intervention in the Community, 17,* 51–64.

MacMahon, I. (Ed.). *Preventive and community medicine.* Boston: Aspen Publishers.

Miller, W.G., & Miller, F.U. (1992). Accidental injuries of children. In U.I. Templer, L.C. Hartlage, & W.G. Cannon (Eds.), *Preventable brain damage: Brain vulnerability and brain health* (pp. 41–57). New York: Springer.

Minkler, M. (Ed.). (1999). *Community organizing and community building for health*. New Brunswick, NJ: Rutgers University Press.

Mohan, D., & Tiwari, G. (Eds.). (2000). *Injury prevention and control*. New York: Taylor & Francis.

Muir Gray, J.A. (1997). *Evidence-based healthcare*. Toronto: Churchill Livingstone.

Mulrow, C., & Cook, D. (Eds.). (1998). *Systematic reviews: Synthesis of best evidence for health care decisions*. Philadelphia: American College of Physicians.

Ontario Neurotrauma Foundation. (1999). *Guide to program design and evaluation planning*. Toronto: Author.

Ontario Public Health Association. (1992). *Priority themes for injury prevention in Ontario*. Toronto: OPHA.

Osborne, D. (1998, January). Two ways to battle spinal injuries. *The Carillon*, 40. Retrieved January 17, 2000 from the World Wide Web: http:// ursu.uregina.ca/~carillon/jan29.98/sports/sports6.html

Øvretveit, J. (1998). *Evaluating health interventions: An introduction to evaluation of health treatments, services, policies and organizational interventions*. Buckingham: Open University Press.

Parsons, W. (1995). *Public policy: An introduction to the theory and practice of policy analysis*. Brookfield, VT: Edward Elgar.

Pederson, A., O'Neill, M., & Rootman, I. (Eds.). (1994). *Health promotion in Canada: Provincial, national and international perspectives*. Toronto: W.B. Saunders Canada.

Plautz, B., Beck, D.E., Selmar, C.S., & Radestsky, M. (1996). Modifying the Environment: A community-based injury reduction program for elderly residents. *American Journal of Preventive Medicine, 12*, 613–618.

Pless, I.B. (2000). Preventing spinal cord injuries: Is this the best we can do? *Canadian Medical Association Journal, 162*, 792–793.

Rivara, F.P. (1995). Developmental and behavioral issues in childhood injury prevention. *Journal of Developmental and Behavioral Pediatrics, 16(5)*, 214–228.

Robert Wood Johnson Foundation. (1999). *National program report: Dissemination of a model injury prevention program for children and adolescents* (pp. 1–51). Author. Retrieved April 19, 2000 from the World Wide Web: http:// www.rjwf.org/health/013396.htm

Robertson, L. S. (1998). *Injury epidemiology: Research and control strategies* (2nd ed.). New York: Oxford University Press.

Rutter, M. (1987). Psychosocial resilience and protective mechanisms. *American Journal of Orthopsychiatry 57*, 316–331.

Sandel, N.E., Bell, K.R., & Michaud, L.J. (1998). Brain injury rehabilitation: Traumatic brain injury, prevention, pathophysiology, and outcome prediction. *Archives of Physical Medicine and Rehabilitation, 79*, S3–S9.

SMARTRISK. (1998). *The economic burden of unintentional injury in Canada.* Toronto: Author.

SMARTRISK. (1999). *The economic burden of unintentional injury in Ontario.* Toronto: Author.

Stover, S.L., De Lisa, J.A., & Whiteneck, C.C. (1995). The epidemiology of spinal cord injury. In S.L. Stover, J.A. De Lisa, & C.C. Whiteneck (Eds.), *Spinal cord injury: Clinical outcomes from the model systems* (pp. 21–55).

Task Force on Community Preventive Services. (2000, January). Introducing the guide to community preventive services: Methods, first recommendations and expert commentary. *American Journal of Preventive Medicine, 18*(1S), 1–2.

Towner, E., Dowswell, T., Simpson, G., & Jarvis, S. (1996). *Health promotion in childhood and young adolescence for the prevention of unintentional injuries.* London: Health Education Authority.

VanLeer Foundation. (1996). *VanLeer Program Evaluation Model.* The Hague: VanLeer Foundation.

Voilmer, U. et al. (1991). Age and outcome following traumatic coma: Why do older people fare worse? *Journal of Neurosurgery, 75*, 37–39.

Volpe, R. (1990). *Life span adaptation projects final report.* Toronto: Laidlaw Foundation.

Volpe, R. (1992, June 5). Human development in context. *International Child Development Centre* (UNICEF), 1–20.

Volpe, R. (1996). The CIPP model and the case study approach. In P. Evans, P. Hurrell, R. Volpe, & M. Stewart (Eds.), *Successful services for our children and families at risk* (Vol. III, pp. 325–330). Paris: OECD.

Volpe, R. (1998). Ontario: Integrating services in Canada's wealthiest province. In P. Evans, P. Hurrell, R. Volpe, & M. Stewart (Eds.), *Coordinating services for children and youth at risk* (Vol. IV). Paris: OECD.

Volpe, R. (1999). Knowledge from evaluation research. In P. Evans, P. Hurrell, R. Volpe, & M. Stewart (Eds.), *Children and families at risk: New issues in integrating services* (Vol. V). Paris: OECD.

Volpe, R., & Tilleczek, K. (1998a). Images of children's rights: A review of Canadian policies. In I. Richardson (Ed.), *Children and youth: An international odyssey.* Edmonton: University of Alberta Press.

Volpe, R., & Tilleczek, K. (1998b). German and Australian youth employment services as forms of social support. In I. Richardson (Ed.), *Children and youth: An international odyssey*. Edmonton: University of Alberta Press.

Walker, B.L. (1995). *Injury prevention for the elderly: A research guide*. Westport, CT: Greenwood.

Watts, C., & Eyster, E.F. (1992). National head and spinal cord injury prevention program of the American Association of Neurological Surgeons and the Congress of Neurological Surgeons. *Journal of Neurotrauma, 9*, S307–S312.

Wilson, D.K., Rodrigue, J.R., & Taylor, W.C. (Eds.). (1997). *Health-promoting and health-compromising behaviors among minority adolescents*. Washington, DC: American Psychological Association.

Wong, C.H. (1999). Leading causes of death, Ontario 1996. *PHERO*, 160–163.

Zigler, J.E., & Capen, D.A. (1998). Epidemiology of spinal cord injury: A perspective on the problem. In A.M. Levine, F. J. Eismont, S.R. Garfin, & J.E. Zigler (Eds.), *Spine trauma* (pp. 2–8). Philadelphia, PA: W.B. Saunders.

2. Prevention of Asphyxiation-Related Injuries

Allen, J. (1998). Around the traps: State and territory news. Prepared for *Injury Issues Monitor, 13*, Retrieved April 16, 2000 from the World Wide Web: http://www.nisu.flinders.edu.au/pubs/monitor13/mon1303.htm

Brenner, R.A., Smith, G.S., Overpeck, M.D. (1994). Divergent trends in childhood drowning rates, 1971 through 1998. *JAMA, 271*, 1606–1608.

Byers, B. (1999). The Ontario drowning report–1999 Edition. *PHERO*, 85–88.

DeVivo, M.J., Sekar, P. (1997). Prevention of spinal cord injuries that occur in swimming pools. *Spinal Cord, 35*, 509–515.

Guidelines for Territorial Authorities on the Fencing of Swimming Pools Act 1987. (1999). *Department of Internal Affairs*, Te Tari Taiwhenua, New Zealand.

Harbourview Injury Prevention Research Center (HIPRC). (1997). *Drowning interventions: Pool fencing*. Retrieved April 3, 2000 from the World Wide Web: http://www.depts.washington.edu/hiprc/childinjury/topic/drowning/fencing.html

Ley, P. (1991). Isolation fencing and drownings in backyard pools. *Medical Journal of Australia, 154*, 711–712.

Lifesaving Society. (1999). *National Drowning Report, 1999*. Retrieved April 25, 2000 from the World Wide Web: http://www.lifesavingsociety.ns.ca/drowning.html

Logan, P., Branche, C.M., Sacks, J.J., Ryan, G., & Peddicord, J. (1994). Childhood Drownings and Fencing of Outdoor Pools in the United States. *Pediatrics, 101*, e3. Retrieved April 5, 2000 from the World Wide Web: http://www.pediatrics.org

Morrison, L., Chalmers, D.J., Langley, J.D., Alsop, J.C., & McBean, C. (1999). Achieving compliance with pool fencing legislation in New Zealand: A survey of regulatory authorities. *Injury Prevention, 5*, 114–118.

Office of Information and Public Affairs. (1998). *How to plan for the unexpected: Preventing child drownings* [Brochure]. Washington, DC: US Consumer Product Safety Commission.

Owens, D.A., Francis, E.L., & Leibowitz, H.W. (1989). Visibility distance with headlights: A functional approach. SAE Technical Paper Series Paper No. 890684. Warrendale, PA: Society of Automotive Engineers.

Pearn, J. (1980). Will fenced pools save lives? A 10-year study from Mulgrave Shire, Queensland. *Medical Journal of Australia, 2*, 510–511.

Pearn, J., & Nixon, J. (1977a). Prevention of childhood drowning accidents. *Medical Journal of Australia, 1*, 616–618. Retrieved April, 2000 from Pubmed database on the World Wide Web: http://www.ncbi.nlm.nih.gov

Pearn, J., & Nixon, J. (1977b). Swimming pool immersion accidents: An analysis from the Brisbane drowning study. *Medical Journal of Australia, 1*, 432–437. Retrieved April, 2000 from Pubmed database on the World Wide Web: http://www.ncbi.nlm.nih.gov

Pitt, W.R. (1986). Increasing incidence of childhood immersion injury in South Brisbane. *Medical Journal of Australia, 144*, 683–685. Retrieved April, 2000 from the PubMed database on the World Wide Web: http://www.ncbi.nlm.nih.gov

Pitt, W.R., & Balanda, K.P. (1991). Childhood drowning and near-drowning in Brisbane: The contribution of domestic pools. *Medical Journal of Australia, 154*, 661–665.

Pitt, W.R., & Balanda, K.P. (1998). Toddler drownings in domestic swimming pools in Queensland since uniform fencing requirements. *Medical Journal of Australia, 169*, 557–578.

Queensland Injury Surveillance Unit (QISU). (2000). Retrieved April 13, 2000 from the World Wide Web: http://www.qisu.qld.gov.au/main.htm

Retting, R.A., Williams, A.F., & Green, M.A. (1996). Red-light running and sensible countermeasures: Summary of research findings. Arlington, VA: Insurance Institute for Highway Safety.

Smith, G.S. (1995). The changing risks of drowning for adolescents in the US and effective control strategies. *Adolescent Medicine, 6*, 153–170.

Smith, G.S. (1995). Drowning prevention in children: The need for new strategies. *Injury Prevention, 1*, 216–217.

State of Queensland, Australia. (1991). *Local Government (Swimming Pool Fencing) Amendment Act of 1991, ss. 49*. Queensland, Australia: Author.

State of Queensland, Australia. (1991). *Standard Building By-Laws (Swimming*

Pool Fencing) Order 1991, ss. 53.1 (Subordinate Legislation 1991, No. 75). Queensland, Australia: Author.

Swimming Pool and Spa Association of Queensland Inc. (SPASA). (1998). Please fence me out. Retrieved April 21, 2000 from the World Wide Web: http://www.deuce.net/cgi-bin/displaypage.asp?id=1295

Thompson, D.C., & Rivara, F.P. (1999). Pool fencing for preventing drowning in children. (Cochrane Review) *The Cochrane Library, 4.* Oxford: Update Software.

Vimpani, G. (1997). *Prevention of childhood injuries: Intentional and unintentional* [prepared for the International Paediatric Association]. Retrieved April 16, 2000 from the World Wide Web: http://www.ipa-france.net/pubs/inches/inch8_3/vim.htm

3. Prevention of Motor and other Road Vehicle–Related Injuries

3M Corporation. (2000a). An overview of ANSI/ISEA 107–99 standard. *Be Safer Be Seen*, 1 (Spring).

3M Corporation. (2000b). Should high-visibility clothing be considered personal protection equipment. *Be Safer Be Seen*, 2 (Summer).

3M Corporation. (2000c). The importance of worker visability in poor weather conditions. *Be Safer Be Seen*, 3 (Winter).

Abbas, K., Mabrouk, I., & El-Araby, K. (1996). School children as pedestrians in Cairo: Proxies for improving road safety. *Journal of Transportation Engineering, 122*, 291–299.

Al-Masaeid, H. (1997). Performance of safety evaluation methods. *Journal of Transportation Engineering, 123*, 364–369.

Al-Masaeid, H., & Sinha, K. (1994). Analysis of accident reduction potentials of pavement markings. *Journal of Transportation Engineering, 120*, 723–736.

Avery, J.G., & Avery, P.J. (1982). Scandinavian and Dutch lessons in childhood road traffic accident prevention. *British Medical Journal, 285*, 621–626.

Baker, S.P., O'Neil, B., Ginsburg, M.J., & Li, G. (1992). Introduction to motor vehicle crashes. In S.P. Baker, B. O'Neil, M.J. Ginsburg, & G. Li (Eds.), *The injury fact book* (pp. 211–232). New York: Oxford University Press.

Barry, S., Ginpil, S., & O'Neill, T. (1999). The effectiveness of air bags. *Accident Analysis and Prevention, 31*, 781–787.

Bateman, M., Howard, I., Johnson, A., & Walton, J. (1999). Model of the performance of a roadway safety fence and its use for design. *Transportation Research Record, 1647*, 122–129.

Billheimer, J. (1999). Evaluation of California motorcyclist safety program. *Transportation Research Record, 1640*, 100–109.

Bowman, B., & Kowshik, R. (1995). Comparative study of glass bead usage in pavement marking reflectorization. *Transportation Research Record, 1442,* 57–64.

Britt, J.W., Bergman, A., & Moffat, J. (1995). Law enforcement pedestrian safety, and driver compliance with crosswalk laws: Evaluation of a four-year campaign in Seattle. *Transportation Research Record, 1485,* 160–167.

Cameron, M.H., Vulcan, A.P., Finch, C.F., & Newstead, S.V. (1994). Mandatory bicycle helmet use following a decade of helmet promotion in Victoria, Australia: An evaluation. *Accident Analysis and Prevention, 26,* 325–337.

Carney, J., III, Faramawi, M., & Chatterjee, S. (1997). Development of reusable high-molecular-weight-high-density polyethylene crash cushions. *Transportation Research Record, 1528,* 11–27.

Carr, D., Skalova, M., & Cameron, M.H. (1997). *Evaluation of the bicycle helmet wearing law in Victoria during its first four years* (Report No. 76 [Abstract]). Melbourne, Australia: Monash University, Accident Research Centre. Retrieved March 4, 2000 from the World Wide Web: http://www.general.monash.edu.au/muarc/rptsum/es76.htm

Carsten, O.M.J., Sherborne, D.J., & Rothengatter, J.A. (1998). Intelligent traffic signals for pedestrians: Evaluation of trials in three countries. *Transportation Research, Part C 6,* 213–229.

Castronovo, S., Dorothy, P., & Maleck, T. (1999). Investigation of the effectiveness of boulevard roadways. *Transportation Research Record, 1635,* 147–154.

Chaudoin, J.H., & Nelson, G. (1985, August). *Interstate routes 15 and 40 shoulder rumble strips* (Report No. Caltrans-08–85–1). California Department of Transportation, Traffic Operations Branch, District 8.

Cote, T.R., Sacks, J.J., Lambert-Huber, D.A., Dannenberg, A.L., Kresnow, M., Lipsitz, M.D., & Schmidt, E.R. (1992). Bicycle helmet use among Maryland children: Effect of legislation and education. *Pediatrics, 89,* 1216–1220.

Cross, D., Stevenson, M., Hall, M., Burns, S., Laughlin, D., Officer, J., & Howat, P. (2000). Child Pedestrian Injury Prevention Project: Student results. *Preventive Medicine, 30,* 179–187.

Cruz, T., & Mickalide, A. (2000). The national Safekids campaign child safety seat distribution program: A strategy for reaching low-income, underserved, and culturally diverse populations. *Health Promotion Practice, 1,* 148–158.

Currie, S.R., DeGagne, T.A., Cwinn, A., Mongeon, S., & Seymour, Y. (1995, July). *A new questionnaire to assess risk for spinal cord injury.* Paper presented at the annual meeting of the American Psychological Association.

Davies, C.H. (1988). *Speed measurements in urban safety project areas* (TRL Working Paper No. WP/RS/66). Crowthorne, UK: Transport Research Laboratory.

Diaz, R., & Cabrera, D. (1997). Safety climate and attitude as evaluation measures of organizational safety. *Accident Analysis and Prevention, 29,* 643–650.

Dorothy, P., Lyles, R., & Narupiti, S. (1998). Michigan's commercial driver's license (CDL) experience. *Journal of Transportation Engineering, 124,* 172–178.

Dowsell, T., Towner, E.M.L., Simpson, G., & Jarvis, S. (1996). Preventing childhood unintentional injuries – What works? A literature review. *Injury Prevention, 2,* 140–149.

Durkin, M., Laraque, D., Lubman, I., & Barlow, B. (1999). Epidemiology and prevention of traffic injuries to urban children and adolescents. *Pediatrics, 103,* 1273–1274.

Eby, D.W., & Kostniuk, L.P. (1999). A statewide analysis of child safety seat use and misuse in Michigan. *Accident Analysis and Prevention, 31,* 555–566.

Ekman, R., Shelp, L., Welander, G., & Svanstrom, L. (1997). Can a combination of local, regional and national information substantially increase helmet wearing and reduce injuries? Experiences from Sweden. *Accident Analysis and Prevention, 29,* 321–328.

Elvik, R., Mysen, A.B., & Vaa, T. (1997). *Trafikksikkerhetshandbok.* (Road Safety Handbook in Norwegian). Oslo, Norway: Transportokonomisk Institutt.

Engel, U., & Thomsen, L.K. (1990). *Effekter af faerdselslovens 40–Sammenfatning* (Report No. 29) (in Danish). Copenhagen, Denmark: Radet for Trafiksikkerhedsforskning.

Engel, U., & Thomsen, L.K. (1992). Safety effects of speed reducing measures in Danish residential areas. *Accident Analysis and Prevention, 24,* 1–28.

Farmer, C., Retting, R., & Lund, A. (1999). Changes in motor vehicle occupant fatalities after repeal of the national maximum speed limit. *Accident Analysis and Prevention, 31,* 537–543.

Finch, D.J. (1999). National practice and experiences in the United Kingdom. In *Speed management: National practice and experiences in Denmark, the Netherlands and in the United Kingdom* (Report No. 167, Annex 2). Copenhagen, Denmark: Danish Road Directorate.

Finch, D.J., Kompfner, P., Lockwood, C.R., & Maycock, G. (1994). *Speed, speed limits and accidents* (Project Report No. 58). Crowthorne, UK: Transport Research Laboratory.

Flannery, A., Elefteriadou, L., Koza, P., & McFadden, J. (1999). Safety, delay, and capacity of single-lane roundabouts in the United States. *Transportation Research Record, 1646,* 63–70.

Fockler, S., Vavrik, J., & Kristiansen, L. (1998). Motivating drivers to correctly adjust head restraints: Assessing effectiveness of three different interventions. *Accident Analysis and Prevention, 30,* 773–780.

Foss, R., & Evenson, K. (1998). Effectiveness of graduated driver licensing in reducing motor vehicle crashes. *American Journal of Preventive Medicine, 16(1S)*, 47–56.

Fur, S. (2000, March 6). PARTY program gives teens a dose of reality. *S&W News, 2 (5)*, 2.

Garder, P. (1998, September). *Little Falls, Gorham: Reconstruction to a modern roundabout* (Final Report, Technical Report 96–2B). Maine Department of Transportation, Bureau of Planning, Research, and Community Services, Transportation Research Division.

Garder, P. (1999). Little Falls, Gorham – reconstruction to a modern roundabout. *Transportation Research Record, 1658*, 17–24.

Gibreel, G., Easa, S., Hassan, Y., & El-Dimeery, I. (1999). State of the art of highway geometric design consistency. *Journal of Transportation Engineering, 125*, 305–313.

Green, L., & Kreuter, M. (1991). *Health promotion planning: An educational and environmental approach*. Mountain View, CA: Mayfield.

Gregersen, N., Berg, H., Engstrom, I., Nolen, S., Nyberg, A., & Rimmo, P. (2000). Sixteen years age limit for learner drivers in Sweden: An evaluation of safety effects. *Accident Analysis and Prevention, 32*, 25–35.

Greibe, P., Nilsson, P.K., & Herrstedt, L. (1999a). Speed management: National practice and experiences in Denmark. In *Speed management: National practice and experiences in Denmark, the Netherlands and in the United Kingdom* (Report No. 167). Copenhagen, Denmark: Danish Road Directorate.

Greibe, P., Nilsson, P.K., & Herrstedt, L. (1999b). *Speed management in urban areas: A framework for the planning and evaluation process* (Report No. 168). Copenhagen, Denmark: Danish Road Directorate.

Grossman, D., & Garcia, C. (1998). Effectiveness of health promotion programs to increase motor vehicle occupant restraint use among young children. *American Journal of Preventive Medicine, 16(1S)*, 12–22.

Guria, J. (1999). An economic evaluation of incremental resources to road safety programmes in New Zealand. *Accident Analysis and Prevention, 31*, 91–99.

Haddon, W. (1972). A logical framework for categorizing highway safety phenomena and activity. *Journal of Trauma, 12(30)*, 193–207.

Haddon, W. (1973). Energy damage and ten countermeasure strategies. *Journal of Trauma 13*, 321–331.

Halldin, P., von Holst, H., & Eriksson, I. (1998). An experimental head restraint concept for primary prevention of head and neck injuries in frontal collisions. *Accident Analysis and Prevention, 30*, 535–543.

Hauer, E., Terry, D., & Griffith, M. (1995). Effect of resurfacing on safety of two-lane rural roads in New York State. *Transportation Research Record, 1467,* 30–37.

Health Education Authority. (1996). *Health promotion in childhood and young adolescence for the prevention of unintentional injuries.* London, UK: Author.

Hearn, G., Barrett, R., & Henson, H. (1995). Development of effective rockfall barriers. *Journal of Transportation Engineering, 121,* 507–516.

Herrstedt, L. (1992). Traffic calming design – A speed management method: Danish experiences on environmentally adapted through roads. *Accident Analysis and Prevention, 24,* 3–15.

Herrstedt, L., Kjemtrup, K., Borges, P., & Anderson, P.S. (1993). *An improved traffic environment: A catalogue of ideas* (Road Data Laboratory Report No. 106). Copenhagen, Denmark: Danish Road Directorate.

Hickey, J., Jr (1997). Shoulder rumble strip effectiveness: Drift-off-road accident reductions on the Pennsylvania Turnpike. *Transportation Research Record, 1573,* 105–109.

Howat, P., Jones, S., Hall, M., Cross, D., & Stevenson, M. (1997). The Precede-Proceed model: Application to planning a child pedestrian injury prevention program. *Injury Prevention, 3,* 282–287.

Hydén, C. (1987). The development of methods for traffic safety evaluation: The Swedish traffic conflicts technique. *Bulletin 70.* Lund, Sweden: Department of Traffic Planning and Engineering, Lund Institute of Technology.

Hydén, C., & Várhelyi, A. (1999). The effects on safety, time consumption and environment of large scale use of roundabouts in an urban area: A case study. *Accident Analysis and Prevention, 32,* 11–23.

Hydén, C., Odelid, K., & Várhelyi, A. (1991). *Traffic safety program for Växjö: Analysis of safety problems and measures* (in Swedish). Lund, Sweden: Lund Institute of Technology.

Introduction to Roundabouts. (1999, November 9). *City of Hutchinson: Roundabouts U.S.A.* Retrieved February 4, 2000 from the World Wide Web: http://www.roundaboutsusA.com/intro.html

Jagger, J. (1992). Prevention of brain trauma by legislation, regulation, and improved technology: A focus on motor vehicles. *Journal of Neurotrauma, 9,* 313–316.

Jakobsson, L., Lundell, B., Norin, H., & Isaksson-Hellman, I. (2000). WHIPS: Volvo's whiplash protection study. *Accident Analysis and Prevention, 32,* 307–319.

Jessie, W., & Yuan, W. (1998). The efficacy of safety policies on traffic fatalities in Singapore. *Accident Analysis and Prevention, 30,* 745–754.

Jones, B. (1997). Age, gender and the effectiveness of high-threat letters: an analysis of Oregon's driver improvement advisory letters. *Accident Analysis and Prevention, 29,* 225–234.

Kimber, R. (1990). Appropriate speeds for different road conditions. In Parliamentary Advisory Council for Transport Safety (Ed.), *Speed accidents and injury: Reducing the risks*. London: PACTS.

Kraan, M., van der Zijpp, N., Tutert, B., Vonk, T., & van Megen, D. (2000). Evaluating networkwide effects of variable message signs in the Netherlands. *Transportation Research Record, 1689*, 60–67.

Lawrence, J., & Siegmund, G. (2000). Seat back and head restraint response during low-speed rear-end automobile collisions. *Accident Analysis and Prevention, 32*, 219–232.

Linderholm, L. (1992). *Traffic safety evaluation of engineering measures*. Lund, Sweden: Lund Institute of Technology.

Lohrey, E., Carney, J., Bullard, L., Jr, Alberson, D., & Menges, W. (1997). Testing and evaluation of Merritt Parkway guiderail. *Transportation Research Record, 1599*, 40–47.

Luoma, J., Schumann, J., & Traube, E.C. (1995). Effects of retroreflector positioning on nighttime recognition of pedestrians. *Accident Analysis and Prevention, 28*, 377–383.

Lynam, D.A. (1987). *Use and effectiveness of speed-reducing measures in urban areas* (TRL Working Paper No. WP/RS/54). Crowthorne, UK: Transport Research Laboratory.

Mak, K., & Hille, R. (1995). Minnesota swing-away mailbox support. *Transportation Research Record, 1468*, 68–75.

Mak, K., Bligh, R., & Falkenberg, P. (1995). Tennessee bridge rail to guardrail transition designs. *Transportation Research Record, 1468*, 75–83.

Malenfant, L., & Van Houten, R. (1989). Increasing the percentage of drivers yielding to pedestrians in three Canadian cities with a multifaceted safety program. *Health Education Research, 5*, 275–279.

Manitoba Public Insurance MPI (December, 1999). *Closing the circle: A strategy of life-long learning for safety* (RoadWise Annual Report 1999).

Margiotta, R., & Chatterjee, A. (1995). Accidents on suburban highways: Tennessee's experience. *Journal of Transportation Engineering, 121*, 255–261.

McArthur, D., & Kraus, J. (1998). The specific deterrence of administrative per se laws in reducing drunk driving recidivism. *American Journal of Preventive Medicine, 16(1S)*, 68–75.

Navin, F., Zein, S., & Felipe, E. (2000). Road safety engineering: An effective tool in the fight against whiplash injuries. *Accident Analysis and Prevention, 32*, 271–275.

Newton, C., Mussa, R., Sadalla, E., Burns, E., & Matthias, J. (1997). Evaluation of an alternative traffic light change anticipation system. *Accident Analysis and Prevention, 29*, 201–209.

Nilsson, G. (1982). *The effect of speed limits on traffic accidents in Sweden* (VTI Report No. 68). Linkoping, Sweden: VTI.

Nordiska Vaegteknisda Foerbundet. (1984). *Rundkjoringer* (Report No. 27). Stockholm, Sweden: Author.

Nuth, J., Mongeon, S., Currie, S.R., & Curran, D.A. (1999, May). *An evaluation of PARTY: A Canadian injury prevention program for teenagers.* Paper presented at the American Society for Academic Emergency Medicine Conference.

O'Neill, B. (2000). Head restraints: The neglected countermeasure. *Accident Analysis and Prevention, 32,* 143–150.

Ogden, K. (1997). The effects of paved shoulders on accidents on rural highways. *Accident Analysis and Prevention, 29,* 353–362.

Ontario Ministry of Transportation. (1997). *Ontario Road Safety Annual Report – 1997.* Retrieved February 20, 2000 from the World Wide Web: http://www.mto.gov.on.ca/english/safety/orsar/

Ontario Ministry of Transportation. (1997). *Ontario Road Safety Annual Report – 1997.* Retrieved May 2, 2000 from the World Wide Web: http://www.mto.gov.on.ca/english/safety/orsar/

Ontario Neurotrauma Foundation (ONF). (1999). *Guide to program design and evaluation planning.* Toronto: Author.

Ourston, L., & Associates. (1993). *Wide nodes and narrow roads.* Paper presented at the 72nd annual meeting of the Transportation Research Board, Santa Barbara, CA.

PARTY Program. (1999). *PARTY program information package.* Toronto, ON: Sunnybrook and Women's College Health Sciences Centre.

Pasanen, E. (1992). *Driving speeds and pedestrian safety: A mathematical model* (Transportation Engineering Publication No. 77). Otaniemi, Finland: Helsinki University of Technology.

Peek-Asa, C. (1998). The effect of random alcohol screening in reducing motor vehicle crash injuries. *American Journal of Preventive Medicine, 16(1S),* 57–67.

Polak, P.H., & Oei, H.L. (1997). National practice and experiences in the Netherlands. In *Speed management: National practice and experiences in Denmark, the Netherlands and in the United Kingdom* (Report No. 167, Annex 2). Copenhagen, Denmark: Danish Road Directorate.

Reeder, A., Alsop, J., Langley, J., & Wagenaar, A. (1999). An evaluation of the general effect of the New Zealand graduated driver licensing system on motorcycle traffic crash hospitalisations. *Accident Analysis and Prevention, 31,* 651–661.

Retting, R., Ulmer, R., & Williams, A. (1998). *Prevalence and characteristics of red light running crashes in the United States.* Arlington, VA: IIHS.

Retting, R., Williams, A., Farmer, C., & Feldman, A. (1999a). Evaluation of red light camera enforcement in Oxnard, California. *Accident Analysis and Prevention, 31,* 169–174.

Retting, R., Williams, A., Farmer, C., & Feldman, A. (1999b, August). Evaluation of red light camera enforcement in Fairfax, Virginia. Prepared for *ITE Journal.*

Retting, R., Williams, A., Preusser, D., & Weinstein, H. (1995). Classifying urban crashes for countermeasure development. *Accident Analysis and Prevention, 21,* 283–294.

Rivara, F.P., Grossman, D.C., & Cummings, P. (1997). Injury prevention (Part 1). *New England Journal of Medicine, 337,* 543–548.

Rivara, F.P., Grossman, D.C., & Cummings, P. (1997). Injury prevention (Part 2). *New England Journal of Medicine, 337,* 613–618.

Rothengatter, T. (1984). A behavioural approach to improving traffic behaviour of young children. *Ergonomics, 27,* 147–160.

Rumblestrips Publications. Pennsylvannia. Rumblestrips. Retrieved February 10, 2000 from the World Wide Web: http://www.rumblestrips.com

SafetyBeltSafe U.S.A. (1998). *Expanding the child passenger safety net.* Project No. OP9914. Torrance, CA. SafetyBeltSafe, U.S.A.

SafetyBeltSafe U.S.A. (1999) *Executive summary: Expanding the child passenger safety net.* Torrance, CA. SafetyBeltSafe, U.S.A.

Salusjärvi, M., 1981. *The speed limit experiments on public roads in Finland* (Publication No. 7/1981). Espoo, Finland: Technical Research Centre of Finland.

Sarkar, S., Nederveen, A.A.J., & Pols, A. (1997). Renewed commitment to traffic calming for pedestrian safety. *Transportation Research Record, 1578,* 11–18.

Sayed, T., Abdelwahab, W., & Nepomuceno, J. (1999). Safety evaluation of alternative signal head design. *Transportation Research Record, 1635,* 140–146.

Sayed, T., Vahidi, H., & Rodriguez, F. (2000). Advance warning flashers: Do they improve safety? *Transportation Research Record, 1692,* 30–38.

Schull, R., & Lange, J. (1990). Speed reduction on through roads in Nordrhein-Westfalen. *Proceedings of the conference, Speed management in urban areas.* Copenhagen, Denmark: Danish Road Directorate.

Segui-Gomez, M. (1998). Evaluating interventions that promote the use of rear seats for children. *American Journal of Preventive Medicine, 16(1S),* 23–29.

Simon, M.J. (1991). Roundabouts in Switzerland. In W. Brilon (Ed.), *Proceedings of an international workshop in Bochum, Germany: II. Intersections without traffic signals.* New York: Springer-Verlag.

Skene, M., Chartier, G., Erickson, D., Mack, G. Kizas, J., Jack, R., & Drdul, R.

(Steering committee). (1998). *Canadian guide to neighbourhood traffic calming*. Transportation Association of Canada.

SMARTRISK. (1999). *The economic burden of unintentional injury in Ontario*. Toronto, ON: Author.

SMARTRISK (1998a). *The economic burden of unintentional injury in Canada*. Toronto, ON: Author.

SMARTRISK. (1998b). *Fact sheet*. Toronto: Author.

SMARTRISK. (1998c). *HEROES program evaluation: Pilot test of a student survey*. Toronto, ON: Author.

SMARTRISK. (1998d). *The stupid line: The line of choice that separates smart risk from stupid risk*. Toronto, ON: Author.

SMARTRISK. (n.d.). *How to host HEROES guide*. [Brochure] Toronto, ON: Author.

South, D., Harrison, W., Portans, I., & King, M. (1988). *Evaluation of the red light camera program and the owner onus legislation*. Victoria, Australia: Victoria Road Traffic Authority.

St John, A., & Glauz, W. (1996). Effect of wide-base tires on rollover stability. *Transportation Research Record, 1485*, 80–89.

Stevenson, M., Iredell, H., Howat, P., Cross, D., & Hall, M. (1999). Measuring community/environmental interventions: The Child Pedestrian Injury Prevention Project. *Injury Prevention, 5*, 26–30.

Stevenson, M., Jones, S., Cross, D., Howat, P., & Hall, M. (1996). The Child Pedestrian Injury Prevention Project. *Health Promotion Journal of Australia, 6*, 32–36.

Teichgraber, W. (1983). Die Bedetund der Geschwindigkeit fur die Verkehrs-sicherheit. *Zeitschrift fur Verkehrssicherheit, 2*, Heft, II Quartal.

Theeuwes, J., & Alferdinck, J. (1997). The effectiveness of side marker lamps: an experimental study. *Accident Analysis and Prevention, 29*, 235–245.

Tombrello, S.M. (1997, November 10). *Piloting an urban child passenger safety education and safety seat voucher distribution program to reach low-income clients in Los Angeles County*. New York: SafetyBelt, Safe, U.S.A.

Tombrello, S.M. (1996, November 19). *Instituting a certification program for child passenger safety specialists in California: A response to a longstanding need*. New York: SafetyBeltSafe, U.S.A.

Toronto Council. (1999). *Red light cameras*. Retrieved April 20, 2000 from the World Wide Web: http://www.city.toronto.on.ca

Towner, E., & Jarvis, S. (1997). The childhood injury prevention and promotion of safety programme (CHIPPS). *Injury Prevention, 3*, 67–68.

U.S. Department of Transportation. (1993). *Traffic safety facts 1992* (Report No. HS-808-022). Washington, DC: Author.

U.S. Department of Transportation. (1994). *Traffic safety facts 1992* (Report No. HS-808-169). Washington, DC: Author.

U.S. Department of Transportation. (1995). *Traffic safety facts 1992* (Report No. HS-808-292). Washington, DC: Author.

U.S. Department of Transportation. (1996). *Traffic safety facts 1992* (Report No. HS-808-471). Washington, DC: Author.

U.S. Department of Transportation. (1997). *Traffic safety facts 1992* (Report No. HS-808-770). Washington, DC: Author.

Van Houten, R., Malenfant, L., & Rolider, A. (1985). Increasing driver yielding and pedestrian signaling with prompting, feedback, and enforcement. *Journal of Applied Behavior Analysis, 18,* 103–110.

Van Minnen, J. (1992, October). *Experiences with new roundabouts in the Netherlands.* Paper presented at the International Workshop on Mini-Roundabouts, Nantes, France.

Várhelyi, A., & Makinen, T. (1998). *Evaluation of in-car speed limiters: Field study.* (Master contract No. RO-96-SC.202).

Várhelyi, A., Comte, S., & Makinen, T. (1998). *Evaluation of in-car speed limiters: Final report* (Master contract No. RO-96-SC.202).

Vernick, J., Li, G., Ogaitis, S., MacKenzie, E., Baker, S., & Gielen, A. (1998). Effects of high school driver education on motor vehicle crashes, violations, and licensure. *American Journal of Preventive Medicine, 16(1S),* 40–46.

Vis, A.A., Dujkstra, A., & Slop, M. (1992). Safety effects of 30 km/h zones in the Netherlands. Accident Analysis and Prevention, 24, 75–86.

Von Kries, R., Kohne, C., Böhm, & Von Voss, H. (1998). Road injuries in school age children: Relation to environmental factors amenable to intervention. *Injury Prevention, 4,* 103–105.

Watanabe, Y., Ichikawa, H., Kayama, O., Ono, K., Kaneoka, K., & Inami, S. (2000). Influence of seat characteristics on occupant motion in low-speed rear impacts. *Accident Analysis and Prevention, 32,* 243–250.

Weber, K. (in press). Child passenger protection. In A.M. Nahum & J.W. Melvin (Eds.), *Biomechanics and prevention* (2nd ed.). New York: Springer-Verlag.

Williams, A. (1998). Comment on occupant and licensing interventions. *American Journal of Preventive Medicine, 16(1S),* 6–8.

Wood, N.E. (1994). *Shoulder rumble strips: A method to alert 'drifting' drivers.* Paper presented at the 73rd annual meeting of the Transportation Research Board, Washington, DC.

Zegeer, C., Huang, H., Stewart, R., & Williams, C. (1999). Investigation of national highway system roadways in the highway safety information system states. *Transportation Research Record, 1635,* 1–9.

Zein, S.R., Geddes, E., Hemsing, S., & Johnson, M. (1997). Safety benefits of traffic calming. *Transportation Research Record, 1578*, 3–10.

Zwerling, C., & Jones, M. (1998). Evaluation of the effectiveness of low blood alcohol concentration laws for younger drivers. *American Journal of Preventive Medicine, 16(1S)*, 76–80.

4. Prevention of Sports, Playground, and Recreation-Related Injuries

American Academy of Neurology. (1997). *Practice parameter: The management of concussion in sports* (Report of the Quality Standards Subcommittee, Summary Statement). *Neurology, 48*, 581–585.

Barth, J.T., Alves, W.M., Ryan, T.V. (1989). Mild head injury in sports: neuropsychological sequelae and recovery of functions. In H.S. Levin, H.M. Eisenberg, & A.I. Bento (Eds.), *Mild head injury* (pp. 257–275). New York: Oxford University Press.

Beach, L., & Robinson, J. (1998/99). *Snowmobile trail officer patrol* (Annual Report). Sudbury, ON: S.T.O.P.

Benson, B.W., Mohtadi, N.G.H., & Meeuwisse, W.H. (1999). Head and neck injuries among ice hockey players wearing full face shields versus half face shields. *Journal of the American Medical Association, 282*, 2328–2332.

Brust, J.D., Roberts, W.O., & Leonard, B.J. (1995). Gladiators on ice: An overview of ice hockey injuries in youth. *Medical Journal of Allina, 5*, 1–4. Retrieved April 13, 2000 from the World Wide Web: http://www. Allina.com/ Allina_Journal/ Winter1996/brust.html

Centers for Disease Control and Prevention. (1995). Injury-control recommendations: Bicycle helmets. *Morbidity and Mortality Weekly Report, 44*, RR–1.

Coleman, P., Munro, J., Nicholl, J.P., Harper, R., Kent, G., & Wild, D. (1996). *The effectiveness of interventions to prevent accidental injury to young persons aged 5–24 years: A review of the evidence.* Sheffield, UK: University of Sheffield Medical Care Research Unit, Centre for Health and Related Research.

Collins, M., Grindel, S., Lovell, M., Dede, D., Moser, D., Phalin, B., Nogle, S., Wasik, M., Cordry, D., Daugherty, M., Sears, S., Nicolette, G., Indelicato, P., & McKeag, D. (1999). Relationship between concussion and neuropsychological performance in college football players. *JAMA, 282 (10)*, 964–970.

Collins, M., Lovell, M., and McKeag, D. (1999). Current issues in managing sports-related concussion. *JAMA, 282 (24)*, 2283–2285.

Doherty, S., Aultman-Hall, L., & Swaynos, J. (2000). Commuter cyclist accident patterns in Toronto and Ottawa. *Journal of Transportation Engineering, 126*, 21–26.

Esselman, P.C., & Uomoto, J.M. (1995). Classification of the spectrum of mild traumatic brain injury. *Brain Injury, 9*, 417–424.

Finch, C., Ferla, J., Chin, G., Maloney, P., & Abeysiri, P. (1997). *Teenagers' attitudes towards bicycle helmets.* (Rep. #64 [Abstract]). Melbourne: Monash University Accident Research Centre. Retrieved April 15, 2000 from the World Wide Web: http://www.general.monash.edu.au/muarc/rptsum/es64.htm

Henderson, M. (1995). *The effectiveness of bicycle helmets: A review* (rev. ed.) [prepared for the Motor Accidents Authority of New South Wales, Australia]. Retrieved March, 2000 from the World Wide Web: http://www.bhsi.org/webdocs/henderso.htm

Hudson, S., Mack, M., & Thompson, D. (2000). How safe are our playgrounds? A national profile of childcare, school and park playgrounds. Cedar Falls, IA: National Program for Playground Safety, University of Northern Iowa.

Kelly, J.P., Nichols J.S., Filley, C.M., Lillehei, K.O., Rubinstein, D., Kleinschmidt-Demasters, J. (1991). Concussion- in sports: guidelines for the prevention of catastrophic outcome. *JAMA, 266 (20),* 2867–2869.

Kelly, James P. (1999). Traumatic brain injury and concussion in sports. *JAMA, 282 (10),* 989–991.

Marcotte, G., & Simard, D. (1993). Fair-play: An approach to hockey for the 1990s. In C.R. Castaldi, P.J. Bishop, & E.F. Hoemer (Eds.), *Safety in ice hockey, 2,* 103–108. Philadelphia, PA: American Society for Testing Materials.

McCrea, M., Kelly, J.P., Kluge, J., Ackley, B., & Randolph, C. (1997). Standardized assessment of concussion football players. *Neurology, 48,* 586–588.

Mölsä, J.J., Tegner, Y., Alaranta, I I., Myllynen, P., & Kujala, U.M. (1999). Spinal cord injuries in ice hockey in Finland and Sweden from 1980 to 1996. *International Journal of Sport Medicine, 20,* 64–67.

Morris, B.A., Trimble, N.E., & Fendley, S.J. (1994). Increasing bicycle helmet use in the community: Measuring response to a wide-scale, 2-year effort [Abstract]. *Canadian Family Physician, 40,* 1126–1131. Retrieved March 12, 2000 from the World Wide Web: http://www.hc-sc.ca/hppb/socialmarketing/publications/smbib98/kids.htm

Reid, S.R., & Losek, J.D. (1999). Factors associated with significant injuries in youth ice hockey players. *Pediatric Emergency Care, 15,* 310–313.

Rivara, F.P. (1995). Developmental and behavioral issues in childhood injury prevention. *Journal of Behavioral Pediatrics,* 16, 362–370.

Rivara, F.P., Thompson, D.C., Thompson, R.S., Rogers, L.W., Alexander, B., Felix, D., & Bergman, A.B. (1994). The Seattle children's bicycle helmet campaign: Changes in helmet use and head injury admissions. *Pediatrics, 93,* 567–569.

Roberts, W.O., Brust, J.D., Leonard, B., & Herbert, B.J. (1996). Fair-play rules and injury reduction in ice hockey. *Archives of Pediatrics and Adolescent Medicine, 150,* 140–145.

Roseveare, C.A., Brown, J.M., Barclay McIntosh, J.M., & Chalmers, D.J. (1999). An intervention to reduce playground equipment hazards. *Injury Prevention, 5,* 124–128.

Rowe, B., Johnson, C., Milner, R., & Bota, G. (1992). Snowmobile fatalities in Ontario: A five year review. *Canadian Medical Association Journal, 146,* 147–152.

Rowe, B.H., Johnson, C., Milner, R., & Bota, G.W. (1994). The association of alcohol and night driving with fatal snowmobile trauma: A case-control study. *Annuals of Emergency Medicine, 24,* 842–848.

Rowe, B.H., Therrien, S.A., Bretzlaff, J., Sahai, V.S., Nagarajan, K.V., & Bota, G.W. (1996). *The effect of a community-based police surveillance program on snowmobile injuries and deaths.* Unpublished manuscript.

Rowe, B.H., Therrien, S.A., Thorsteinson, K., & Bota, G.W. (1994). *A preliminary comparison of snowmobile injuries and deaths in the Sudbury Region: The Effect of the STOP officer and police education programs.* Unpublished manuscript.

Safety Towards Other Players (S.T.O.P.). (1999). *Ontario Minor Hockey Association worldwide purchasing program outline and order form.* Retrieved April 13, 2000 from the World Wide Web: http://www.omha.net/stop/index.html

Sosin, D.M., Keller, P., Sacks, J.J., Kresnow, M., & Van Dyck, P.C. (1993). Surface-specific fall injury rates on Utah school playgrounds. *American Journal of Public Health, 83,* 733–735.

SMARTRISK. (1998). *The economic burden of unintentional injury in Canada.* Toronto: Author.

Thompson, D.C., & Hudson, S. (2000). National Action Plan for the Prevention of Playground Injuries. Cedar Falls, IA: National Program for Playground Safety, University of Northern Iowa.

Thompson, D.C., Rivara, F.P., & Thompson, R. (1999). Helmets for preventing head and facial injuries in bicyclists (Cochrane Review). *The Cochrane Library, 4.* Oxford: Update Software.

Torg, J.S., Vegso, J.S., Jennett, B., & Das, M. (1985). The national football head and neck injury registry: Fourteen-year report on cervical quadriplegia, 1971 through 1984. *Journal of the American Medical Association, 254,* 3439–3443.

Vaz, E. (1982). *The Professionalization of Young Hockey Players.* Lincoln, Nebraska: University of Nebraska Press.

Wood, T., & Milne, P. (1988). Head injuries to pedal cyclists and the promotion of helmet use in Victoria, Australia. *Accident Analysis and Prevention, 20,* 177–185.

5. Prevention of Farm-Related and Occupational Injuries

Becker, W.J. (1991). *Agricultural accident prevention.* Agricultural Engineering

Department. Miami: University of Florida. Retrieved February 14, 2000 from the World Wide Web: http://www.cdc.gov/niosh.nasd/docs/as02500.html

Canadian Agricultural Injury Surveillance Program (CAISP). (1997). *Fatal farm injuries in Canada, 1991–1995*. Kingston, ON: Queen's University, Author.

Canadian Agricultural Injury Surveillance Program (CAISP). (1999). *Hospitalized farm injuries in Canada, 1990–1996*. Kingston, ON: Queen's University, Author.

Day, L.M. (1999). Farm work related fatalities among adults in Victoria, Australia: The human cost of agriculture. *Accident Analysis and Prevention, 31*, 153–159.

Day, L.M. (1999). *Evaluation of the tractor rollover protective structure rebate scheme, 1997/98*. Retrieved March 8, 2000 from the World Wide Web: http://www.general.monash.edu.au/muarc/rptsum/es155.htm

Day, L.M., & Rechnitzer, G. (1999). *Evaluation of the tractor rollover protective structure rebate scheme, 1997/98*. Australia: Monash University Accident Research Center.

Farm Safety Association. (1999). Farm Safety Association 1999 executive. *Farmsafe, 24(3)*, 3.

Haddon, W. (1980). Advances in epidemiology of injuries as a basis for public health policy. *Public Health Reports 95(5)*, 411–421.

Kelsey, T. W. (1994). The agrarian myth and policy responses to farm safety. *American Journal of Public Health, 84*, 1171–1177.

Local Government Focus. *Falls prevention for small business*. January, 2000 edition.

Lockinger, L., Hillier, T., Hagel, L., Chen, Y., McDuffie, H., & Dosman, J. (1997). Farm response: An accident preparedness course for farm families. *Agricultural Health and Safety: Recent advances*, 387–390.

North American Guidelines for Children's Agricultural Tasks. (1999). National Farm Medicine Centre: Marshfield, Wisconsin.

Ontario Agricultural Human Resource Committee. (1999). *Agricultural safety audit program: A management tool for employers*. Canada: Ontario Agricultural Human Resource Committee.

Ontario Agricultural Human Resource Committee. (1999, November). *Agricultural safety audit program: A management tool for all farms*. Guelph, ON: Farm Safety Association.

Picket, W., Hartling, L., Dimich-Ward, H., Guernsey, J.R., Hagel, L., Voaklander, D.C., & Brison, R.J. *Patterns of hospitalized farm injury in Canada*. Kingston, ON: Queen's University, Canadian Agricultural Injury Surveillance Program.

Randall, R., & Tormoehlen, K. (1998). *Tractor operation: Gearing up for safety*. U.S.A.: American Society of Agricultural Engineers.

Shutske, J., Gilbert, B., Chaplin, J., & Gunderson, P. (1997). *Sensor evaluation for human presence detection*. Department of Biosystems and Agricultural Engineering, University of Minnesota. Retrieved March 8, 2000 from the World Wide Web: http://gaie.bae.umn.edu/~fs/sensweb/

Small Business Falls Prevention Project. (2000). *Tips to prevent slips, trips, and falls in the workplace* [Project Brochure]. Hume, Australia: Hume City Council, Safe Living.

Small Business Research Unit. (2000, April). *Small business falls prevention evaluation brief*. Footscray, Australia: Victoria University.

Small Business Research Unit. (2000, February). *Small business falls prevention project evaluation plan for Hume city council*. Footscray, Australia: Victoria University.

SMARTRISK. (1999). *The economic burden of unintentional injury in Ontario*. Toronto: Author

Thelin, A. (1990). Epilogue: Agricultural, occupational and environmental health policy strategies of the future. *American Journal of Industrial Medicine, 18*, 523–526.

Tormoehlen, R., Reeder, R., & Sheldon, E. (1999). *Evaluation of tractor safety educational strategies*. Paper No. 99–15 presented at the 1999 summer conference of the National Institute for Farm Safety, Inc.

Williams, D.L., Hull, D.O., & Silleto, T.A. (1979). *Safe operation of agricultural equipment*. U.S.A.: American Society of Agricultural Engineers.

Wilson, P. (2000). *Small business falls prevention project* (executive summary). Hume, Australia: Hume City Council, Safe Living.

6. Prevention of Fall-Related Injuries

Barlow, B., Niemirska, M., Gandhi, R.P., & Leblanc, W. (1983). Ten years of experience with falls from a height in children. *Journal of Pediatric Surgery, 18(4)*, 509–511.

Buchner, D.M., Hornbrook, M.C., Kutner, N.G., Tinetti, M.E., Ory, M.G., Mulrow, C.D., Schechtman K.B., Gerety, M.B., Fiatarone, M.A., & Wolf, S.L. (1993). Development of the common data base for the FICSIT trials. *Journal of the American Geriatric Society, 41*, 297–308.

Campbell, A.J., Robertson, M.C., Gardner, M.M., Norton, R.N., & Buchner, D.M. (1999). Falls prevention over 2 years: A randomized control trial in women 80 years and older. *Age and Ageing, 28*, 513–518.

Campbell, A.J., Robertson, M.C., Gardner, M.M., Norton, R.N., & Buchner, D.M. (1999). Psychotropic medication withdrawal in a home-based exercise program to prevent falls: A randomized, control trial. *Journal of the American Geriatric Society, 47,* 850–853.

Campbell, A.J., Robertson, M.C., Gardner, M.M., Norton, R.N., Tilyard, M.W., & Buchner, D.M. (1997). Randomised control trial of a general practice programme of home based exercise to prevent falls in elderly women. *British Medical Journal, 315,* 1065–1069.

Coogler, C.E., & Wolf, S.L. (1999). Falls. In W. Hazzard, E. Bierman, J. Blass, W. Ettinger Jr, J. Halter, & J. Oslander (Eds.), *Principles of geriatric medicine and gerontology* (pp. 1535–1546). New York: McGraw-Hill.

Gillespie, L.D., Gillespie, W.J., Cummings, R., Lamb, S.E., & Rowe, B.M. (1999). Interventions to reduce the incidence of falling in the elderly (Cochrane Review) *The Cochrane Library, 4,* 1–31. Oxford: Software Update.

Haddon, W. Jr (1980). Advances in the epidemiology of injuries as a basis for public policy. *Public Health Reports, 95(5),* 411–421.

Healthy Ageing Research Unit. (1998). *No falls! No fear! Falls prevention project.* Australia: University of Queensland.

Horan, M.A., & Little, R.A. (1998). *Injury in the aging.* New York: Cambridge University Press.

Hornbrook, M.C., Stevens, V.J., Wingfield, D.J., Hollis, J.F., Greenlick, M.R., & Ory, M.G. (1994). Preventing falls among community-dwelling older persons: Results from a randomized trial. *The Gerontologist, 34(1),* 16–23.

Hyde, A.S. (1996). *Accidental falls: Their causes and their injuries.* Key Biscayne, FL: HAI.

Kutner, N.G., Barnhart, H., Wolf, S.L., McNeely, E., & Xu, T. (1997). Self-report benefits of tai chi practice by older adults. *Journal of Gerontology: Psychological Sciences, 52B,* 242–246.

New York City Department of Health, Bureau of Window Falls Prevention. (1999, February). *Understand the basics: The window guard law.* Retrieved March, 2000 from the World Wide Web: http://www.ci.nyc.ny.us/html/doh/html/win/winbas2.html

New York City Department of Health, Bureau of Window Falls Prevention. *Window guards required: Lease notice to tenant.* Retrieved March, 2000 from the World Wide Web: http://www.ci.nyc.ny.us/html/doh/html/win/winapa.html

People's Republic of China. (1983). *Preliminary study of reducing aging with taijiquan* (People's Sport and Exercise Publication). People's Republic of China.

Province, M.A., Hadley, E.C., Hornbrook, M.C., Lipsitz, L.A., Miller, J.P., Mulrow, C.D., Ory, M.G., Sattin, R.W., Tinetti, M.E., & Wolf, S.L. (1995). The effects of exercise on falls in elderly patients: A preplanned meta-analysis of the FICSIT trials. *Journal of the American Medical Association, 273,* 1341–1347.

Rizzo, J.A., Baker, D.I., McAvay, G., & Tinetti, M.E. (1996). The cost-effectiveness of a multifactorial targeted prevention program for falls among community elderly persons. *Medical Care, 34,* 954–969.

Robson, E., Edwards, J., Lightfoot, P., & Bursey, R. (1999). *Steady as you go: A falls prevention program for seniors in the community.* Edmonton: Capital Health, Regional Public Health.

SMARTRISK. (1998). *The economic burden of unintentional injury in Canada.* Toronto: Author.

SMARTRISK. (1999). *The economic burden of unintentional injury in Canada.* Toronto: Author.

Spiegel, C.N., & Lindaman, F.C. (1977). Children can't fly: A program to prevent childhood morbidity and mortality from window falls. *American Journal of Pediatric Health, 67(12),* 1143–1147.

Steinberg, M., Cartwright, C., Peel, N., & Williams, G. (2000). A sustainable programme to prevent falls and near falls in community dwelling older people: Results of a randomised trial. *Journal of Epidemiology and Community Health, 54,* 227–232.

Tinetti, M.E., Baker, D.I., Garrett, P., Gottschalk, M., Koch, M.L., & Horwitz, F.I. (1993). Yale FICSIT: Risk factor abatement strategy for fall prevention. *Journal of the American Geriatric Society, 41,* 315–320.

Tinetti, M.E., Baker, D.I., McAvay, G., Claus, E.B., Garrett, P., Gottschalk, M., Koch, M.L., Trainor, K., & Horwitz, F.I. (1994). A multifactorial intervention to reduce the risk of falling among elderly people living in the community. *New England Journal of Medicine, 331,* 821–827.

Tinetti, M.E., McAvay, G., & Claus, E. (1996). Does multiple risk factor reduction explain the reduction in fall rate in the Yale FICSIT trial? *American Journal of Epidemiology, 144,* 389–399.

Wat-Klein, G.P., Silverstone, F.A., Busavaraja, N., Foley, C.J., Pascaru, A., & Ma, P.-H. (1988). Prevention of falls in the elderly population. *Archives of Physical Medicine and Rehabilitation, 69,* 689–691.

Wolf, S.L., Barnhart, H.X., Ellison, G.L., & Coogler, C.E. (1997). The effect of tai chi quan and computerized balance training on postural stability in older subjects. *Physical Therapy, 77,* 371–384.

Wolf, S.L., Barnhart, H.X., Kutner, H.G., McNeely, E., Coogler, C., & Xu, T. (1996). Reducing frailty and falls in older persons: An investigation of tai chi and computerized balance training. *Journal of the American Geriatric Society, 44,* 489–497.

Wolf, S.L., Coogler, C.E., Green, R.C., & Xu, T. (1993). Novel interventions to prevent falls in the elderly. In H.M. Perry III, J.E. Morley, & R.M. Coe (Eds.),

Aging and musculoskeletal disorders: Concepts, diagnosis, and treatment (pp. 178–195). New York: Springer.

Wolf, S.L., Coogler, C., & Xu, T. (1997). Exploring the basis for tai chi chuan as a therapeutic exercise approach. *Archives of Physical Medicine and Rehabilitation, 78,* 886–892.

Wolf, S.L., Kutner, H.G., Green, R.C., & McNeely, E. (1993). The Atlanta FICSIT study: Two exercise interventions to reduce frailty in elders. *Journal of the American Geriatric Society, 41,* 329–332.

7. Comprehensive Community-Based Prevention Strategies

Appy, M. (1997). Taking safety seriously. *NFPA Journal,* 33–34.

Baker, S.P., O'Neil, B., Ginsburg, M.J., & Li, G. (1992). Overview of injury mortality. In S.P. Baker, B. O'Neil, M.J. Ginsburg, & G. Li (Eds.), *The injury fact book* (pp. 17–38). New York: Oxford University Press.

Black, D. (1998, June). Program teaches kids to think before leaping. *Toronto Star,* pp. F1–F2.

Damba, C., Sam, E., Edmonds, V., Tator, C., & Cusimano, M. (in press). *Evaluation of behaviour, knowledge of injury, and knowledge gained by senior elementary and high school students participating in a school based injury prevention program.* Manuscript submitted for publication.

Davidson, L., Durkin, M., Kuhn, L., O'Connor, P., Barlow, B., & Heagarty, M. (1994a). The role of city and state agencies in injury prevention. *American Journal of Public Health, 84,* 1853–1855.

Davidson, L., Durkin, M., Kuhn, L., O'Connor, P., Barlow, B., & Heagarty, M. (1994b). The impact of the Safe Kids/Healthy Neighborhoods injury prevention program in Harlem, 1988 through 1991. *American Journal of Public Health, 84,* 580–586.

Durkin, M., Laraque, D., Lubman, I., & Berlow, B. (1999). Epidemiology and prevention of traffic injuries to urban children and adolescents. *Pediatrics, 103,* 1273–1274.

Gresham, L., & Zirkle, D. (1999). *Partnering for Injury Prevention: Outcomes of the Think First for Kids curriculum-based injury prevention program for elementary school children.* National Think First Conference.

Guba, E.C., & Lincoln, Y.S. (1989). *Fourth generation evaluation.* London: Sage.

Haddon, W. Jr (1980). Advances in epidemilogy of injuries as a basis for public policy. *Public Health Reports, 95(5),* 411–421.

Interwest Applied Research. (1998, November). *Evaluation report 1: Adequacy of current knowledge tests to measure growth.*

Interwest Applied Research. (1999, March). *Evaluation report 2: Results from the first four Risk Watch sites.*

Interwest Applied Research. (1999, August). *Evaluation report 3: Results from the first year of Risk Watch.*

Laraque, D., Barlow, B., Davidson, L., & Heagarty, M. (1994). The Central Harlem Playground Injury Prevention Project: A model for change. *American Journal of Public Health, 84,* 1691–1692.

Lee-Han, H. (1998, May 29). Home alone?: A review of safety issues among unsupervised 10–14 year old children. *Public Health and Epidemiology Report of Ontario,* 116–122.

National Fire Protection Association & Lowe's Home Safety Council. (n.d.) *It's time for Risk Watch: A comprehensive injury prevention curriculum for children in preschool through grade 8* [Brochure]. Quincy, MA: Author.

National Fire Protection Association (NFPA), & Lowe's Home Safety Council. (1998). *Safety program grade 3 and 4: Risk Watch.* Quincy, MA: Author.

Robertson, L.S. (1998). *Injury epidemiology: Research and control strategies.* New York: Oxford University Press.

Sharman, A., & Cusimano, M.D. (2000). Think First! Are there such things as "accidents"? *OPHEA Journal, winter,* 26–27.

SMARTRISK. (1998). *The economic burden of unintentional injury in Canada.* Toronto: Author.

Think First Foundation. (n.d.-a). *National injury prevention programs: Think First Oregon.* [Leaflet].

Think First Foundation. (n.d.-b). *National injury prevention programs: Think First for teens.* [Leaflet].

Think First Foundation. (1999). *Think First of Canada.* Retrieved January 8, 2000 from the World Wide Web: http://www.medi-fax.com/thinkfirst/thinkcan.html

Valsiner, J., & Lightfoot, C. (1987). Process structure of parent-child-environment relations and the prevention of children's injuries. *Journal of Social Issues, 43(2),* 61–72.

VanLeer Program Evaluation Model. (1996). The Hague: VanLeer Foundation.

Volpe, R. (1995). Another face of child abuse prevention. *Connection, (3)* Winter/Spring, 1–5.

Volpe, R. (1996). Foreword to B. Flint, *Hope rewarded: Deprivation, recovery, and adaptation.* Toronto: University of Toronto Press.

Volpe, R. (1996). New South Wales, Australia: How integrated services can be used to address broad ranging problems, from bad behaviour to violent crime. In P. Evans, P. Hurrell, R. Volpe, & M. Stewart (Eds.), *Successful programs for children and families at risk* (Vol. III, pp. 209–220). Paris: OECD.

Volpe, R. (1996). Ontario, Canada: Integrating services in Canada's wealthiest province. In P. Evans, P. Hurrell, R. Volpe, & M. Stewart (Eds.), *Successful programs for children and families at risk* (Vol. III, pp. 175–183). Paris: OECD.

Volpe, R. (1997). Ontario, Canada: Integrating services in Canada's wealthiest province. In P. Evans, P. Hurrell, R. Volpe, & M. Stewart (Eds.), *Successful programs for children and families at risk* (Vol. III). Paris: OECD.

Volpe, R. (1998). Four OECD city integrated service case studies: Duisburg, Germany; Hamilina, Finland (with P. Hurrell), Lisbon, Portugal (with P. Hurrell), and St Louis, Missouri (with P. Hurrell). In P. Evans, P. Hurrell, R. Volpe, & M. Stewart (Eds.), *Coordinating services for children and youth at risk* (Vol. IV). Paris: OECD.

Volpe, R., Clancy, C., Buteau, C., & Tilleczek, K. (1998). *Effective Ontario initiatives to retain secondary students at risk of dropping out of school*. Toronto: Ministry of Education.

Volpe, R., & Tilleczek, K. (1998). German and Australian youth employment services as forms of social support. In I. Richardson (Ed.), *Children and youth: An international odyssey*. Edmonton: University of Alberta Press.

Volpe, R., & Tilleczek, K. (1998). Images of children's rights: A review of Canadian policies. In I. Richardson (Ed.), *Children and youth: An international odyssey*. Edmonton: University of Alberta Press.

Wolf, A. (1997). According to Risk Watch cofounders NFPA and Lowe's Home Safety Council, safe fun isn't only possible it's essential. *NFPA Journal, 2(4)*, 58–63.

Wolf, A. (1998). Don't miss the bus. *NFPA Journal, 3(1)*, 85–91.

Zigler, J.E., & Capen, U.A. (1998). Epidemiology of spinal cord injury: A perspective on the problem. In A.M. Levine, F.J. Fismont, S.R. Garfin, & J.E. Zigler (Eds.), *Spine trauma* (pp. 2–8). Philadelphia, PA: W.B. Saunders.

Index

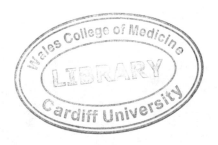